T0188878

Peptide Research Protocols
Endothelin

METHODS IN MOLECULAR BIOLOGY™

John M. Walker, SERIES EDITOR

METHODS IN MOLECULAR BIOLOGY™

Peptide Research Protocols

Endothelin

Edited by

Janet J. Maguire

and

Anthony P. Davenport

*Clinical Pharmacology Unit, University of Cambridge,
Cambridge, UK*

Humana Press ✳ Totowa, New Jersey

© 2002 Humana Press Inc.
Softcover reprint of the hardcover 1st edition 2002
999 Riverview Drive, Suite 208
Totowa, New Jersey 07512

www.humanapress.com

The content and opinions expressed in this book are the sole work of the authors and editors, who have warranted due diligence in the creation and issuance of their work. The publisher, editors, and authors are not responsible for errors or omissions or for any consequences arising from the information or opinions presented in this book and make no warranty, express or implied, with respect to its contents.

This publication is printed on acid-free paper. ∞
ANSI Z39.48-1984 (American Standards Institute) Permanence of Paper for Printed Library Materials.

Production Editor: Jessica Jannicelli.

Cover design by Patricia F. Cleary.

For additional copies, pricing for bulk purchases, and/or information about other Humana titles, contact Humana at the above address or at any of the following numbers: Tel.: 973-256-1699; Fax: 973-256-8341; E-mail: humana@humanapr.com; or visit our Website: www.humanapress.com

Photocopy Authorization Policy:

10 9 8 7 6 5 4 3 2 1

Library of Congress Cataloging in Publication Data

ISBN 978-1-61737-291-9   e-ISBN 978-1-59259-289-0

Preface

The endothelins are a remarkable family of signaling peptides: molecular biology predicted the existence of their receptors and synthetic enzymes prior to both the identification of the encoded proteins and the synthesis of antagonists and inhibitors for use as pharmacological tools. Although considerable advances have been made, culminating in the design of endothelin antagonists with therapeutic potential in cardiovascular disease, much remains to be discovered.

Tantalizingly, new research frontiers are emerging. To support further progress, *Peptide Research Protocols: Endothelin* encompasses experimental protocols that interrogate all facets of an endogenous mammalian peptide system, from peptide and receptor expression through synthetic pathway to peptide function and potential role in human disease.

Chapters describe the use of molecular techniques to quantify the expression of mRNA for both endothelin receptors and the endothelin-converting enzymes. Peptides, precursors, receptors, and synthetic enzymes may be localized and quantified in plasma, culture supernatants, tissue homogenates, and tissue sections using antibodies, while additional information on receptor characterization may be obtained using radioligand binding techniques. Several protocols cover in vitro assays that determine the function of the endothelin peptides in isolated preparations, that characterize new endothelin receptor ligands, or provide information on the tissue-specific processing of endothelin precursor peptides. Finally, in vivo protocols illustrate the role of the endothelin peptides in healthy human individuals, describe animal models that reveal the alteration of the endothelin system in cardiovascular disease, and therefore predict the therapeutic potential of drugs that manipulate endothelin synthesis or function. A particular strength of *Peptide Research Protocols: Endothelin* is that, although each protocol may be used independently, many of the techniques are written to be complementary. The sequencing of the human genome presents new challenges in understanding the role in human physiology and pathophysiology of novel encoded proteins and peptides. The protocols described in this book have proved successful in endothelin research and the experimental strategies described have a wider relevance for determining the functional importance of the emerging orphan receptors and their cognate peptidic ligands.

Janet J. Maguire
Anthony P. Davenport

Contents

Contributors

MICHAEL J. ASHBY • *Clinical Pharmacology Unit, University of Cambridge, Cambridge, UK*

STEWART BARKER • *Department of Experimental Therapeutics, William Harvey Research Institute, St. Bartholomew's and the Royal London School of Medicine and Dentistry, Queen Mary University of London, London, UK*

ROGER CORDER • *Department of Experimental Therapeutics, William Harvey Research Institute, St. Bartholomew's and the Royal London School of Medicine and Dentistry, Queen Mary University of London, London, UK*

ANTHONY P. DAVENPORT • *Clinical Pharmacology Unit, University of Cambridge, Cambridge, UK*

GILLIAN A. GRAY • *Endothelial Cell Biology and Molecular Cardiology Group, Centre for Cardiovascular Sciences, Division of Biomedical and Clinical Laboratory Sciences, University of Edinburgh, Edinburgh, UK*

CAROLYN D. JACKSON • *School of Biochemistry and Molecular Biology, University of Leeds, Leeds, UK*

NOORAFZA Q. KHAN • *Department of Experimental Therapeutics, William Harvey Research Institute, St. Bartholomew's and the Royal London School of Medicine and Dentistry, Queen Mary University of London, London, UK*

RHODA E. KUC • *Clinical Pharmacology Unit, University of Cambridge, Cambridge, UK*

DELPHINE M. LEES • *Department of Experimental Therapeutics, William Harvey Research Institute, St. Bartholomew's and the Royal London School of Medicine and Dentistry, Queen Mary University of London, London, UK*

JANET J. MAGUIRE • *Clinical Pharmacology Unit, University of Cambridge, Cambridge, UK*

JUAN CARLOS MONGE • *Terence Donnelly Heart Centre, Division of Cardiology, St. Michael's Hospital, University of Toronto, Canada*

KAREN E. PORTER • *Integrated Molecular Cardiology Group, Institute for Cardiovascular Research, University of Leeds, Leeds, UK*

LORCAN SHERRY • *Research and Development, Organon Laboratories Ltd., Newhouse, Lanarkshire, UK*

PAULA J. W. SMITH • *Department of Neuroscience, University of Edinburgh, Edinburgh, UK*

FIONA E. STRACHAN • *Scottish Poisons Information Bureau, Lothian University Hospital NHS Trust, Edinburgh, UK*

ANTHONY J. TURNER • *School of Biochemistry and Molecular Biology, University of Leeds, Leeds, UK*

DAVID J. WEBB • *Clinical Pharmacology Unit and Research Centre, University of Edinburgh, Western General Hospital, Edinburgh, UK*

J. RUTH WU-WONG • *Abbott Laboratories, Santa Clara, CA*

I

ENDOTHELIN PEPTIDE PROTOCOLS

1

Immunocytochemical Localization of Endothelin Peptides, Precursors, and Endothelin-Converting Enzymes

Rhoda E. Kuc

1. Introduction

This chapter will describe the protocol used for the immunocytochemical (ICC) visualization of endothelin (ET) peptides, precursors and endothelin converting enzymes (ECEs) in both frozen cryostat tissue sections and cultured cells using polyclonal primary antisera raised in rabbits. We have raised antisera against the ET-1 carboxy-terminal heptapeptide, ET-1 $_{(15-21)}$, which is conserved in all three ET isoforms, (thus, the antibody does not distinguish between the three mature peptides); big ET-1 $_{(31-38)}$, big ET-2 $_{(31-37)}$ and big ET-3 $_{(31-42)}$ *(1)*, the ECE-1 isoforms *(2,3)* and ECE-2 *(4)* (*see* **Fig. 1**). The specificity of these antisera have been characterized using radioimmunoassays (RIA, *[5]*, *see* Chapter 2), enzyme-linked immunosorbant assays (ELISA, *see* Chapter 2) and in a comprehensive range of human and animal tissues using ICC, including comparisons with commercially available antibodies, although in most cases the staining achieved with these was less intense *(1,6)*.

In this protocol, visualization of the primary antibody is achieved using the immunoperoxidase (PAP) method, with DAB as the chromogen. This is the method of choice, as the amplification steps give greater sensitivity over direct staining methods and the production of an insoluble, brown reaction product at the site of the antigen results in a permanent record. Alternatively, a fluorescein conjugated secondary antibody that results in a green fluorescence product under UV illumination may be used. Interpretation of results is possibly the most difficult part of immunocytochemistry; it requires an understanding of the complete process from tissue selection and processing, through the infinite

From: *Methods in Molecular Biology, vol. 206: Peptide Research Protocols: Endothelin*
Edited by: J. Maguire and A. Davenport © Humana Press Inc., Totowa, NJ

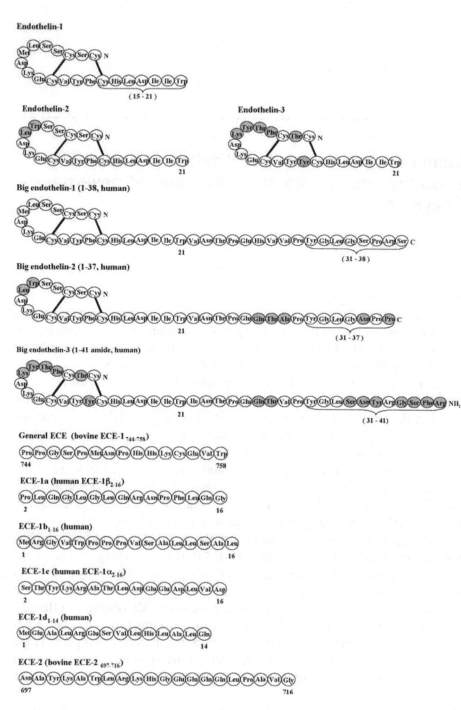

Fig. 1. Amino acid sequences used to generate site-directed antisera in endothelin peptides and endothelin-converting enzyme (ECE) proteins.

variables of antibody dilution and incubation times to the choice of revealing steps. Consideration must be given to each of these steps, along with the various controls included in the protocol, when viewing the final result. Histological knowledge of the tissue or cells under investigation is essential in identifying the apparent distribution of the antigen.

Using the protocol described here, we have found immunoreactive mature ET, and the precursor peptides to be widely expressed within the human vascular endothelium, although not in the underlying smooth muscle cells. Their presence has also been identified in many nonvascular tissues *(1,5–10)*. While big ET-1 is known to be released by endothelial cells, it has little biological activity at physiological concentrations so must be converted to the mature peptide to cause vasoconstriction *(11)*. The conversion of the big ETs to the mature peptides, by the unique cleavage of the Trp^{21}-Val^{22} or Trp^{21}-Ile^{22} bond *(12,13)*, is achieved via one or more of the endothelin converting enzymes *(14–17)*. Using antisera against the ECEs, we have demonstrated the co-localization of the converting enzymes *(18)* with the endothelin peptides and their precursors in a range of human tissues *(2)*, as summarized in **Table 1**. We have determined the subcellular localization *(19)* of ECE-2 within cultured HUVECs, previously predicted by the detection of ECE-2 mRNA *(17)*. In addition, ICC has allowed us to demonstrate, for example in human kidney *(20)*, the localization of the ECE-1α enzyme, to confirm biochemical studies demonstrating the conversion of ET-1 from big ET-1. ICC can therefore be an invaluable tool in its own right determining the anatomical localization of both peptides and enzymes, as well as in combination with other techniques in understanding complex biological mechanisms such as the endothelin system.

2. Materials

1. Liquid nitrogen, Dewer (or thermos flask), iso-pentane (2-methyl butane), beaker, tongs (dry ice may also be used, placing tissue onto a piece of foil over the pellets of dry ice).
2. Single-edged razor blades.
3. Cryostat-chucks and cork discs, if used.
4. Mounting medium, OCT compound Gurr® (361603E Merck/BDH, Poole, Dorset, UK).
5. Cryostat with motorized microtome, to cut frozen sections of 10–30 μm (e.g., Bright Instrument Co. Ltd., Huntingdon, Cambs., UK).
6. Slide racks (metal with handle[s], to hold 24 slides).
7. Slide baths (400–500 mL, note glass baths with lids should be used for paraformaldehyde, acetone and xylene, for other solutions small plastic lunch/freezer boxes are ideal).

Table 1
Immunocytochemical Localization of Endothelin Peptides and Converting Enzymes in Human Tissues

	Mature ET	Big ET-1	Big ET-2	Big ET-3	ECE-1	ECE-2
Umbilical (1,2,6,10,19)						
HUVECS	+	+	+	+	+gen,a,b,c[a]	+gen
Umbilical vein	+				+gen	+gen
Umbilical artery	+				+gen	+gen
Heart (1,5)						
Myocytes	–	–	–	–	–	–
Endocardial endothelial	+	+	+	–	+gen	+gen
Vessels (1,2,8,18)						
Intra–myocardial	+	+	+	–	+gen	+gen
Epicardial coronary artery	+	+	+	–	+gen,a,c	+gen,2
Saphenous vein	+	+	+	–	+	+
Saphenous vein graft	+	+	+	–	+gen	+gen
Internal mammary artery	+	+	+	–		
Mesenteric artery/ vein	+/+	+/–	+/+	–/–		
Aorta	+					
Lung (2,3,7,18)						
Airway epithelial cells	+	–	+	+	+gen,a,b,c	+gen
Sub mucosal glands	+	+	+	+	–	–
Parenchyma	+	+	–	–	–	–
Pulmonary vessels	+	+	+/–	?	+b,c	+gen

(Continued)

Tissue / cell type					
Kidney (2,18,20)					
Collecting ducts				+a,b,c	+
Distal convoluted tubules				+a,b,c	
Glomeruli				+a,b,c	
Resistance vessels,	+			+a,b,c	+
Renal vein/ artery	+			+a,b,c	+
Adrenal (2,10)					
Supply arteries	+	+	+	+gen	+gen
Resistance vessels	+	+	+	+gen	+gen
Capillary sinusoids	+	–	–	–	–
Medulla	–	–	+	–	–
Zona glomerulosa	+	–	–	–	–
Zona fasiculata	+	–	–		
Zona reticularis	+	–	–	–	–
Brain (2,18,19)					
Pial vessels, <50 μm	+			+gen,b,c	+gen,2
Cortex					
Glial limitans				+gen,b,c	+gen,2
Neurones and processes				+gen,b,c	+gen,2
Astrocytes	+/–*			+gen,b,c	+gen,2
Endometrium/Myometrium (6,9)					
Glandular and luminal epithelial	+	+	+		
Vascular endothlial cells	+	+	+		

[a]ECE antisera raised against a sequence common to the ECE-1 isoforms and ECE-2 (*see* **ref. 2**). a,b,c, ECE-1 isoform detected using the appropriate ECE-1 antisera (*18*); 2, ECE-2 isoform (*19*).

8. Microscope slides: (1) Our preferred treatment for ICC is to coat slides with poly-L-lysine (P-8920 Sigma-Aldrich Co. Ltd, Poole, Dorset, UK, Sigma, St. Louis, MO). Place a small drop onto the slide and distribute evenly, using the end of another slide, allow to air-dry. (2) Gelatin-subbed slides may also be used in ICC, although they are less effective in retaining tissue sections. Wash slides in racks in a detergent solution, rinse in deionized water, then dip into a gelatin solution (5 g gelatin, 0.25 g chromium potassium sulfate, dissolved by heating to 45°C in 500 mL deionized water) then air-dry and store at room temperature. These are our preferred choices for radioligand binding. Alternatively pretreated slides are available (e.g., Polysine 406/0178/00 or Superfrost plus 406/0179/00, Merck/BDH, Poole, Dorset, UK).

9. Coverslips, rectangular for slides, circles for cultured cells.

10. 12-Well sterile culture plates.

11. Sterile gelatin solution for coating coverslips (0.5 g gelatin/200 mL deionized water, autoclave and store at 4°C).

12. Methanol, acetone, ethanol, industrial methylated spirits (IMS), xylene, (all analytical grade, from a general laboratory supplier). A series of alcohol baths are prepared for dehydrating sections, 30%, 70%, and 100% IMS (balance deionized water), 100% ethanol (×2) and acid alcohol (100% ethanol + 1 mL concentrated HCl). With the exception of 100% ethanol, these may be stored and reused several times.

13. Phosphate buffered saline (10X stock solution): 400 g NaCl, 10 g KCl, 10 g KH_2PO_4, 57.5 g Na_2HPO_4, dissolved in 5 L of deionized water and stored at room temperature). A 1:10 dilution in deionized water is made from the stock as required. PBS-T is made by a 1:10 dilution of the stock solution (1 L + 9 L deionized water) and the addition of 1 mL/L Tween-20 to give a final concentration of 0.1%. PBS-T is stored at 4°C. Other buffers such as Tris or a Tris-PBS combination may be used, however it is important that they do not contain sodium azide (often found in commercially prepared buffers) as this may inhibit the binding of peroxidase to its substrate thus leading to a false negative result.

14. Paraformaldehyde stock made at 8% w/v, i.e., dissolve 40 g paraformaldehyde in 500 mL of deionized water, heat on a hotplate stirrer in a fume hood to 80°C. Clear the solution by adding 1 mL of glacial acetic acid, allow to cool, filter, and store at 4°C. A 400 mL, freshly prepared working solution is made by adding 200 mL of 8% paraformaldehyde to 200 mL of 2X PBS, i.e., 1:5 dilution of the 10X PBS stock.

15. Hydrophobic pen, "Immedge" pen (Vector Laboratories, Peterborough, UK).

16. Incubation trays. 24 × 24 cm NUNC bioassay dishes (Gibco BRL) are modified "in-house" by the addition of four perspex rods, fixed with adhesive to the bases in two pairs, to give support to two rows of 6–7 slides per tray (*see* **Fig. 2**).

17. Antisera/normal sera and conjugates. The primary antisera against the endothelin peptides, receptors and enzymes are all designed and produced "in house". Commercial antisera are also available (e.g., Peninsula Laboratories, St. Helens, UK

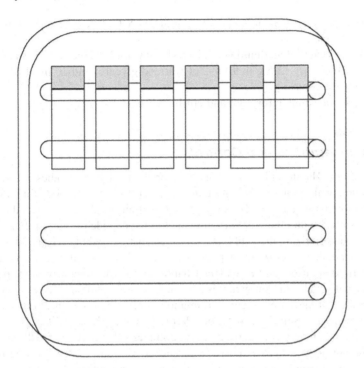

Fig. 2. Tray design for incubation of microscope slides.

or Peptide Institute, Osaka, Japan). Other reagents are obtained from commercial suppliers (e.g., DAKO Ltd, Ely, Cambs., UK). This company is our preferred supplier, providing high quality of reagents, preabsorbed against human antigens, to reduce nonspecific staining, and they provide excellent technical support. The fluorescence reagents were purchased from Vector Laboratories (Peterborough, UK), from whom instructions for handling and storage, as well as suggested use, may be obtained.

18. DAB (3,3' diaminobenzidine tetrahydrochloride, D-5637, Sigma-Aldrich, Poole, Dorset, UK). DAB is carcinogenic; care should be taken to avoid breathing in the powder when handling it. To avoid weighing out the powder, in a fume cupboard add sufficient deionized water to dissolve the entire contents of the supplied vial to a concentration of 24 mg/mL. The DAB solution may then be stored in 2.5 mL aliquots at −20°C. To prepare the final incubation solution, add a thawed 2.5 mL aliquot to 100 mL of 0.05 M Tris-HCl buffer, pH 7.6, immediately prior to use add 1 mL 0.3% hydrogen peroxide (this should give a final DAB concentration of 0.6 mg/mL, this solution will remain stable for 1–2 h).

19. Hematoxylin solution (e.g., Harris' modified hematoxylin solution, HHS-16, Sigma-Aldrich, Poole, Dorset, UK and Scott's tap water (3.5 g sodium bicarbonate, 20 g magnesium sulfate added to 1 L of deionized water).

20. Xylene-based permanent mountant (e.g., DePeX-Gurr®, 361254D, Merck/BDH, Poole, Dorset, UK).
21. DABCO (triethylenediamine; 1,4-Diazabicyclo[2.2.2]octane, Sigma-Aldrich D-2522), dissolve 2.5 g in 90 mL of warmed glycerol and 10 mL PBS, store at room temperature.
22. Microscope suitable for light and epifluoresce.

3. Methods
3.1. Considerations and Controls

1. Specificity: Having either raised in house, or obtained the antibodies of choice from a commercial supplier, it is important to characterize each antibody for its specificity for the target antigen. To confirm the specificity of the antibodies, they can be preabsorbed with other peptides unrelated to the peptide of interest. For example, when characterizing the antibodies raised against ET and big ET peptides, a range of nonendothelin vasoactive peptides were used. These specificity checks may also be carried out using an ELISA (*see* Chapter 2). In order to enhance the specificity of the antisera for the antigen, it is advisable, where possible, to affinity purify the antisera to remove nonspecific immunoglobulins and any interfering peptides (e.g., using the SulfoLink Kit from Perbio Science UK Ltd., Cheshire, UK) this has usually already been carried out for commercial antisera. Once the specificity of the antibody is known, positive and negative tissue controls can be included routinely to monitor the assay system. For a novel peptide, this requires the processing of a range of tissues to first determine the distribution of the antigen and thus identify suitable negative and positive tissue controls.
2. Negative controls: The ideal negative control is demonstrated by the preabsorption of the primary antibody with the purified antigen to achieve the attenuation or complete loss of staining in a tissue. In this procedure, the primary antibody, at the working dilution, is preincubated with an excess of the purified antigen before use (this should already be done for a commercial antibody, and indeed may not be possible in the laboratory where a source of the antigenic peptide may not be available). Another negative control is to substitute a serum, known not to contain antibodies to the antigen, for the primary antibody. Ideally this would be a preimmune serum sample taken from the same animal prior to challenge with the antigen (with antiserum from a commercial source this may again not be possible). Where a preimmune is not available a nonimmune serum can be substituted, i.e., serum from the same species in which the primary antibody is generated.
3. Positive controls: When determining the distribution of the peptide antigens in a range of human and animal tissues, comparisons with other known cell markers, e.g., von Willebrand factor, smooth muscle α-actin, glial fibrillary acidic protein and macrophage staining, can be used as positive controls for the assay procedure and also to confirm localization of the antigen to specific cell types. Once the distribution of the antigen is determined, known positive tissues should be included in the protocol when investigating "new" tissues.

A Link antibody vs PAP complex

PAP complex	Link antibody (e.g. SAR)			
	1:50	1:100	1:150	1:200
1:100				
1:200				
1:300				
1:400				

B Primary antibody

PAP complex	Primary antibody			
	1:100	1:300	1:500	1:1000
1:100				
1:200				
1:300				
1:400				

Fig. 3. Titration checkerboard. The optimum dilutions for more than one reagent are determined simultaneously. First (**A**), the link antibody and PAP complex are titrated, as they are interdependent. Keeping the conditions for these constant (**B**), the optimum dilution of the primary antibody is then determined. For each example (**A**) and (**B**) 16 slides/tissue sections are required.

4. In ICC the concentration of antigens and antibodies is crucial in achieving a reliable result, too high a concentration of antibody can result in a false negative (a similar phenomenon to that seen in agglutination testing) or in the more easily predicted over staining and increase in nonspecific background staining. The ideal ICC protocol is one that achieves a balance, giving the highest possible specific staining with the least background staining. It is advisable when using a new antibody or investigating the distribution of a known antibody in a new tissue, to use a range of dilutions not only for the primary antibody but also for the secondary or "link" antibody, as well as the peroxidase conjugate. A titration checkerboard is a useful example of how such dilutions might be organized (*see* **Fig. 3**).

5. Finally, to demonstrate the localization of the antigen within a tissue section, it is possible to counterstain the sections. The DAB product is insoluble in alcohol and organic solvents; it is therefore possible to use a Hematoxylin stain prior to the alcohol dehydration and xylene steps and the mounting of the slides. Development of the counterstain should be monitored to avoid overstaining, which may result in obliteration of the antigen specific staining.

3.2. Tissue Preparation

3.2.1. Preparation of Tissues and Cryostat Sections

1. Tissues for ICC should be as fresh as possible and processed within minutes of removal. Tissue should be cut into blocks of 1–2 cm^3 using a single-edged razor blade, frozen over dry ice, isopentane or liquid nitrogen, wrapped loosely in foil, labeled and stored at −80°C until required (*see* **Note 1**). Alternatively, the tissue may be frozen directly onto cryostat chucks, or cork discs, by embedding in OCT mounting medium either over dry ice or on the cold shelf of the cryostat. The mounted tissue may be sectioned immediately or stored, wrapped in foil, at −80°C (*see* **Note 2**).

2. Allow tissue, whether previously stored at −80°C or freshly mounted, to equilibrate to cutting temperature, i.e., −20 to −30°C depending on tissue type (*see* **Note 3**). For ICC, cut cryostat sections at 30 μm and thaw mount onto microscope slides pretreated with poly-L-lysine to aid adhesion of the tissue section (*see* **Note 4**). Allow cut sections to air-dry before either commencing ICC or storing slides in sealed boxes at −80°C until required.

3.2.2. Preparation of Cultured Cells for ICC (e.g., HUVECs)

1. Cultured human umbilical vein endothelial cells (HUVECs), at primary passage (*see* **Note 5**), are seeded into 12-well culture dishes containing gelatin coated coverslips and incubated for up to 7 d until almost confluent (*see* **Note 6**).

2. Remove culture plates from the incubator and wash (2 × 5 min) with PBS to remove incubation media and immediately process for ICC. If cells can not be processed immediately, fix with a 1:1 mixture of acetone and methanol and freeze at −80°C until required (*see* **Subheading 3.3.2.** and **Note 7**).

3.3. Immunocytochemistry

3.3.1. Tissue Sections

1. Transfer air-dried sections (dried for between 3 and 24 h) into slide racks. Fix by immersion in 400 mL baths of freshly prepared 4% paraformaldehyde in 0.1 *M* phosphate buffered saline (PBS), for 30 min at 4°C (*see* **Note 8**).

2. Wash slides by immersing, in racks, into 400 mL baths of PBS (3 × 5 min), remove excess buffer by carefully wiping around each section, encircle the section with a hydrophobic pen, and label each slide using a pencil (*see* **Note 9**). Place the slides horizontally into incubation trays humidified by the addition of PBS to the bottom of the trays (*see* **Fig. 2** and *see* **Note 10**).

3. Block nonspecific staining by covering sections with 200–500 μL of 10% "normal" swine serum in PBS (*see* **Note 11**). Incubate sections, in the trays with lids on to maintain humidity, for up to 2 h at room temperature.

4. Tip off the blocking reagent and gently tap the slides on the base of the incubation tray. Any excess is carefully wiped from around the sections. Then add a volume (typically 100–300 μL) of the primary antibody against the antigen under investigation (also positive and negative controls), diluted appropriately in PBS-TSS

(i.e., PBS, 0.1% Tween-20, + 1% swine serum, 3.3 mg/mL BSA), onto each section, and incubate the slides at 4°C overnight (*see* **Note 12**).

5. Return the slides to the slide-racks and wash, as in **step 2**, return slides to the trays and incubate with the appropriately diluted secondary antibody (swine anti-rabbit at 1: 200 in PBS/TSS) for 1 h at room temperature (*see* **Note 13**).

6. Wash slides by immersing, in racks, into 400 mL baths of PBS containing 0.1% Tween-20 (PBS-T) (3 × 5 min), remove excess buffer by carefully wiping around each section and incubate for a further 1 h at room temperature with the appropriately diluted (1:400 in PBS-TSS) rabbit peroxidase-anti-peroxidase (PAP) reagent.

7. Wash slides again as in **step 6** above, then incubate for up to 4 min with a freshly prepared solution of the chromogenic substrate DAB. Monitor slides for development of the brown reaction product. Stop the reaction, by gently flooding the sections with deionized water from a wash bottle or pipet and transfer them to slide racks in a bath of deionized water. At this point, the slides may be counterstained with Hematoxylin to aid in the interpretation of antigen distribution (*see* **Note 14**).

8. Transfer the slide racks through the series of alcohol baths (1–2 min each) to dehydrate the sections, then into a bath of xylene for at least 1 h to clear. Mount the slides using DePeX and coverslips, allow them to dry, and remove excess mountant before viewing under a light microscope.

3.3.2. Cultured Cells

1. To fix cells (freshly prepared as in **Subheading 3.2.2.** above, or if frozen cells are used allow to thaw) on coverslips, carefully add 2 mL of acetone: methanol (1:1 mix) to each well and incubate for 5 min. Aspirate to remove the fixative and allow cells to dry.

2. Carry out the ICC procedure as described for tissue sections (*see* **Subheading 3.3.1.**) with the following modifications: The incubation volume used is 1 mL/well. Wash cells by aspirating the incubation solutions, and replace 2–3× with PBS-TSS (*see* **Note 7**).

3. Following incubation with DAB, aspirate the wells and fill with deionized water to stop the reaction. Remove each coverslip individually from the wells and dip through an alcohol series to dehydrate. Mount each coverslip, cell side down, onto a microscope slide with DePeX and allow to dry before viewing under a light microscope (*see* **Note 15**).

3.3.3. Immunocytochemistry with Immunofluorescence Visualization

1. Process tissue sections or cells to the end of the primary antibody incubation step and wash (*see* **Subheadings 3.3.1.** and **3.3.2.** above) with the following changes: Fix tissue sections in acetone for 10 min at 4°C. The primary incubation may be reduced to 1–2 h at room temperature (*see* **Note 16**).

2. To visualize the primary antibody, incubate with swine anti-rabbit fluorescein conjugated secondary antibody (1:30 dilution in PBS-TSS), for 1 h at room temperature (*see* **Note 17**).

3. Wash as described above and mount with DABCO mounting medium before examining under epifluorescent illumination (*see* **Note 18**).

4. Notes

1. Ideally, tissues should be frozen as soon as possible after surgery for human tissues or euthanasia of animals. Keeping delays to a minimum is essential in preserving tissue integrity, i.e., to minimize the activity of degradative enzymes, and to preserve antigen availability. If tissues are cut into small blocks and quickly frozen, the need for repeated freeze thaw cycles is reduced, the formation of ice crystals which may disrupt tissue morphology will be limited and smaller blocks will be less likely to crack during the freezing process. When storing tissues care should be taken to wrap the tissue loosely in foil, to prevent it sticking to the foil. The appropriately labeled tissue can then be placed into a sealable bag, to minimize dehydration, and then preferably into a box to prevent crushing, before storing at $-80°C$.

2. The cryostat chuck should be cooled either over dry ice or on the cold shelf of the cryostat; larger pieces of tissue may be mounted directly onto the chuck with mounting medium. For smaller tissues, a layer of mounting medium may be applied to the chuck and allowed to freeze before mounting the tissue, this will allow a greater proportion of the tissue to be sectioned without fear of the blade coming into contact with the chuck. Also, for smaller tissues, more than one piece of tissue may be mounted on the same chuck. In some laboratories, tissues are preferentially mounted onto cork discs for storage and then the discs mounted onto the cryostat chucks for sectioning and then removed. This is not recommended, as the inherent "sponginess" of the cork can lead to its compression during sectioning. This allows movement of the tissue while sectioning, producing inconsistencies in the thickness and quality of the sections obtained. In addition the repeated freeze-thawing of the mounting medium used to "glue" the disc to the chuck may add to this variability, as we have found that when mounting medium has been through a freeze-thaw cycle it fails to solidify adequately. In mounting tissues onto cryostat chucks, consideration should be given to the orientation of the tissue. For example, keeping the tissue parallel to the chuck surface will ensure less trimming of the tissue is required before achieving a complete section. Small tissues such as blood vessels may require support, e.g., holding the vessel upright using fine forceps until the mounting medium has frozen. Once mounted, the tissue may be stored at $-80°C$.

3. The temperature for optimal sectioning of a tissue will vary and should be determined empirically. When positioning the chuck onto the tissue holder within the cryostat the orientation of the tissue should be considered, depending upon the shape of the tissue. An irregular piece of tissue, for example, would be better sectioned with the longest "side" rather than the irregular aspect or "point" as the leading edge, as this may result in the tissue section rotating as the section is cut, giving a creased or torn section. Good quality sections are imperative in interpreting results, sections of irregular thickness, or containing tears or folds, may

result in entrapment of the antibody or edge effects, resulting in a falsely high signal being seen. Once the orientation is decided it is a good idea to mark the chuck, to enable subsequent sectioning of the same tissue to be achieved more easily and without loss of tissue due to trimming.

4. Sections (30 μm for ICC, 10 μm for radioligand binding) are thaw-mounted onto slides, pretreated to increase adhesion of the sections. For ICC of frozen sections, poly-L-lysine is the preferred option. For radioligand binding, a chrome alum-gelatin coating is preferred. There are also several commercially available sources of pretreated slides.

5. Use primary or first passage cultures only, as subsequent subcultures may exhibit an increased pleomorphism and decreased capacity to form confluent monolayers of cells.

6. We routinely use 12-well plates, this allows a combination of treatments to be performed (including duplicates, dilution ranges, negative controls-preimmune sera, preabsorption of antisera, positive controls-antisera with known characteristics, e.g., von Willebrand factor) within a plate. HUVECs are not easily grown in culture and require prior treatment of the support in order for them adhere. In a laminar flow hood, alcohol and flame 12 round coverslips. Dip each one into a solution of 0.25% gelatin, remove excess by touching the edge to a sheet of absorbent tissue paper and place one in each well of a 12-well culture plate, allow to dry in laminar flow cabinet. As a precaution against contamination, irradiate with UV light (10 min) prior to storage at room temperature. Seeded plates are incubated at 37°C in a humidified incubator gassed with 5% CO_2 until confluence is approached. Using the cells just before they are fully confluent avoids cells piling up, which would encourage sheets of cells to lift off during further manipulations.

7. Cells are washed by tipping the plate at an angle and carefully aspirating off the incubation buffer from the bottom corner at the edge of the coverslip with a Pasteur pipet. PBS, 2 mL/well, is then added slowly with the pipet angled to the side of the well rather than directly onto the cells to prevent the cells lifting off. This is repeated 1–2×. If cells are not to be used immediately they may be fixed (1:1 mix of acetone:methanol) and allowed to dry before freezing at −80°C.

8. Fixation is an important step in the processing of tissues, if the antigen in question is not fixed, it may be washed away. The aim in fixation of tissues is to preserve both tissue morphology and antigen availability. Mild or underfixation may preserve the antigen, but result in a loss of morphology of the surrounding tissues, making interpretation of the staining difficult. Conversely overfixation, while maintaining morphology of the tissue, may result in masking or denaturation of the antigen, i.e., reducing the availability or altering the presentation of the antigen, and as the antibody can only bind to that antigen presented, this would result in low levels of staining. For small antigens, frozen tissue sections are the preferred option, and for endothelin peptides the fixation of choice in our hands has been found to be a mild formaldehyde solution, whereas for characterization of the endothelin receptors and endothelin-converting enzymes (ECE), an acetone

fixation is used. It is therefore essential for the individual researcher to spend some time in optimising the conditions to be used. For the endothelin peptides, we routinely use 4% paraformaldehyde buffered in PBS, however when visualizing the endothelin receptors and converting enzymes this was found to diminish the staining, therefore following optimization we found fixation for 10 min in acetone at 4°C to be the preferred method. Endogenous peroxidases within certain tissues such as red blood cells, liver, kidney and brain can produce nonspecific staining via a direct reaction with the H_2O_2 of the chromogen solution. Incubation of the sections with a methanolic H_2O_2 solution (1 : 4, mix of 3% H_2O_2:methanol) may be used to suppress the endogenous activity, however, this treatment may also result in a decrease in adhesion of the section to the microscope slide, thus requiring the investigator to treat the sections more carefully during subsequent protocol steps.

9. When manipulating slides, it is crucial to limit damage of the sections as much as possible. After each incubation and wash step, the excess buffer must be removed to prevent dilution of the next reagent. Care must be used in wiping buffer from around the sections to prevent damage to the tissue. Using a hydrophobic pen to ring the tissue sections is recommended. It provides a guide when wiping excess liquid from the slide, preventing the section from being accidentally wiped off, by providing surface tension it also allows smaller incubation volumes of antisera to be used without the solutions running off the slides. It is important not to allow the sections to dry out at any stage of the staining protocol as this may result in uninterpretable results. Therefore, when processing a large number of slides, it is advisable to wipe only up to six slides at a time before adding the incubation solution. Pencil (or a diamond pen) should be used to label slides, as inks will be solubilized and lost during the alcohol dehydration and xylene stages.

10. For the fixation and wash stages, baths of reagents are the easiest and least labor-intensive method to use. However, for incubations with antisera only small volumes of reagent are used because of the limitations of cost and availability of reagents. The sections are therefore incubated horizontally with 100–300 μL incubation volume/slide, in incubation trays humidified to prevent the sections drying out.

11. The nonimmune or "normal" blocking serum chosen is usually from the same species that is providing the secondary antibody, i.e., if, as in this case, the second antibody is raised in swine, swine nonimmune sera is used. Following incubation, this reagent is not washed off but is tipped off, therefore, care must be taken to ensure that only a thin layer remains to prevent further dilution of the primary antibody.

12. The combination of antibody dilution, incubation time and incubation temperature used are interdependent and will all have a bearing on the final nonspecific background staining and specific staining intensity achieved within a particular tissue. It is therefore necessary to determine the optimum conditions empirically. Commercial antisera are often supplied with suggested conditions for use, however, these may not necessarily be appropriate for every application. For example, we routinely chose to incubate the primary antibody at 4°C overnight, however a

shorter incubation at room temperature or even 37°C may work better for other antibodies.

13. Since the antisera against the endothelin peptides were raised in rabbits, the secondary antibody chosen for this system is Swine anti-rabbit (at a dilution of 1:200). This provides the "link" between the primary antibody and the PAP complex as both are raised in the same animal species. The PAP complex (used at a 1:400 dilution) consists of the enzyme peroxidase and an antibody against peroxidase. The peroxidase complexes with the substrate, hydrogen peroxide (H_2O_2), this in turn reacts with the chromogen (an electron donor) to produce a colored product. It may be noted that in this reaction the enzyme is not depleted and therefore each molecule of enzyme bound is available to react with further hydrogen peroxide and therefore produce more molecules of colored product, providing further amplification in signal. This is an advantage of the immunoperoxidase method over immunofluorescence techniques in which one fluorescent molecule binds with no amplification step. Each visualization method has its own drawbacks, for example, the PAP method produces a permanent and intense staining, however, endogenous peroxidase activity may be a problem in some tissues, e.g., kidney and brain, giving an increased background signal. In fluorescence staining, while endogenous peroxidase activity is less important, the staining produced will fade over time.

14. DAB is potentially carcinogenic, therefore it is advisable to avoid contact with the powder. It is important to prepare the solution of DAB immediately prior to use, as solutions will deteriorate within 1–2 h. The colored product is insoluble in alcohol and organic solvents, thus allowing for counterstaining with the alcohol-based stain Hematoxylin (following wash in water bath incubate for 5 min, wash in tap water, 30 s, followed by Scott's Tap water for 1 min, then wash again before continuing with protocol), dehydration through a series of baths of increasing alcohol concentration and permanent mounting in xylene-based mountants such as DePeX.

15. The cultured cells should be manipulated gently to prevent them lifting from the coverslips. A pair of forceps with curved fine tips may be used to lift each coverslip in turn from the wells and to dip them through the series of alcohol baths. Excess alcohol is removed by touching the edge of the coverslip onto absorbent paper, and the coverslip is lowered, cell side down, onto a pool of DePeX on a microscope slide.

16. Incubating tissues overnight at 4°C allows for a more dilute primary antibody to be used and will produce less nonspecific background staining. This is very useful when supplies of a primary antisera are limited. When using fluorescence conjugated antibodies, background staining is less of a problem, and as these are usually commercially available antibodies, limited supplies are not an issue, therefore, more concentrated solutions may be used.

17. Fluorescein is the choice of conjugated dye as it produces the most intense fluorescent yield. This fluoresces in the green wavelength range; others are available which fluoresce in the red (rhodamine and Texas Red) and the blue (phycoeryth-

rin) ranges. This difference allows dual (or even multiple) labeling of different antigens simultaneously visualized as different colored signals within the same cells or tissue sections.

18. DABCO scavenges free radicals produced by excitation of fluorochromes and is added to nonpermanent mountants to reduce fading of the fluorescence signal, the major drawback of using immunofluorescent dyes. If immediate viewing is not possible, storage times may be increased by keeping slides wrapped in foil and refrigerated. If necessary, the sections can be restained.

Acknowledgments

Supported by grants from the British Heart Foundation.

References

1. Howard, P. G., Plumpton, C., and Davenport, A. P. (1992) Anatomical localization and pharmacological activity of mature endothelins and their precursors in human vascular tissue. *J. Hypertens.* **10,** 1379–1386.
2. Davenport, A. P., Kuc, R. E., Plumpton, C., Mockridge, J. W., Barker, P. J., and Huskisson, N. S. (1998) Endothelin-converting enzyme in human tissues. *Histochem. J.* **30,** 359–374.
3. Mockridge, J. W., Kuc, R. E., Huskisson, N. S., Barker, P. J., and Davenport, A. P. (1998) Characterization of site-directed antisera against endothelin-converting enzymes. *J. Cardiovasc. Pharmacol.* **31,** S35–S37.
4. Russell, F. D. and Davenport, A. P. (1999) Evidence for intracellular endothelin-converting enzyme-2 expression in cultured human vascular endothelial cells. *Circ. Res.* **84,** 891–896.
5. Plumpton, C., Ashby, M. J., Kuc, R. E., O'Reilly, G., and Davenport, A. P. (1996) Expression of endothelin peptides and mRNA in the human heart. *Clin. Sci.* **90,** 37–46.
6. Cameron, I. T., Davenport, A. P., van Papendorp, C., Barker, P. J., Huskisson, N. S., Gilmour, R. S., et al. (1992) Endothelin-like immunoreactivity in human endometrium. *J. Reprod. Fertil.* **95,** 623–628.
7. Marciniak, S. J., Plumpton, C., Barker, P. J., Huskisson, N. S., and Davenport, A. P. (1992) Localization of immunoreactive endothelin and proendothelin in the human lung. *Pulm. Pharmacol.* **5,** 175–182.
8. Bacon, C. R. and Davenport, A. P. (1996) Endothelin receptors in human coronary artery and aorta. *Br. J. Pharmacol.* **117,** 986–992.
9. Cameron, I. T., Plumpton, C., Champeney, R., van Papendorp, C., Ashby, M. J. and Davenport, A. P. (1993) Identification of endothelin-1, endothelin-2 and endothelin-3 in human endometrium. *J. Reprod. Fertil.* **98,** 251–255.
10. Davenport, A. P., Hoskins, S. L., Kuc, R. E., and Plumpton, C. (1996) Differential distribution of endothelin peptides and receptors in human adrenal gland. *Histochem. J.* **28,** 779–789.

11. Plumpton, C., Haynes, W. G., Webb, D. J., and Davenport, A. P. (1995) Phosphoramidon inhibition of the in vivo conversion of big endothelin-1 to endothelin-1 in the human forearm. *Br. J. Pharmacol.* **116**, 1821–1828.
12. Opgenorth, T. J., Wu-Wong, J. R., and Shiosaki, K. (1992) Endothelin-converting enzymes. *FASEB J.* **6**, 2653–2659.
13. Turner, A. J. and Murphy, L. J. (1996) Molecular pharmacology of endothelin converting enzymes. *Biochem. Pharmacol.* **51**, 91–102.
14. Xu, D., Emoto, N., Giaid, A., Slaughter, C., Kaw, S., Dewit, D., and Yanagisawa, M. (1994) ECE-1: a membrane-bound metalloprotease that catalyzes the proteolytic activation of big endothelin-1. *Cell* **78**, 473–485.
15. Shimada, K., Matsushita, Y., Wakabayashi, K., Takahashi, M., Iijima, Y., and Tanzawa, K. (1995a) Cloning and functional expression of endothelin-converting enzyme cDNA. *Biochem. Biophys. Res. Commun.* **207**, 807–812.
16. Shimada, K., Takahashi, M., Ikeda, M., and Tanzawa, K. (1995b) Identification of two isoforms of an endothelin-converting enzyme-1. *Febs. Lett.* **371**, 140–144.
17. Emoto, N. and Yanagisawa, M. (1995) Endothelin converting enzyme-2 is a membrane bound, phosphoramidon-sensitive metalloprotease with acidic pH optimum. *J. Biol. Chem.* **270**, 15,262–15,268.
18. Davenport, A. P. and Kuc, R. E. (2000) Cellular expression of isoforms of endothelin converting enzyme (ECE-1c, ECE-1b and ECE-1a) and Endothelin-converting enzyme-2. *J. Cardiovasc. Pharmacol.* **36**, S12–S14.
19. Russell, F. D. and Davenport, A. P. (1999) Evidence for intracellular endothelin-converting enzyme-2 expression in cultured human vascular endothelial cells. *Circ. Res.* **84**, 8, 891–896.
20. Russell, F. D., Coppell, A. L., and Davenport, A. P. (1998) In vitro enzymatic processing of radiolabeled big ET-1 in human kidney. *Biochem. Pharmacol.* **55**, 697–701.

2

Analysis of Endothelins by Enzyme-Linked Immunosorbent Assay and Radioimmunoassay

Anthony P. Davenport and Rhoda E. Kuc

1. Introduction

This chapter describes procedures for the measurement of endothelin peptides by antibodies, focusing on the two main immunoassay techniques that are widely used. In a two-site "sandwich" enzyme-linked immunosorbent assay (ELISA) one antibody is immobilized to a solid phase and captures the endothelin (ET) peptide(s), which is quantified by the binding to this complex of a second, enzyme-labeled antibody in the liquid phase. In a radioimmunoassay (RIA), the ET peptide(s) to be measured competes for the binding of a fixed concentration of radiolabeled peptide to a fixed concentration of antibody in the liquid phase. In contrast to the ELISA, the immune complex measured in a RIA does not contain the analyte and therefore inverse (falling) standard curves of peptide concentration vs bound labeled peptide are produced. For a more detailed discussion of the two techniques, **refs.** *1* and *2* are recommended.

Both immunoassay techniques are characterized by limited purification of the analyte and may therefore be susceptible to interference by unrelated molecules or crossreact with structurally-related peptides. Where the precise identification of the ET peptides present in the tissue samples is required, these immunoassays can be preceded by chromatographic separation (*see* Chapter 3). ELISAs can also be used to test the specificity of antisera used to visualize, but not to quantify, ET peptides in tissue sections by immunocytochemistry (*see* Chapter 1).

From: *Methods in Molecular Biology, vol. 206: Peptide Research Protocols: Endothelin*
Edited by: J. Maguire and A. Davenport © Humana Press Inc., Totowa, NJ

1.1. ET-1 and Big ET-1

ET-1 is the principal isoform in the human cardiovascular system and remains the most potent constrictor of human vessels discovered. ET-1 is unusual amongst the mammalian bioactive peptides in being released from a dual secretory pathway *(3,4)*. The peptide is continuously released from vascular endothelial cells by the constitutive pathway, producing intense constriction of the underlying smooth muscle and contributing to the maintenance of endogenous vascular tone *(5)*. The peptide is also released from endothelial cell-specific storage granules (Weibel-Palade bodies) in response to external physiological, or perhaps pathophysiological, stimuli producing further vasoconstriction *(3,4)*. Thus, ET-1 functions as a localy released, rather than circulating, hormone and concentrations are comparatively low in plasma and other tissues.

In pathophysiological conditions, tissue levels of ET-1, and its precursor big ET-1, are significantly increased, e.g., within the wall of human vessels containing atherosclerotic lesions *(6)*. Increases in the plasma levels of immunoreactive ET have been measured in number of pathophysiological conditions including coronary vasospasm and congestive heart failure *(7,8)*. Raised plasma levels of big ET-1 appear to be particularly predictive of disease severity and prognosis *(9)*.

1.2. ET-2 and Big ET-2

ET-2 has been less extensively studied than other ET peptides. We detected ET-2 mRNA *(10)* and mature peptide *(11)* in human cardiovascular tissues and ET-2 was as potent a vasoconstrictor as ET-1 in human arteries and veins *(12)*. Big ET-2 has been detected in the cytoplasm of endothelial cells *(13)* and, surprisingly, in normal human plasma, big ET-2 levels are higher than big ET-1 *(14)*. ET-2 has also been identified in failing hearts from humans *(15)*. A specific ELISA has been developed for big ET-2, giving plasma levels of 0.85 ± 0.03 pmol/L, $n = 42$ (unpublished observations). However, the physiological or pathophysiological role of this isoform remains to be discovered.

1.3. ET-3 and Big ET-3

Endothelial cells do not synthesize ET-3, but the mature peptide and big ET-3 are detectable in plasma *(14,16,17)* and other tissues including heart *(11)* and brain *(18)*. ET-3 is unique in that it is the only endogenous isoform that distinguishes between the two endothelin receptors. It has the same affinity at the ET_B receptor as ET-1 but, at physiological concentrations, has little or no affinity for the ET_A sub-type. In humans, ET_A receptors predominate in the human vasculature and the low density of ET_B receptors ($<15\%$) present on the smooth muscle of the vasculature contribute little to vasoconstriction *(12)*. ET_B receptors are the principal sub-type in the kidney, localizing to nonvascular tissues. Evidence is emerging that the ET_B sub-type functions as a clearing receptor to remove ET from the circulation. Blockade of the ET_B receptor results in a rise in circulating immunoreactive ET. Blockade of the ET_B receptor by receptor antagonists results in a corresponding rise in circulating levels of ET-3 *(17)*. A selective ET-3 ELISA can be used to measure the extent of ETB receptor blockade *(17)*.

ET-3 levels are also altered in disease *(16)*. ET-3 may play a beneficial role in human disease by activating ET_B receptors to release opposing vasodilators, thus limiting unwanted vasoconstriction.

1.4. Species Differences

The majority of published immunoassays have been developed to measure ET in human tissue and plasma. However, there are no reported differences in the predicted amino-acid sequences in other mammalian species where the ET-1 (dog, bovine, pig, guinea pig, rat, mouse, rabbit) or ET-3 (mouse, rat) genes have been sequenced. Vasoactive intestinal contractor, the rodent (mouse and rat) equivalent of human ET-2, differs by only one amino acid. The assays described below would be expected to detect the mature peptides in most, if not all, mammalian species. In other vertebrates (e.g., fish), the N-terminus is reported to vary from the human ET-1 sequence but the C-terminus is conserved; selecting antisera directed to the C-terminus should therefore ensure 100% crossreactivity. The C-terminus of big ET precursors can also vary between species.

1.5. Two-Site "Sandwich" ELISA or Radioimmunoassay?

Quantification of endogenous levels of ET peptides in plasma, other tissues, in cell cultures and following the fate of exogenously applied peptides in vitro or in vivo represents a challenge because of the potential for crossreactivity between the three isoforms and their precursors. Although ET-1 is the predominant isoform in many tissues, the term immunoreactive endothelin (IR-ET) is used to reflect that some assays may detect and therefore measure ET-2 and/or ET-3 together with precursors. It is not surprising that there is variation in the absolute amounts of "immunoreactive ET" measured, e.g., in human plasma, reflecting variation in recovery following the method of solid-phase extraction, the type of immunoassay employed, and the specificity of the antisera. This limitation must be considered in the design of experiments to ensure appropriate control to allow measurement of relative changes rather than absolute levels of immunoreactivity.

Sandwich ELISAs are available from a number of commercial sources including the Biotrak™ endothelin-1 ELISA from Amersham Pharmacia Biotech *(19)*. This kit, one of the first to be developed, is recommended because of excellent intra- and inter-assay coefficients of variation and good recovery following solid phase extraction *(19)*. In this assay, samples are incubated in microtiter wells that are precoated with an antibody against the C-terminus of ET to which ET isoforms in the sample bind specifically. Unrelated molecules are removed during a subsequent washing step. Bound ET is measured using a peroxidase-labeled Fab' fragment of an anti-N-terminal ET-1 antibody conjugate (creating the sandwich), which catalyzes the conversion of a chromogenic substrate to a visible reaction product. This assay has been well characterized for crossreactivity against ET peptides and their precursors and the lack of crossreactivity with pharmacological tools used in ET research, such as receptor antagonists, has been demonstrated. The main advantages of the sandwich ELISAs are speed, they avoid the use of radioactivity, and they can be more specific than the more commonly used RIAs, as two antibody binding sites are required on the same molecule for a signal to be obtained. Sandwich ELISAs are the method of choice for most applications. The sensitivity of an ELISA can be comparable to a RIA when making direct measurements of comparatively small volumes of conditioned tissue culture media or physiological saline. However, owing to potential interference in the ELISA, it is not yet possible to measure plasma or tissue ET levels without solid-phase extraction, as it is with RIA.

Radioimmunoassay kits are also widely available from several sources; those from Amersham Pharmacia Biotech have been well characterized *(20)*. For large studies, it may be more economical to purchase antisera suitable for RIA separately or to generate antisera "in house" and then combine these with commercially available tracers.

1.6. RIA for ET-1/ET-2 & Precursors (N-Terminus)

Two kits are available using antisera directed to the N-terminus of ET-1 and ET-2 (RPA535 and the high sensitivity assay, RPA545) that have virtually no crossreactivity with ET-3. As expected these antisera crossreact with, and would therefore detect, big ET-1 and big ET-2. These kits will detect peptides (ET-1 and ET-2) selective for the ET_A receptor but cannot be used to monitor the conversion of big ET-1 to ET-1.

1.7. RIA for ET-1/ET-2/ET-3 (C-Terminus)

Antisera directed to the common C-terminus of the ET isopeptides (e.g., RPA555) display the expected crossreactivity for ET-1, ET-2 and ET-3 with little crossreactivity for the precursor peptides *(20)*. This assay is recommended to quantify all the mature, and therefore biologically active, peptides and can also be used to measure the conversion of big ET to ET-1.

1.8. RIA for the Separate Measurement of ET-1, Big ET-1, and CTF

More than 90% of ET-1 synthesized by endothelial cells is thought to be released towards the smooth muscle cells, where it immediately binds to its receptors. Only a small fraction escapes into the circulation and plasma levels may not accurately reflect potential increases in ET-1 as a result of disease or following treatment with ET receptor antagonists. Synthesis of ET-1 from big ET-1 also results in the formation of the biologically inactive C-terminal fragment (CTF) in an equimolar ratio. Since this peptide does not bind to ET receptors, it can provide a better measure of the conversion of big ET-1 *(21–23)*. In the solid phase extraction method described below, the CTF fragment elutes differentially from the biologically active ET-1 and big ET-1 peptides, allowing all three components of the ET-1 synthetic pathway to be measured.

2. Materials

2.1. Preparation of Biological Samples for Solid Phase Extraction

2.1.1. Preparation of Solid Tissues

1. Homogenizer (Polytron or similar).
2. 0.5 *M* Acetic acid containing 0.1% Triton X-100 solution.
3. Boiling water bath.
4. Polypropylene centrifuge tubes.
5. Centrifuge.

2.1.2. Preparation of Plasma for Solid-Phase Extraction

1. Blood collection tubes containing EDTA at a final concentration of 1.2–2 mg/mL of blood. These can be either commercial evacuated tubes (Monovette—Sarstedt, Leicester, UK; Vacutainer—Becton Dickinson, London, UK) or polypropylene screw-capped tubes (K10pp—LIP, Keighley, UK).
2. Polypropylene tubes (e.g., Sarstedt, Leicester, UK).
3. 2 *M* Hydrochloric acid.

2.2. Solid Phase Extraction of Biological Samples

1. Silica mini-columns, e.g., Amprep 500 mg C2 or C18 columns (Amersham Pharmacia Biotech, Little Chalfont, Bucks., UK) or C8 SPE-ED (Applied Separations, Allentown, PA).
2. Hydrochloric acid, trifluoroacetic acid, methanol, deionized water.
3. Vacuum manifold and centrifugal sample concentrator, e.g., Savant Speedvac, Thermoquest Life Sciences Ltd., Basingstoke, Herts, UK.

2.3. Detection of ET Peptides Using ELISA Kits

1. ELISA kit, e.g., Biotrak endothelin-1 ELISA (Amersham Pharmacia Biotech, Little Chalfont, Bucks., UK).
2. Pipets (ideally multichannel) and tips to dispense between 50–200 µL vol.
3. Polypropylene tubes.
4. 37°C Incubator.

5. Microtiter plate shaker (e.g., Wellmixx 2, ThermoDenley, Basingstoke, Hants., UK).
6. Microtiter plate washer (e.g., Biotrak Microtiter plate washer, Amersham Pharmacia Biotech, Little Chalfont, Bucks., UK).
7. Microtiter plate reader (e.g., Biotrak Microtiter plate reader, Amersham Pharmacia Biotech, Little Chalfont, Bucks., UK).
8. Deionized water.
9. 1.0 *M* Sulphuric acid.

2.4. Detection of ET Peptides Using RIA Kits

1. RPA535 or high sensitivity assay, RPA545 for ET-1/ET-2 and precursors. RPA555 for ET-1/ET-2/ET-3 (Amersham Pharmacia Biotech, Little Chalfont, Bucks., UK).
2. Polypropylene assay tubes (12 × 75 mm, 55.526, Sarstedt, Leicester, UK).
3. Magnetic separation racks (e.g., Amerlex-M Separator, Amersham Pharmacia Biotech, Little Chalfont, Bucks., UK).

2.5. RIA for the Separate Measurement of ET-1, Big ET-1 and CTF

Materials as for **Subheading 2.4.** with the following additions/modifications.

1. $[^{125}I]$-ET-1 and $[^{125}I]$-big ET-1 (2200 Ci/mmol), (Amersham Pharmacia Biotech, Little Chalfont, Bucks., UK).
2. ET-1(1-21, human) and big ET-1(1-38, human) peptides, (Peptide Institute, Osaka, Japan).
3. Assay buffer (per liter): 5.74 g Na_2HPO_4, 1.14 g NaH_2PO_4 2.5 g BSA, 0.5 g sodium azide and 100 μL Tween-20, at pH 7.2–7.4.
4. Antisera. The primary antisera against the endothelin peptides were all designed and produced "in house". Commercial antisera are also available (e.g., Bachem, St. Helens, UK or Peptide Institute, Osaka, Japan).

3. Methods

3.1. Preparation of Biological Samples for Solid Phase Extraction

Cell culture media and physiological saline can be assayed directly in both the ELISA and RIA. However, solid tissues and plasma require solid phase extraction.

3.1.1. Homogenization of Solid Tissues

1. Cut tissue (typically 1–3 g wet weight) into small pieces, transfer to polypropylene tubes and homogenize with 10 vol of ice-cold 0.5 *M* acetic acid/0.1% Triton X-100, for 30 s on the maximum setting.
2. Heat the homogenates in a water bath at 100°C for 15 min, cool and clarify by centrifugation at 48,000*g* for 20 min at 4°C, prior to solid phase extraction (*see* **Subheading 3.2.**).

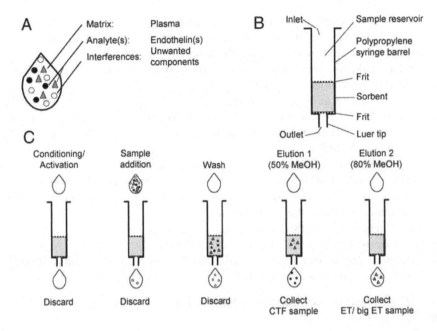

Fig. 1. Schematic diagram illustrating the differential solid phase extraction of IR-ET, big ET-1, and CTF.

3. Retain a portion of each homogenate for the measurement of protein concentration if the results are to be expressed as the amount of IR-ET/mg protein (*see* **Note 1**).

3.1.2. Collection and Preparation of Plasma

1. Collect whole blood into EDTA tubes, mix well, (but do not shake) and centrifuge at 2000*g* for 10 min at 4°C. Remove the plasma into polypropylene tubes. If necessary, samples of plasma may be stored at −80°C (*see* **Note 2**).
2. If samples are to be processed immediately, measure 5 mL of plasma into fresh polypropylene tubes and acidify by adding 1.25 mL of 2 *M* HCl (*see* **Note 3**). Cap the tube, mix by inversion, and then centrifuge for 10 min at 2000*g* to remove any precipitate.

3.2. Solid Phase Extraction of Plasma or Tissue Homogenates

3.2.1. Extraction of Tissue for Measurement by ELISA and RIA Kits

1. Attach the silica mini-columns (appropriately labeled with sample details) to the vacuum manifold and precondition by adding 2 mL of methanol. Allow this to pass completely onto the column before adding 2 mL of deionized water. It is important not to allow the columns to dry out before addition of the sample. If they do dry out, repeat the preconditioning step (*see* **Fig. 1**, **Note 4**).

2. Add the prepared plasma or homogenate samples (typically 2–5 mL) to the conditioned columns and allow these to pass through the column under gravity (do not use vacuum). If necessary, top the column up as the sample passes through until all of the sample is on the column. At this stage apply the vacuum carefully until no more sample drips through.

3. Wash the column through to waste (i.e., do not collect the eluate) with 2 × 2.8 mL vol of 0.1% TFA in water using vacuum to produce a flow-through rate of approx 1 mL/min. Continue to apply vacuum until no more wash drips through the column (*see* **Note 5**).

4. Place labeled tubes into the manifold to collect eluate.

5. Add 2 × 2 mL of 80% MeOH/0.1% TFA in deionized water. Allow both 2 mL aliquots to pass onto the column under gravity. Only then apply vacuum until no more eluate drips into the collection tubes.

6. Dry all tubes overnight in an evacuated centrifuge.

7. Cap tubes and store at −80°C, or process immediately.

8. Extracted samples, tissue culture media and physiological saline can be stored at −80°C until studies are complete.

3.2.2. Extraction of Samples for Detection of ET-1, Big ET-1, and CTF by RIA

1. Use C8 mini-columns for this extraction and carry out **steps 1–4** as described in **Subheading 3.2.1.** Continue as follows.

2. Elute the CTF fragment by adding 2 × 2 mL 50% MeOH/0.1% TFA in deionized water. Allow the solution to pass through, under gravity, until all of the solution is on the column. Only then apply vacuum until no more eluate drips into the collection tubes.

3. Place a new set of tubes into the manifold to collect the mature ET/big ET-1 fraction.

4. To elute the mature ET and big ET-1 fraction add 2 × 2 mL 80% MeOH/0.1% TFA, in deionized water, and proceed as described in **steps 5–8** under **Subheading 3.2.1.**

3.3. ELISA Protocol

1. Reconstitute and dilute kit reagents (buffers, standards, and antibody) as instructed.

2. Prepare a standards curve over the concentration range of 1–32 fmol/mL ET-1 by serial dilution in assay buffer.

3. Reconstitute the lyophilized samples by vortexing them in assay buffer (typically 250 μL) to allow duplicate aliquots of 100 μL to be used in the assay. It is crucial that the sample is thoroughly dissolved.

4. The recommended format of the 96-well plate precoated with anti-ET-1[15–21] comprises the first two wells for the blank, the second two for the nonspecific binding (NSB), 12 for the standards curve leaving 80 wells for the determination of 40 unknown samples in duplicate.

5. Pipet assay buffer (100 μL) into each NSB well and then the standards (2 × 100 μL aliquots from six standards of 1, 2, 4, 8, 16, and 32 fmol ET-1/well) and samples (2 × 100 μL of reconstituted sample or culture media used directly). Use new pipet tips for each duplicate.

6. Cover and incubate the microtiter plates for 16–24 h at 4°C.

7. To remove unbound material, wash and aspirate all wells 4× with 400 μL wash buffer using a 96-well microtiter plate washer. Blot the plate on tissue paper to remove any remaining liquid.

8. Detect bound ET-1 by pipeting 100 μL of the detection reagent (horseradish peroxidase [EC. 1.11.1.7] conjugated FAb' fragment of anti-ET-1 antibody reconstituted in assay buffer) into all wells, except the blank. Incubate for exactly 30 min at 37°C in a humidified container.

9. Repeat the washing and blotting step (**step 6** above).

10. Immediately add 100 μL of the chromogenic substrate (TMB, 3,3',5,5'-tetramethylbenzidine) into all wells. Cover and mix on a plate shaker at ambient temperature for exactly 40 min.

11. Add of 100 μL of 1.0 M sulfuric acid to each well to stop the development of the blue color reaction and produce a yellow color, which is more optically dense. Immediately mix, and measure the absorbance at 450 nm (within 30 min to avoid fading) using a 96-well microtiter plate reader.

12. Calculate the average absorbance for duplicate wells and subtract the mean NSB. Plot, mean absorbance (y-axis) vs ET-1 standard per well (x-axis) and interpolate unknown values from the standards curve. Alternatively, use the quadratic curve fitting programs that are supplied with plate readers that interpolate sample values from the standard curves automatically (*see* **Note 7** and **Fig. 2**).

3.4. RIA Kit Protocol

1. Reconstitute lyophilized samples by vortexing in assay buffer (typically 250 μL) to allow duplicate aliquots of 100 μL to be used in the assay. It is crucial that the sample is thoroughly dissolved and this may require several hours with sonication and/or trituration (*see* **Note 6**).

2. Prepare kit reagents as instructed (assay buffer, standards, antisera, and tracer).

3. Prepare the working standards by serial dilution of the stock solution provided to produce a standards curve for ET-1 over the concentration range 0.5–256 fmol/tube ET-1.

4. Aliquot samples, standards and blanks into labeled tubes according to the format suggested in the kit instructions. Briefly, use the first two tubes for the total count (Total, T), the second two for the nonspecific binding (Blank, NSB—add 200 μL assay buffer), the next two for the Zero standard (B_0—add 100 μL assay buffer). The next 16 tubes are for the standards curve (8 standards in duplicate, 100 μL of standard/tube, starting with the most dilute) and up to 40 samples in duplicate (80 tubes, 100 μL sample/tube). Use a new pipet tip for each duplicate.

5. Pipet 100 μL of the diluted primary antisera into all tubes except the Totals and Blank tubes. Vortex to mix thoroughly.

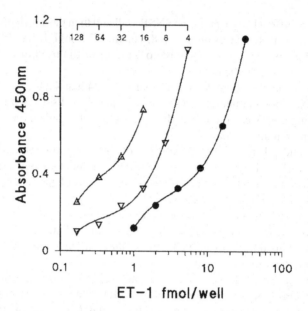

Fig. 2. An example of a standards curve for an ET-1 ELISA (•). The concentration of IR ET-1 in conditioned medium (Δ,∇) from human umbilical vein endothelial cells has been diluted as shown in the scale above the curves to illustrate parallelism with authentic standards.

6. Cover tubes with foil to prevent evaporation and incubate at 4°C for 16–24 h (i.e., overnight).
7. Prepare the radioligand tracer, [^{125}I]-ET-1 as instructed (*see* **Note 8**). Pipet 100 μL into all tubes, mix well, seal the Total tubes with caps, recover with foil and incubate for a further 16–24 h at 4°C.
8. Bring the Amerlex M separation reagent (donkey anti-rabbit antisera linked to magnetizable beads) to room temperature and aliquot 250 μL into all tubes (except the Total tubes). Vortex to mix and then incubate at room temperature for 10 min.
9. Separate the antibody bound fraction by transferring the tubes (except Totals) to the magnetic separation racks. Make sure that all tube bases are in contact with the magnetic base plate and that the racks fit the magnetic bases and are not loose.
10. Incubate the tubes for 15 min at room temperature. After this time the reagent should change from an opaque green mixture to a clear blue solution covering a small brown pellet that contains the bound counts. Invert the magnetic racks sharply over a sink (make sure it is suitable for the disposal of radioactive material), tipping the blue solution and unbound counts to waste (*see* **Note 8**). Do not reinvert the racks, leave inverted and place immediately onto absorbent paper, over foil, to drain for 5–30 min. Tap the bases of racks once or twice during this time. If magnetic racks are not available then the tubes can be

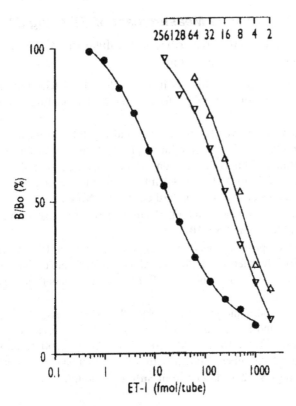

Fig. 3. An example of a standards curve for an ET RIA (•). The concentration of IR ET in extracts from human heart (∇,Δ) has been diluted as shown in the scale above the curves to illustrate parallelism with authentic standards.

centrifuged at 4°C for 10 min at 1500g or higher and the solution decanted to leave a pellet.

11. Transfer all tubes to gamma counter racks and measure radioactivity in each tube, including the Totals. Count each tube for at least 60 s.

12. Calculate the average CPM for each duplicate and subtract the background. Calculate %B_0/T:

$$\%B/\text{Total} = (B_0 \text{ cpm} - \text{NSB cpm})/(\text{Total cpm} - \text{NSB cpm}) \times 100$$

13. Calculate %B/B0 for each standard and sample:

$$\%B/B_0 = (\text{Standard or sample cpm} - \text{NSB cpm})/(B_0 \text{ cpm} - \text{NSB cpm}) \times 100$$

Plot mean %B/B_0 (*y*-axis) vs log ET-1 standard fmol/tube (*x*-axis) and interpolate unknown values from the standards curve (*see* **Fig. 3**). Alternatively quadratic curve fitting programs supplied with gamma counters can be used and sample values interpolated from the standard curves automatically.

3.5. RIA for the Separate Measurement of ET-1, Big ET-1, and CTF

The RIA is carried out as described in **Subheading 3.4.** with the following modifications/additions to each step.

1. Reconstitute samples by the addition of 250 μL of RIA buffer for the 50% MeOH, CTF fraction and 500 μL for the 80% MeOH, mature ET/ big ET fraction (*see* **Note 6**).
2. Prepare standard curves for both ET-1 and big ET-1 from the stocks of each peptide. Dilute the ET-1 stock solution (10^{-4} M) in RIA buffer to give 2 mL of a 10^{-8} M solution. This is the top concentration of the standard curve. From this, perform serial dilutions of 1 mL + 1 mL eleven times, each in RIA buffer, to give a total of 12 concentrations/standard curve (*see* **Note 9**).
3. Aliquot samples, standards and blanks into labeled tubes according to the format given in **Table 1** (*see* **Note 10**).
4. Dilute the appropriate primary antibody for each assay in RIA buffer to the previously empirically determined dilution. Aliquot 100 μL into each tube (*see* **Table 1**), vortex to mix, cover the tubes with foil to prevent evaporation, and incubate at 4°C overnight.
5. Prepare the radioligand tracer (*see* **Note 8**) for each assay, [^{125}I]-ET-1 for the mature assay and [^{125}I]-big ET-1 for the big ET-1/CTF assay, by dilution into RIA buffer to achieve 10–15,000 cpm/100 μL. Aliquot 100 μL into all tubes, mix well, cap the Total tubes, recover with foil and incubate overnight at 4°C.
6. Continue **steps 6–12** as described in **Subheading 3.4.**

4. Notes

1. There are a variety of methods for protein determination commercially available. When measuring protein levels in sections of tissue we solubilize the proteins in 0.5 M NaOH/1% SDS (heated to 80°C for 30 min and centrifuged to remove any precipitate). Therefore, our protein assay of choice is the Bio-Rad DC assay (500-0116, Bio-Rad, Hemel Hempstead, Herts, UK), which is specifically designed to be compatible with detergents.
2. The tubes containing whole EDTA blood can be spun at speeds equating to 1200–2000*g*, for 6–10 min, (i.e., less *g*—more time). Excessive *g*-force will result in hemolysis, which is undesirable. Too low a speed results in poor volume recovery and low plasma ET estimation. Polypropylene tubes are recommended for storage of plasma samples as they exhibit low peptide binding and are structurally competent at −80°C.
3. The ratio of plasma to 2 M HCl is 4:1 v/v, smaller volumes of plasma may be extracted but the final sensitivity of the assay will be lower. With a 5 mL plasma volume, reconstituted after extraction to 250 μL and assayed (2 × 100 μL) for a single analyte, each assay tube will contain the equivalent of 2 mL of plasma and the detection limit of plasma will be approx 0.5 pmol/L. Where the extracted

Table 1
Format for Radioimmunoassay

Tubes	Standard/sample (μL)	Buffer (μL)	1° Antibody (μL)	Label (μL)	Amerlex (μL)
1–2	TOTAL	–	–	100	–
3–4	BLANK/NSB	200	–	100	250
5–6	REF/B0	100	100	100	250
7–8	0.488*	100	100	100	250
9–10	0.977	100	100	100	250
11–12	1.95	100	100	100	250
13–14	3.91	100	100	100	250
15–16	7.81	100	100	100	250
17–18	15.63	100	100	100	250
19–20	31.25	100	100	100	250
21–22	62.5	100	100	100	250
23–24	125	100	100	100	250
25–26	250	100	100	100	250
27–28	500	100	100	100	250
29–30	1000	100	100	100	250
31–32	sample 1	100	100	100	250
33–200	samples 2–85	100	100	100	250

*Tubes 7–30 are standard curve dilutions (pmol/L) in duplicate.

sample is reconstituted in 500 µL and assayed in duplicate, e.g., for mature ET (2 × 100 µL) and big ET-1 (2 × 100 µL), each assay tube will contain the equivalent of 1 mL of plasma, making the lowest plasma concentration of ET-like immunoreactivity detectable to be 1 pmol/L. This assumes an assay detection limit (sensitivity) of 1.0 fmol/tube (100 µL).

4. Vacuum can be used to speed up the various stages of solid-phase extraction, however, it is essential that the column does not dry out during the conditioning or sample application stages. During sample application, only apply vacuum to the columns such that the flow rate through the column does not exceed 1 mL/min.

5. The columns in routine use in our laboratory have a volume above the sorbent bed of 2.8 mL. We therefore normally fill the columns to the brim twice in the washing stages, as this is both quicker, and ensures that all traces of sample are washed through the column. If robotic systems are being used, 5 mL of 0.1% TFA is a sufficient wash.

6. It is essential that the lyophilized, solid-phase extracted samples are allowed to fully dissolve in the ELISA/RIA buffer. The inclusion of Tween-20 (0.1%) in the RIA buffer facilitates this. Careful choice of the conditions of vacuum centrifugation (minimized time and applied heat) will assist this. Sometimes the samples will need to be left overnight at 4°C to redissolve completely.

7. Validation of the two-site ELISA: The sensitivities of detection for this assay (defined as two standard deviations above mean zero dose absorbance) are 0.5 fmol/well with ED_{50} values of 13 fmol/well. Intra- and interassay are <6.6% and <20.3%. The ELISA crossreacted with ET-1 (defined as 100%) and ET-2 (>100%). Crossreactivity with big ET-1 was very low (0.07%), and was undetectable with the C-terminal fragment of big ET-1, ET-3, big ET-2 and big ET-3 at the highest concentrations tested. There was no detectable crossreactivity with unrelated vasoactive peptides such as atrial natriuretic factor and porcine brain natriuretic peptide. Importantly, the ET_A selective antagonist FR139317 and the ET_B selective agonist BQ3020 did not crossreact, indicating that this assay can be used to measure IR ET in the presence of these compounds. Dilution curves of the conditioned medium from human umbilical vein endothelial cell cultures, known to secrete mature ET peptide, paralleled those of the standard ET-1 (*see* **Fig. 1**). This confirmed that the immunoreactivity detected in the tissue culture supernatants was the expected endogenous ET-1.

8. Follow local rules for the use of ionizing radiation in your laboratory. Dispose of aqueous radioactive waste in a designated sink.

9. We have found that 200 tubes are the optimum number that can be processed in one batch at the precipitating antibody stage. Each batch of 200 tubes must contain a full standard curve, which occupies 30 tubes, leaving 170 tubes, which is sufficient for the assay of 85 samples in duplicate. It may therefore be necessary to increase volumes of standards produced, as there should be at least one standard curve included per 200 tubes (i.e., per 85 samples in duplicate).

10. The big ET-1 RIA will have twice as many tubes as the mature ET assay as the 50% MeOH fractions (containing CTF) are assayed in this RIA.

Acknowledgments

Supported by grants from the British Heart Foundation, Royal Society, and Isaac Newton Trust.

References

1. Gosling, J. P. (ed.) (2000) *ELISA Immunoassays.* OUP, Oxford, UK.
2. Chard, T. (1990) An Introduction to Radioimmunoassay and Related Techniques. (Burton, R. H. and van Knippenberg, P. H., eds.) Elsevier, Amsterdam, The Netherlands.
3. Davenport, A. P. and Russell, F. D. (2001) Endothelin converting enzymes and endothelin receptor localization in human tissues, in *Handbook Exp. Pharmacol. vol. 152* (Warner, T. D., ed.), Springer-Verlag, Berlin, Germany, pp. 209–237.
4. Russell, F. D., Skepper, J. N., and Davenport, A. P. (1998) Human endothelial cell storage granules: a novel intracellular site for isoforms of the endothelin converting enzyme. *Circ. Res.* **83,** 314–321.
5. Haynes, W. G. and Webb, D. J. (1994) Contribution of endogenous generation of endothelin-1 to basal vascular tone. *Lancet* **344,** 852–854.
6. Bacon, C. R., Cary, N. R. B., and Davenport, A. P. (1996) Endothelin peptide and receptors in human atherosclerotic coronary artery and aorta. *Circ. Res.* **79,** 794–801.
7. Kurihara, H., Yoshizumi, M., Sugiyama, T., Yamaoki, K., Nagai, R., Takaku, F., Satih, H., Inui, J., Yanagisawa, M., and Masaki, T. (1989) The possible role of endothelin-1 in the pathogenesis of coronary vasospasm. *J. Cardiovasc. Pharmacol.* **13(Suppl 5),** S132–S137.
8. Wei, C. M., Lerman, A., Rodeheffer, R. J., McGregor, C. G., Brandt, R. R., Wright, S., et al. (1994) Endothelin in human congestive heart failure. *Circ.* **89(4),** 1580–1586.
9. Monge, J. C. (1998) Neurohormonal markers of the clinical outcome of cardiovascular disease: is endothelin the best one? *J. Cardiovasc. Pharmacol.* **32(Suppl 2),** S36–S42.
10. O'Reilly, G., Charnock-Jones, D. S., Morrison, J. J., Cameron, I. T., Davenport, A. P., and Smith, S. K. (1993) Alternatively spliced mRNA's for human endothelin-2 and their tissue distribution. *Biochem. Biophys. Res. Commum.* **193,** 834–840.
11. Plumpton, C., Ashby, M. J., Kuc, R. E., O'Reilly, G., and Davenport, A. P. (1996) Expression of endothelin peptides and mRNA in the human heart. *Clin. Sci.* **90,** 37–46.
12. Maguire, J. J. and Davenport, A. P. (1995) ET_A receptors mediate the constrictor responses to endothelin peptides in human blood vessels in vitro. *Br. J. Pharmacol.* **115,** 191–197.
13. Howard, P. G., Plumpton, C., and Davenport, A. P. (1992) Anatomical localization and pharmacological activity of mature endothelins and their precursors in human vascular tissue. *J. Hypertens.* **10,** 1379–1386.

14. Matsumoto, H., Suzuki, N., Kitada, C., and Fujino, M. (1994) Endothelin family peptides in human plasma and urine: their molecular forms and concentrations. *Peptides* **15**, 505–510.

15. Plumpton, C., Champeney, R., Ashby, M. J., Kuc, R. E., and Davenport, A. P. (1993) Characterisation of endothelin isoforms in human heart: Endothelin-2 demonstrated. *J. Cardiovasc. Pharmacol.* **22(Suppl 8)**, 26–28.

16. Suzuki, N., Matsumoto, H., Miyauchi, T., Goto, K., Masaki, T., Tsuda, M., and Fujino, M. (1990) Endothelin-3 concentrations in human plasma: increased concentrations in patients undergoing haemodialysis.*Biochem. Biophys. Res. Commum.* **169**, 809–815.

17. Davenport, A. P., Plumpton, C., Ferro, C. J., Webb, D. J., and Horton, J. (1998) Systemic infusion of an endothelin receptor antagonist increases plasma ET-3 in humans. *Br. J. Pharmacol.* **123**, 290P.

18. Takahashi, K., Ghatei, M. A., Jones, P. M., Murphey, J. K., Lam, H. C., O'Haloran, D. J., and Bloom, S. R. (1991) Endothelin in human brain and pituitary gland: presence of immunoreactive endothelin, endothelin messenger ribonucleic acid, and endothelin receptors. *J. Clin. Endocrinol. Metab.* **72**, 693–699.

19. Plumpton, C., Horton, J., Kalinka, K. S., Martin, R. and Davenport, A. P. (1994) Effects of phosphoramidon and pepstatin A on the secretion of endothelin-1 and big endothelin-1 in human umbilical vein endothelial cells: Measurement by two-site ELISAs. *Clin. Sci.* **87**, 245–251.

20. Davenport, A. P., Ashby, M. J., Easton, P., Ella, S., Bedford, J., Dickerson, C., et al. (1990) A sensitive radioimmunoassay measuring endothelin-like immunoreactivity in human plasma: comparison of levels in essential hypertension and normotensive controls. *Clin. Sci.* **78**, 261–264.

21. Plumpton, C., Haynes, W. G., Webb, D. J., and Davenport, A. P. (1995) Phosphoramidon inhibition of the in vivo conversion of big endothelin-1 to endothelin-1 in the human forearm. *Br. J. Pharmacol.* **115**, 1821–1828.

22. Plumpton, C., Haynes, W. G., Webb, D. J., and Davenport, A. P. (1995) Measurement of C-terminal fragment of big endothelin-1: A novel method for assessing the generation of endothelin-1 in human. *J. Cardiovasc. Pharmacol.* **26(Suppl 3)**, S34–S36.

23. Plumpton, C., Ferro, C. J., Haynes, W. G., Webb, D. J., and Davenport, A. P. (1996) The increase in human plasma immunoreactive endothelin but not big endothelin-1 or its C-terminal induced by systemic administration of the endothelin antagonist TAK-044. *Br. J. Pharmacol.* **119**, 311–314.

3

Separation of Endothelin Isoforms by High Performance Liquid Chromatography and Detection by Radioimmunoassay

Michael J. Ashby

1. Introduction

All three isoforms of endothelin (ET) have been detected in human and animal plasma and tissues *(1–4)*. As described in Chapter 2, radioimmunoassay (RIA) and enzyme-linked-immunosorbent assay (ELISA) are the methods of choice to quantify immunoreactive ET peptides. However, ET-1, ET-2 and ET-3 share a common C-terminal sequence and indeed ET-1 and ET-2 differ by only two amino acids in the N-terminal region. Thus, it is usually not possible to distinguish between the different isoforms using available antibodies *(see* **Note 1**). In order to determine which isoforms are present in, e.g., tissue, plasma, or cell culture extracts, it is necessary to carry out high performance liquid chromatography (HPLC) separation of the samples. As the levels of ET peptides in biological samples are too low to be detected by ultraviolet (UV) spectrophotometry and would be masked by the presence of other peptides, fractions are collected from the HPLC analytical column for subsequent analysis by RIA as previously described *(see* Chapter 2). Using this technique, we have identified mature ET-1, ET-2, ET-3 and the precursor, big ET-1, in tissue extracts of human heart *(5)*. We have shown that ET-1 is the major isoform, confirmed by mass spectrometry *(6)* *(see* **Note 2**), present in cultured human endothelial cells from a number of sources, including umbilical vein and the endocardium, whereas levels of ET-2 and ET-3 were below the level of detection in these cells. Absence of ET-2 in endothelial cells is surprising as mRNA encoding this isoform is present in human endothelial cells *(7)* and the mature peptide is present in plasma *(3)*. The source of ET-2 remains unclear, but it is

From: *Methods in Molecular Biology, vol. 206: Peptide Research Protocols: Endothelin*
Edited by: J. Maguire and A. Davenport © Humana Press Inc., Totowa, NJ

possible that this peptide is synthesized only under certain, as yet unspecified, physiological or pathophysiological conditions.

The method described for HPLC separation of ET isoforms has other applications. HPLC can be used to follow the fate of exogenous peptides, added in vitro or injected in vivo, to monitor for example the conversion of big ET precursors to the mature peptide or the degradation of the mature peptides. The technique may also be used to purify ET peptides that have been labeled with biotin or a radioisotope.

The method outlined below can be used for many other peptides using a C18 column and a simple gradient of water:acetonitrile:trifluoroacetic acid (TFA), e.g., 94.9:5:0.1 v/v increasing to 19.9:80:0.1 v/v over 60 min. Once the elution position of the peptide of interest is established, the gradient conditions for that peptide can be optimized.

The protocol in use in our laboratory utilizes two identical batch-matched HPLC columns. One is used to standardize the HPLC conditions with real-time UV detection of micromolar concentrations of ET peptide standards. The second column is used with nanomolar concentrations of the ET peptide standards to separate extracts of physiological samples for analysis of the collected fractions using RIA. Using this technique, following solid-phase extraction (*see* Chapter 2), we have successfully analyzed a range of human tissues, including heart ventricle and atria *(4,5)*, kidney *(9)*, endometrium *(8)*, in addition to plasma, cell lysates, and tissue culture supernatants *(6)*.

2. Materials

2.1. Sample Preparation

Materials for solid phase extraction of biological samples for HPLC are as described in Chapter 2 (*see* **Subheadings 2.1.** and **2.2.**), except that C18 Seppak Vacs (Waters, Watford, UK) should be used instead of Amprep C2 minicolumns.

2.2. HPLC

1. Binary Gradient HPLC system and injector with 100 µL loop.
2. UV detector set at 214 nm and chart recorder or data acquisition system.
4. Polypropylene 75 × 12 mm test tubes (5 mL) or suitable tubes for the fraction collector above.
5. 2X Batch-matched Spherisorb ODS II 5µm 250 × 4.6 mm HPLC columns.
6. Acetonitrile (CH_3CN).
7. Trifluoroacetic acid (TFA, CF_3CO_2H).
8. Sodium phosphate (dibasic) (Na_2HPO_4) (*see* **Note 3**).
9. Solvent A: 50 mM Na_2HPO_4 in H_2O 75.9% (*see* **Note 4**).
   Acetonitrile   24%
   Trifluoroacetic acid   0.1%

10. Solvent B: 50 mM Na$_2$HPO$_4$ in H$_2$O   59.9%
    Acetonitrile   40%
    Trifluoroacetic acid   0.1%
11. 10^{-4} M stock solutions of ET peptides (e.g., Peptide Institute, Osaka, Japan), made up according to manufacturers' instructions.
12. Evacuated centrifuge, e.g., Savant sample concentration system (Thermo Life Sciences, Basingstoke, UK).
    All solvents and chemicals must be HPLC grade or purer, all buffers must be filtered (0.2 μm) and degassed before use.

3. Methods

3.1. Sample Preparation

Prepare solid tissue, cell lysates and plasma samples for HPLC analysis as described in Chapter 2 (*see* **Subheadings 3.1.** and **3.2.**). Although cell culture media and physiological buffers can be analyzed directly by RIA, these samples must be extracted before loading on to the HPLC column. This removes salts, concentrates the relatively dilute solutions, and allows reconstitution in Solvent A for injection. Therefore acidify the samples with 2 M HCl (4:1, sample: 2 M HCl v/v) and extract as described in Chapter 2, **Subheading 3.2.**

3.2. HPLC

1. Program the following gradient: flow rate 1 mL/min, 0–10 min 100% A, 10–50 min linear gradient to 100% B, 50–80 min 100% A. This equilibrates the column ready for the next run (*see* **Note 5**).
2. Optimize the system as follows using one of the columns (*see* **Note 6**).
3. Ensure that the HPLC system is fully purged with Solvent A before use.
4. All samples or standards for injection should be reconstituted or diluted in Solvent A.
5. Make a 10^{-5} M mix of ET-1, ET-2, ET-3 and big ET-1 from the 10^{-4} M peptide standards in Solvent A: e.g., 40 μL of each isoform + 240 μL of Solvent A.
6. Inject 100 μL of this solution (containing 1 nmol of each ET peptide) onto the column and monitor the UV absorbance at 214 nm in real time. Four peaks should be seen with retention times of approx 24, 28, 31, and 35 min. Ensure that there is baseline separation between the peaks. If there is not, then adjust the gradient until there is separation. This can usually be achieved either by lengthening the time period over which the gradient is run or by reducing the percentage of acetonitrile in Solvent A.
7. Flush the system extensively (with, e.g., Solvent A) to remove any trace of the relatively large amounts of ET peptides used to standardize the system using UV detection.
8. Exchange the column to the other batch-matched column (*see* **Note 7**).
9. Make a 10^{-8} M mix of the ET peptides (physiological amounts) in Solvent A and inject 100 μL of this mix (containing 1 pmol of each peptide) onto the column. Collect the eluent in 1 mL fractions for 50 min.

10. Lyophilize the fractions in a Savant Sample Concentrator (or equivalent) system.
11. Reconstitute each fraction in 500 μL of RIA buffer, and analyze duplicate 100 μL aliquots using the mature ET RIA and big ET-1 RIA (*see* Chapter 2, **Subheading 3.5.**) to elucidate the ET peptide profile (fraction number vs ET-IR, *see* **Fig. 1**).
12. Repeat **steps 9–11** with a blank injection (100 μL of Solvent A). This is the negative control for both the chromatography and the RIA (*see* **Note 8**).
13. Once the system has been optimized following the above procedure, and the specific chromatography system used has been demonstrated to be able to separate ET isoforms, samples may be analyzed. Reconstitute the extracted samples in 100 μL of Solvent A and follow **steps 9–11** to elucidate the relative proportions of ET isoforms occurring in each one (*see* **Note 9**).

4. Notes

1. There are now antibodies available that can distinguish ET-3 from ET-1/ET-2 and these form the basis of ET-3 specific ELISAs *(10)*.
2. If it is intended to couple the HPLC system to a mass spectrometer, then all compounds used must be volatile, therefore, mobile phases composed of ammonium acetate: acetic acid: acetonitrile *(6)* are commonly used.
3. Sodium Phosphate is used in the mobile phase as, if absent, ET-3 elutes in a broad band, often obscuring ET-1.
4. It is possible with some HPLC systems to have 50 mM Na$_2$HPO$_4$, 0.1% TFA in H$_2$O as Solvent A, and acetonitrile, 0.1% TFA as Solvent B, and create the required gradient conditions using the system's gradient programmer. However, we have found that a more reproducible and stable gradient is formed if the formulations described in **steps 9** and **10** of **Subheading 2.2.** above are followed.
5. It is essential to fully equilibrate the gradient system before applying the next sample, or variable elution times will result. The UV absorbance of the mobile phase usually increases with the percentage of acetonitrile, and so equilibrating with 100% Solvent A until the absorbance has returned to baseline is recommended. This time will vary from system to system and should be tested and optimized for each HPLC setup.
6. Mark this column UV, or similar, to note that it has been used with micromolar concentrations of ET solutions. Ensure that the system has been fully flushed before changing columns. This avoids any possibility of carryover of micromolar standards into a physiological sample run, where the expected levels will be nanomolar or less.
7. Mark this column RIA or similar to note that only nanomolar ET levels have been injected.
8. With every session of HPLC runs, standards (100 μL of 10^{-8} M mix of ET-1, ET-2, ET-3 and Big ET-1) and blanks (100 μL of Solvent A) must be run. It is advisable to run a standard and blank injection every 5–10 sample runs.
9. After each series (40–50 runs) of sample, standard and blank runs has been completed it is advisable to run 20 column volumes of acetonitrile:TFA:water 20:0.1:79.9 followed by 20 column volumes of acetonitrile:TFA:water

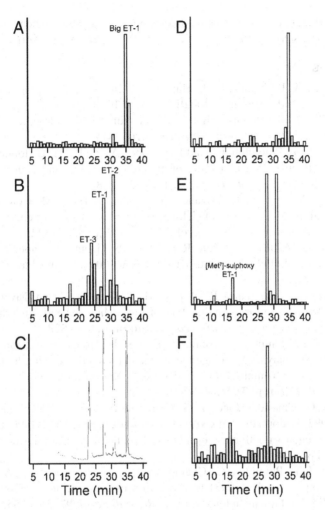

Fig. 1. Representative HPLC profiles of ET peptide standards and tissue extracts. The UV trace (**C**) was obtained using the column reserved for injection of micromolar concentrations of ET peptides. The other panels show the results of radioimmunoassay of 1-min fractions collected from the column used for separation of tissue extracts and nanomolar concentrations of ET peptide standards. The elution order is ET-3 (24 min), ET-1 (28 min), ET-2 (31 min) and big ET-1 (35 min). The peak at 17 min is [met[7]]-sulphoxy ET-1 *(6,9)*. (**A**) Mix of 1 pmol (100 μL of 10^{-8} *M* solution) each of authentic ET-1, ET-2, ET-3 and big ET-1, fractions assayed for big ET-1. (**B**) Mix of 1 pmol each of authentic ET-1, ET-2, ET-3 and big ET-1, fractions assayed for mature ET. (**C**) UV absorbance trace at 214 nm of 1 nmol (100 μL of 10^{-5} *M* solution) of each of authentic ET-1, ET-2, ET-3 and big ET-1. (**D**) Extract of human right atrium, fractions assayed for big ET-1. (**E**) Extract of human left ventricle, fractions assayed for mature ET. (**F**) Extract of human renal medulla, fractions assayed for mature ET.

80:0.1:19.9, to remove extremely hydrophobic compounds. Then repeat the 20% acetonitrile step and finally recondition with Solvent A (*see* **Note 5**).

References

1. Davenport, A. P., Nunez, D. J., Hall, J. A., Kaumann, A. J., and Brown, M. J. (1989) Autoradiographical localization of binding sites for porcine [^{125}I] endothelin-1 in humans, pigs and rats: functional relevance in humans. *J. Cardiovasc. Pharmacol.* **13(Suppl 5)**, S166–S170.
2. Howard, P. G., Plumpton, C., and Davenport, A. P. (1992) Anatomical localization and pharmacological activity of mature endothelins and their precursors in human vascular tissue. *J. Hypertens.* **10**, 1379–1386.
3. Suzuki, N., Matsumoto, H., Miyauchi, T., Kitada, C., Tsuda, M., Goto, K., Masaki, T., and Fujino, M. (1991) Sandwich-enzyme immunoassays for endothelin family peptides. *J. Cardiovasc. Pharmacol.* **17(Suppl 17)**, S420–S422.
4. Plumpton, C., Ashby, M. J., Kuc, R. E., O'Reilly, G., and Davenport, A. P. (1996) Expression of endothelin peptides and mRNA in the human heart. *Clin. Sci.* **89**, 37–46.
5. Plumpton, C., Champeney, R., Ashby, M. J., Kuc, R. E., and Davenport, A. P. (1993) Characterisation of endothelin isoforms in human heart: Endothelin 2 demonstrated. *J. Cardiovasc. Pharmacol.* **22(Suppl 8)**, S26–S28.
6. Ashby, M. J., Plumpton, C., Teale, P., Kuc, R. E., Houghton, E., and Davenport, A. P. (1995) Analysis of endogenous human endothelin peptides by high performance liquid chromatography and mass spectrophotometry. *J. Cardiovasc. Pharmacol.* **26(Suppl 3)**, S247–S249.
7. O'Reilly, G., Charnock-Jones, D. S., Cameron, I. T., Smith, S. K., and Davenport, A. P. (1993) Endothelin-2 mRNA splice variants detected by RT-PCR in cultured human vascular smooth muscle and endothelial cells. *J. Cardiovasc. Pharmacol.* **22(Suppl 8)**, S18–S21.
8. Cameron, I. T., Plumpton, C., Champeney, R., van Papendorp, C., Ashby, M. J., and Davenport, A. P. (1993) Identification of Endothelin-1, endothelin-2 and endothelin-3 in human endometrium. *J. Reprod. Fertil.* **97**, 251–255.
9. Karet, F. E. and Davenport, A. P. (1993) Human kidney: Endothelin isoforms revealed by HPLC with radioimmunoassay, and receptor sub-types detected using ligands BQ123 and BQ3020. *J. Cardiovasc. Pharmacol.* **22(Suppl 8)**, S29–S33.
10. Davenport, A. P., Plumpton, C., Ferro, C. J., Webb, D. J., and Horton, J. (1998) Systemic infusion of an endothelin receptor antagonist increases plasma ET-3 in humans. *Br. J. Pharmacol.* **123**, 290P.

II

ENDOTHELIN RECEPTOR PROTOCOLS

4

Radioligand Binding Assays and Quantitative Autoradiography of Endothelin Receptors

Anthony P. Davenport and Rhoda E. Kuc

1. Introduction

1.1. Endothelin Receptors

Endothelin (ET) receptors belong to the G-protein-linked seven transmembrane spanning family of receptors, located in the plasma membrane. Receptors can be identified by their amino acid structure and provide unambiguous evidence for expression of a gene encoding a particular sub-type in specific cells or tissues (*see* Chapter 6).

To date, only two ET receptor sub-types have been isolated and cloned from mammalian tissues, ET_A *(1)* and ET_B *(2)*. ET receptors are unusual in being isolated and cloned before the discovery of sub-type selective antagonists. However, receptor function cannot be predicted from the amino acid sequence alone. The two sub-types were originally distinguished, using functional studies, by their rank order of affinity for the endogenous peptides: ET-3 typically displays at least two orders of magnitude lower affinity for the ET_A receptor than ET-1, whereas both peptides are equipotent at the ET_B receptor (*3, see* **Table 1**). Characterizing the functional role of ET receptor subtypes by in vitro assays and establishing whether synthetic compounds are selective agonists or antagonists is described in Chapters 5 and 11. While functional studies can provide quantitative measurement of affinities, ligand-binding assays are needed to measure a second key parameter, receptor density, and combined with quantitative autoradiography, can be used to visualize the distribution of receptors within tissue. The combination of molecular techniques with ligand binding in the same tissue can provide compelling evidence for receptor expression *(4,5)*.

From: *Methods in Molecular Biology, vol. 206: Peptide Research Protocols: Endothelin*
Edited by: J. Maguire and A. Davenport © Humana Press Inc., Totowa, NJ

Table 1
Cloned Mammalian Endothelin Receptors

	ET_A (mammalian)	ET_B (mammalian)	ET_{B2} (avian)	ET_C (amphibian)
Potency	ET-1 = ET-2 > ET-3	ET-1 = ET-2 = ET-3	ET-1 = ET-3 >> S6c	ET-3 > ET-1
Human	427	442	436	444
Bovine	427	441		
Rat	426	442		
Mouse	–	442		
Porcine	427	–		

Bracketed homology annotations: 94% (within ET_A), 59% (between human ET_A 427 and ET_B 442), 89% (ET_B group), 91%, 88%.

Values are numbers of amino acids in cloned receptor protein. Percentages indicate sequence homology between receptor subtypes and species.

This chapter focuses on ligand-binding techniques that can be used to measure the affinity and amount of ET_A and ET_B receptor protein, together with the ratio of the two sub-types in tissues or cells. Changes in these parameters can be measured following experimental treatment in animal models (6) or in response to disease processes (7). More detailed information about the general theory of receptor binding can be found in **refs. 8–10**.

1.2. Endothelin Receptor Distribution

ET receptors are widely expressed in all tissues (11,12), consistent with the physiological role of endothelins as ubiquitous, potent, long-lasting, endothelium-derived vasoactive peptides, contributing to the maintenance of normal vascular tone. In human vessels, ET_A receptors (>85%) are mainly located on vascular smooth muscle cells (13) and are the principal sub-type mediating vasoconstriction (14). ET_B receptors are present on the endothelial cells lining the vessel wall and on activation by ET are thought to release endothelium-derived relaxing factors such as nitric oxide, limiting the vasoconstrictor actions of other peptides. The functional role of ET-1 is discussed in more detail in **refs. 15–17**. While ET_A receptors present on smooth muscle cells are mainly responsible for constriction in humans, in animals this can vary depending on the species and vascular bed. For example, ET-1 mediates contraction only via ET_A receptors in rat aorta, by ET_B receptors in rabbit saphenous vein, but by both sub-types in porcine coronary artery (14). ET receptors are also localized to nonvascular tissue. High densities are often present on epithelial cells such as those present in the lungs and kidney. The human kidney is rich in ET_B receptors (comprising about 70%) and this sub-type may have a role in sodium excretion as well as functioning as "clearing" receptors, removing ET from the plasma. Regions of the brain, such as the cerebellum, express some of the highest densities of ET receptors *(11)*. Less than 10% are ET_A receptors and these are mainly present on intracerebral vessels. ET_B receptors predominate on glial cells and to a lesser extent on neurones. Intriguingly, unlike the periphery, endothelial cells from the cerebral microvasculature express ET_A receptors *(18)*. Because ET does not normally cross the blood-brain barrier, most of these receptors will only respond to peptide synthesized and released within the brain.

1.3. Splice Variants

Alternative splice variants of both ET_A and ET_B receptors have been reported but to date these variants either show no change in binding characteristics or do not bind ET-1 at all and their physiological or pathophysiological significance is unclear. Intriguingly, a gene encoding a truncated (109 amino acids deleted) ET_A receptor was more abundant than the wild type in melanoma cell lines and tissue. The expressed receptor did not bind ET-1, suggesting reduced responsiveness to ET-1 in these tumors *(19)*. A variant ET_B receptor displaying an increase in the length of the second cytoplasmic domain by 10 amino acids did not result in any change in ligand affinities *(20)*. A splice variant consisting of 436 amino acids with 91% sequence similarity to the known human ET_B receptor (442 amino acids) showed the same ligand-binding properties of the wild-type but no functional response was detected *(21)*.

1.4. Other Sub-Types

Functional studies have suggested that the peptide PD142893 can block the vasodilator actions of ET-1 at endothelial ET_B receptors but not constrictor responses mediated by ET_B smooth muscle receptors. However, in the ET_B receptor gene knockout mouse, both the PD142893-sensitive vasodilator response and the PD142893-resistant contractile response to the ET_B agonist Sarafotoxin 6c (S6c) were completely absent. These results demonstrate that the pharmacologically heterogeneous responses to S6c are mediated by ET_B receptors derived from the same gene *(22)*. In native human tissue, using a combination of selective ligands, we have been unable to detect further sub-types *(23–26)*. A very detailed binding study (including PD142893) was unable to distinguish between ET_B receptors expressed by human isolated endothelial cells compared with smooth muscle cells in culture *(27)*.

The cloning by RT-PCR of an avian sub-type of the ET_B receptor has been reported, called *EDNRB2*. The expression pattern differs from that of the established gene *EDRB*, because it is strongly expressed in melanoblasts and melanocytes. The expressed receptor bound ET-1, ET-2 and ET-3 with similar affinity consistent with the pharmacological profile for an ET_B receptor but differs from the ET_B receptor by displaying a low affinity for the ET_B agonist, S6c (*28, see* **Table 1**).

1.5. Amphibian ET-3 Receptor

An ET-3 specific receptor (ET-3 > ET-1) has been cloned from *Xenopus laevis* dermal melanophores, with 47% sequence similarity to the bovine ET_A and 52% with the rat ET_B receptor (*see* **Table 1**). No mammalian homolog has yet been reported *(29)*.

1.6 Characterization of ET Receptors

In binding assays, it is not possible to distinguish between agonists and antagonists, and both classes of compounds will be referred to as ligands. This chapter will follow the convention that the affinity of a ligand for a receptor, the K_D, is the equilibrium dissociation constant and is a measure of the strength of interaction of a ligand to its receptor. The reciprocal of the K_D is the association constant, K_A. ET-1 and related synthetic ligands typically bind with K_D values in the nanomolar or sub-nanomolar range. By definition, the K_D is the concentration of ligand that will occupy 50% of the receptors. The K_D can be used to calculate the concentration of a radiolabeled ligand needed to occupy a desired proportion of receptors. The fraction of receptors occupied is equal to $L/K_D + L$, where L is the free ligand concentration. For example, a radioligand with a K_D of 0.2 nM would occupy 9% of the receptors at a concentration of 0.02 nM. The second parameter that can be calculated is the maximum density of receptors or B_{max}. This is usually corrected using the amount of protein present in the binding assay and expressed as amount of ligand bound/mg protein. The determination of the maximum density of receptors in a particular tissue is unique to ligand binding and cannot be determined in a functional assay.

1.7. ET Receptor Ligands

Most studies characterizing and localizing ET receptors use [^{125}I]-ET-1, directly labeled via the Tyr[13] (*see* **Table 2**). This ligand binds with the same affinity to both sub-types and is stable under nonphysiological binding conditions with little or no degradation of labeled ET-1 being detected. [^{125}I]-ET-2, [^{125}I]-VIC (vasoactive intestinal contractor, the murine isoform of ET-2) and [^{125}I]-Sarafotoxin 6b have also been labeled and used in saturation assays where

Table 2
Radiolabeled and Unlabeled Ligands Commercially Available
for the Study of the Endothelin System

	ET_A/ET_B	ET_A	ET_B
Labeled	$[^{125}I]$-ET-1	$[^{125}I]$-PD151242	$[^{125}I]$-BQ3020
	$[^{125}I]$-ET-2	$[^{125}I]$-PD164333	$[^{125}I]$-IRL1620
	$[^{125}I]$-S6b	$[^3H]$-BQ123	
Unlabeled	ET-1	PD151242	BQ788
	ET-2	FR139317	BQ3020
	S6b	BQ123	IRL1620 S6c

they also bind to both sub-types (30–32). ET-3 can be labeled at Tyr^6, Tyr^{13} and Tyr^{14}. Tyr^6 is generally used, as it is more difficult to separate $[^{125}I]$-ET-3 labeled at the latter two Tyr residues, although all three ET-3 ligands have similar affinities. The selectivity of ET-3 for ET_B vs ET_A receptors is often only about two orders, and it is difficult to precisely delineate the two sub-types using this labeled peptide in saturation assays. For saturation assays and autoradiography using a fixed concentration of ligand, $[^{125}I]$-PD151242 is rec-ommended to localize ET_A receptors. This linear tetrapeptide binds with sub-nanomolar affinity to the ET_A receptor and has about 10,000-fold selectivity for this sub-type in human and animal tissues (33). A nonpeptide ET_A selective ligand is also available, $[^{125}I]$-PD164333 (34), with comparable affinity as well as a tritiated ligand, $[^3H]$-BQ123 (35). The above ligands are available com-mercially either as catalog items or as custom syntheses from Amersham Pharmacia Biotech (http://www.apbiotech.com).

ET_B receptors can be characterized using $[^{125}I]$-BQ3020, a truncated linear analog of ET-1, where the disulfide bridges have been removed by substitution of Ala for Cys residues (23). This ligand binds with sub-nanomolar affinity to the ET_B receptor, with at least 1500-fold selectivity for this sub-type over the ET_A receptor. Alternatively, the truncated analog, $[^{125}I]$-IRL1620 can also be used, particularly in animal tissues (36). $[^{125}I]$-IRL1620 is available from NEN Life Science Products (http://www.lifesciences.perkinelmer.com).

For characterizing ET receptors in competition binding assays, ET_A selec-tive antagonists BQ123 (37), FR139317 (38) or PD151242 (32) are recom-mended and for ET_B receptors, unlabeled agonists Sarafotoxin 6c (39), BQ3020 (23), IRL1620 (36) or the antagonist, BQ788 (40). The above, unlabeled ligands have been chosen for their selectivity and commercial availability from a number of sources. Nonpeptide ligands have also been developed by pharma-ceutical companies and these are described in detail in **ref. 41**.

2. Materials

2.1. Ligand Binding Assays

1. Slide mounted cryostat sections (10–30 μm) from fresh-frozen tissue or cultured cells grown on coverslips (*see* Chapter 1, **Notes 1–6**).
2. [^{125}I]-labeled radioligands, unlabeled ET-1 to define NSB and competing ligands for competition assays.
3. Assay buffer: 0.05 *M* HEPES, 5 m*M* MgCl$_2$, 0.3% BSA fraction V, pH 7.4.
4. Ice-cold wash buffer (0.05 *M* Tris-HCl, pH 7.4, at 4°C).
5. Polypropylene assay tubes (12 × 75 mm, 55.526, Sarstedt, Leicester, UK).
6. Slide incubation trays with lids (*see* Chapter 1).
7. Metal slide racks.
8. Slide baths.
9. Filter paper to wipe sections from slides.
10. Gamma counter.

2.2. Quantitative Autoradiography and Image Analysis

1. Radiation-sensitive film (Kodak BioMax MR-1).
2. Autoradiography standards (^{125}I-Microscales, RPA 523, Amersham Pharmacia Biotech, Little Chalfont, Bucks., UK).
3. Autoradiography cassettes, boards, and adhesive tape.
4. Kodak D19 developer and Kodak Unifix.
5. Dark room with safelight for processing films.
6. Image analyzer.

3. Methods

3.1. Saturation Binding

3.1.1. Saturation Binding Assay

Receptor affinity and density can be readily determined by saturation analysis. In this assay, a number of tissue preparations can be used: partially purified plasma membrane fractions from tissue homogenates, cells transfected with cloned receptors, or freshly isolated or cultured cells. The method described below uses fresh frozen tissue sections (usually 10–30 μm thick) cut on a microtome and mounted on microscope slides. The latter method has the advantage that radioactivity can be determined in the whole section by wiping the tissue from the slide or by apposing to Radiation-sensitive film for autoradiography. It avoids lengthy homogenization procedures that can result in degradation of receptor protein and permits the visualization of anatomical regions, which can be important in comparing normal with diseased or control vs experimental tissue. This is particularly important for characterizing ET ligands binding to discrete regions within tissue sections, such as blood vessels.

Saturation assays will be illustrated using [^{125}I]-PD151242, an ET_A selective ligand, in slide mounted tissue sections of human heart *(42)*. An initial starting point is to label sections with radioligand concentrations that are selected to span a range at least an order of magnitude above and below the K_D of the ligand, if this is already known *(see* **Note 1**). Nonspecific binding is determined at each concentration of [^{125}I]-PD151242 by co-incubation of sections with a 1000-fold excess of unlabeled peptide over the K_D. The sections are incubated for a defined period of time at a constant temperature in order to ensure equilibrium conditions; these conditions will have been determined previously in association experiments *(see* **Subheading 3.3.1.**). For [^{125}I]-PD151242, a 2 h incubation at 23°C is sufficient to reach equilibrium. Equilibrium is rapidly broken by washing to separate bound from free ligand and conditions for this should be examined to find an optimal compromise between retention of bound label and a high percentage of specific binding. Sections are wiped from the slide, and the amount of radioactivity bound to the tissue is measured. For homogenates, separation of the bound from the free ligand can be achieved by rapid filtration of the incubation mixture through a filter or by centrifugation.

1. Cut consecutive cryostat sections (typically 10–30 μm) of fresh-frozen tissue and thaw mount onto gelatin coated microscope slides *(see* Chapter 1 for more details). Allow to air-dry briefly and store at –70°C until required. Typically, 20 sections (10 total and 10 NSB) are required for each saturation curve together with a further three sections collected into microcentrifuge tubes to measure protein *(see* **Note 2**).
2. Dilute the stock solution [^{125}I]-PD151242 (5×10^{-8} *M*) to give the highest concentration of 1×10^{-9} *M* by adding 20 μL of stock solution to 980 μL of assay buffer (1 in 50).
3. Using the highest concentration, prepare a serial dilution (500 μL label + 500 μL assay buffer) to give a total of 10 concentrations over the range 1.95×10^{-12} – 1×10^{-9} *M*. Vortex, and use a new pipet tip between each dilution.
4. Remove 250 μL from each of the serial dilutions to determine the NSB, leaving 250 μL to measure total binding (totals). Add 2.5 μL of 1×10^{-4} *M* unlabeled ET-1 to each NSB tube to give a final concentration of 1×10^{-6} *M* to define the NSB.
5. Count 20 μL aliquots of each total concentration in a gamma counter to determine the amount (DPM) of radioligand added for each dilution. These values are required in subsequent analysis of the data *(see* **Subheading 3.1.4.**).
6. In an incubation tray, preincubate 20 microscope slides bearing consecutive tissue sections (10 total, 10 NSB) with 200 μL assay buffer for 15 min at room temperature to remove endogenous ligand and degradative enzymes.
7. Tip off preincubation buffer into the tray and replace with 200 μL of each total or NSB solutions. Cover with a lid to maintain the humidity and incubate for 120 min at room temperature to reach equilibrium.

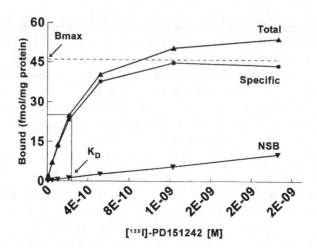

Fig. 1. Saturation isotherm for the binding of increasing concentrations of the ET_A selective ligand, [^{125}I]-PD151242, to sections of human ventricle. The amount of radioactivity bound to the tissue, measured in DPM by gamma counting, has been converted to fmol of [^{125}I]-PD151242 per mg of protein present in the incubation mixture. Nonspecific binding (NSB), which is linear and not saturable, was subtracted from the total to give the amount of specific binding. The specific binding saturates and an approximate value for the B_{max} can be estimated from the ordinate. An approximate value for the K_D can be obtained the abscissa, corresponding to 50% of the B_{max}.

8. Break equilibrium by transferring slides to racks and washing in 400 mL baths containing ice cold 0.05 *M* Tris-HCl buffer, pH 7.4, at 4°C (3 × 5 min).
9. Drain and wipe each section from the slide with a filter paper circle, transfer to a counting tube, and count in a gamma counter to measure DPM.
10. For autoradiography following **step 8**, rinse sections once in deionized water to remove buffer salts, and dry rapidly in a stream of cold air prior to apposing to radiation-sensitive film.

3.1.2. Graphical Analysis

An example of a saturation isotherm for the binding of [^{125}I]-PD151242 to human heart is shown in **Fig. 1**. The total, specific and nonspecific binding has been plotted against increasing concentrations of the radiolabeled ligand. Nonspecific binding occurs because the ligand may also bind to other proteins and lipids. This is linear and not saturable. The amount of specific binding observed where the isotherm plateaus is an approximation of the B_{max}. An estimate of the K_D can also be derived from the concentration of [^{125}I]-PD151242 that labels half of the target receptors (50% of the B_{max}). However, a better estimate can be achieved by linearizing the data using a Scatchard plot

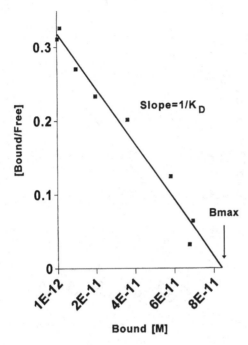

Fig. 2. Scatchard transformation of the data from Fig.1.. The slope of the line is equal to the negative reciprocal of the K_D (approx 0.3 nM) and the intercept of the line with the abscissa is an estimate of B_{max} (approx 55 fmol/mg protein). These values were then used as initial estimates in the computer program LIGAND, which uses nonlinear curve fitting to calculate the final binding parameters for [^{125}I]-PD151242; K_D = 0.24 nM, B_{max} = 50.6 fmol/mg protein in this tissue.

(**Fig. 2**). Here the ratio of bound and free radioligand (B/F) is plotted on the ordinate against the amount of bound radioligand (B) on the abscissa. The slope of the line through the points is equal to the negative reciprocal of the K_D and the intercept of the line with the abscissa is an estimate of B_{max}. This latter parameter is generally standardized against a suitable reference that allows a direct comparison of receptor density in different tissues and in different studies (*see* **Note 2**).

A linear Scatchard plot indicates that the radioligand binds with a single affinity. Under certain circumstances, the Scatchard plot yields a concave line indicating either that the ligand binds to multiple populations of sites with differing affinities for the radioligand or negative co-operativity. A curvi-linear convex line may indicate positive co-operativity. The Hill plot of log (Bound/ B_{max}-Bound) vs log [Free] is used to interpret these possible anomalous binding

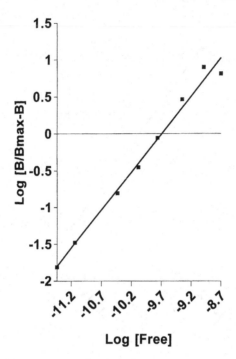

Fig 3. Hill plot of the data from **Fig. 1.** The slope of the line = the Hill coefficient (nH). For [^{125}I]-PD15242, the Hill slope (nH) was close to a value of one (1.03), indicating that the radioligand was binding with a single affinity to receptors within the heart tissue, consistent with the linear Scatchard plot.

interactions (**Fig. 3**). The Hill coefficient (the slope of the line through the points) will be approx 1 when the ligand binds to a single population of sites or when the ligand is binding to multiple populations of sites with similar affinity for the radioligand. A value less than one may indicate either negative co-operativity or multiple populations of binding sites with differing affinities for the radioligand. However, in saturation experiments, radiolabeled ET-1, ET-2 and sub-type selective ligands are expected to bind with Hill slopes close to 1.

3.1.3. Nonlinear Curve Fitting Programs

In practice nonlinear iterative curve fitting programs are used to calculate final estimates of the binding parameters. Nonlinear regression analysis utilizes equations that can define curves. KELL (Biosoft, http:///www.Biosoft.com) contains EBDA (Equilibrium Binding Data Analysis) and LIGAND programs (*43,44*). This suite is recommended because a number of saturation curves can be co-analyzed simultaneously. EBDA performs the preliminary analysis of both saturation and competition binding experiments, converting radioactivity in DPM into molar concentrations of ligand. Hill slopes are calculated separately and a Scatchard transformation is used to provide initial estimates of K_D and B_{max}. LIGAND uses the files created by EBDA, together with initial estimates of the binding parameters, to fit the data to a specified model of the radioligand binding, which may be to one, two, or more sites. A weighted, nonlinear curve fitting routine is iteratively refined to provide more accurate estimates of the K_D and B_{max} values than those obtained with linear (Scatchard) transformations alone.

A runs test is used to determine whether the data points differ significantly from the fitted curve. A good fit will have points randomly distributed around the fitted line, whereas a run of consecutive points, appearing either above or below the fitted line, may provide evidence for a significant lack of fit. In a saturation assay over a limited concentration range, many radioligands will bind with a single affinity, and a one-site fit is an appropriate model. However, curvilinear Scatchard plots, displayed in the EBDA results (or a significant departure of the data from the fitted curve in the runs test), may suggest that the ligand is binding with different affinities to more than one population of receptors. Therefore, a two- (or possibly three-) site fit should be tested, and compared with the one site model within the LIGAND program. LIGAND calculates an F value, taking into account the improvement in the goodness of fit that accompanies an increase in the number of parameters to be fitted in the two-site model compared with a one-site fit. The program will indicate which of the two models is statistically the better fit.

3.1.4. Analysis of Saturation Binding Data: Running EBDA and LIGAND

1. Run the EBDA program, enter assay type (HOT), data type (DPM), specific activity of the label in dpm/pmol (typically 4440000 for a label with specific activity of ~2000 Ci/mmol), volume of incubation in mL (0.2 mL in above assay) and calculation type (specific bound).
2. For each concentration, enter values (in DPM) for total and NSB from the gamma counter and press ESC to initiate calculations.
3. Check raw data input for accuracy prior to analysis and save data as an EBDA file.
4. Select curve fitting and select the model to be fitted (one-site, two-site, etc.) starting with a one-site model. Examine the initial estimates for a one site model and if these are reasonable begin curve fitting. The program calculates initial estimates of the K_D and B_{max}. Print these results to be used as initial estimates by the Ligand program and create a Ligand file (*see* **Note 3**).
5. Run the Ligand program and load the Ligand file created in EBDA. Up to 10 files from separate saturation assays can be loaded and co-analyzed. In this program, the following notation is used for fixed parameters:
   N—B/F ratio at infinite free concentration and used to calculate NSB.

C—This is a conversion factor used to adjust the amount of protein in different experiments if required, but is not used in the following example.

The following parameters are calculated:

K—This is the association constant of the radioligand ($[^{125}I]$-PD151242), K_A, being calculated and is the reciprocal of the K_D value. LIGAND uses K_A instead of K_D.

R—B_{max}, the maximum density of binding sites. This value is corrected using the amount of protein per section(s) mounted on the microscope slide in the incubation volume (*see* **Note 4**).

6. Start curve fitting by selecting the number of sites to be fitted (one-site, two-site, etc.).
7. Nominate the fixed values: for the NSB, the constant N1 is zero because the individual NSB values have been entered and C1 is set to 1.
8. Set the initial estimates for the floating parameters: K11, the initial estimate obtained from EBDA of the K_D (entered as the reciprocal of the K_D) and R1, the initial estimate from EBDA of the B_{max}.

   The program iteratively refines the initial estimates and upon convergence display the final estimates for the K_D (K11) and B_{max} (R1) together with the standard error (*see* **Note 4**).
9. Rerun EBDA and under Saturation select Hill analysis in order to calculate the Hill slope together with the standard error.

3.2. Competition Binding

3.2.1. Competition Binding Assays

Having determined the K_D of a radiolabeled ligand for a target receptor in a saturation assay, this information can be used to determine the ability of other unlabeled compounds, tested over a much wider concentration range (typically 10 pM–100 μM), to compete for the binding of a fixed concentration of the labeled ligand. Competition binding experiments can also be used to determine the selectivity (if any) of a particular ligand for ET_A or ET_B receptors and thus allow determination of the density and proportion of each sub-type in the tissue. Competition curves are obtained by plotting specific binding as a percentage of total binding (binding in the absence of competitor) against the log concentration of the competing ligand. Both ET receptor sub-types are present in left ventricle of the human heart in a ratio of about 60% ET_A:40% ET_B allowing ligands to be characterized against both receptors in the same tissue. In **Fig. 4**, $[^{125}I]$-ET-1 has been used to label all of the ET receptors in this tissue *(23,25,26)* since the peptide has equal affinity for both the ET_A and ET_B subtype. A steep competition curve is usually indicative of binding to a single population of receptors. However, increasing concentrations of unlabeled PD151242 inhibited the binding of $[^{125}I]$-ET-1 biphasically. A shallow curve or a curve with clear inflection points is indicative of multiple populations of binding sites. The partial F-test and the runs test can again be used to differen-

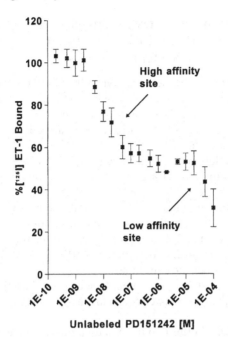

Fig. 4. Competition binding curve for the inhibition of a fixed concentration of [^{125}I]-ET-1 (0.1 n*M*) binding to ET receptors by increasing concentrations of unlabeled PD151242 in sections of human ventricle. Over the concentration range tested, PD151242 competed in a biphasic manner and a two-site fit was preferred to a one-site or three-site model using LIGAND. The high affinity site corresponded to the endothelin ET$_A$ receptor (K$_D$ = 7.2 + 2.8 n*M*), the low affinity site to the ET$_B$ receptor, K$_D$ = 104 + 23 μ*M*. Each value represents the mean ± s.e.m. of three individuals.

tiate single and multiple populations of binding sites. In this case, a two-site fit was preferred, consistent with PD151242 binding with high affinity to the ET$_A$ site but low, micromolar, affinity to the ET$_B$ receptors, giving about 15,000-fold selectivity for the ET$_A$ receptor.

The plot of log (%B/[100−%B]) against log [L*], where %B is the percentage of radioligand bound and [L*] is the concentration of the competing ligand, gives a line through the points with slope equal to the pseudo Hill coefficient. This approximates unity for a one-site fit and is less than unity if negative co-operativity is indicated or if two or more populations of receptors with differing affinities for the competing ligand are present. However, binding constants for multiple receptor populations is difficult to determine accurately by graphical means. EBDA uses an equation that allows interpretation of a heterogeneous population of binding sites and provides estimates of the pseudo Hill coefficient and receptor affinity. LIGAND is then used to test for one, two, or more binding sites as described for the analysis of saturation data.

1. Cut 25 consecutive cryostat sections (typically 10–30 μm) of fresh-frozen tissue per competition assay. Two sections are used to measure total binding, two sections for the NSB leaving 21 sections for construction of the competition curve by the unlabeled ligand. A further three sections are collected into microcentrifuge tube to measure protein.

2. Dilute the stock solution of radiolabeled [^{125}I]-ET-1 (5×10^{-8} M) in assay buffer to give a concentration of 1.1×10^{-10} M (1:454.5 dilution equivalent to 13.2 μL in 6 mL of assay buffer).

3. Prepare a stock concentration (1×10^{-3} M) of the competing ligand. Dilute this in assay buffer to give three further stock solution solutions (1×10^{-4}, 2×10^{-4} and 5×10^{-4} M) as shown in **Table 3**. From each of three solutions, prepare a series of dilutions to give a concentration range $1 \times 10^{-3} - 2 \times 10^{-10}$ M. Vortex, and use a new pipet tip between each dilution.

4. Pipet 225 μL of [^{125}I]-ET-1 into 2 tubes labeled total, 2 labeled NSB and a further 21 labeled with each final concentration of competing ligand ($1 \times 10^{-4} -2 \times 10^{-11}$ M).

5. Pipet 25 μL of assay buffer into the two total tubes to give a final concentration of [^{125}I]-ET of 1×10^{-10} M. Vortex.

6. Pipet 25 μL of 1×10^{-5} M unlabeled ET-1 into the two NSB tubes to give a final concentration of 1×10^{-6} M. Vortex.

7. Pipet 25 μL of each prepared concentration of competing ligand into the appropriately labeled tube. Vortex, and use a new pipet tip between each solution.

8. In incubation trays, preincubate 25 microscope slides bearing consecutive tissue sections (2 total, 2 NSB, 21 competing ligand) with 200 μL assay buffer for 15 min at room temperature to remove endogenous ligand and degradative enzymes.

9. Tip off preincubation buffer into tray and replace with 200 μL of total, NSB, or competing ligand dilution. Cover with lid to maintain humidity and incubate for 120 min at room temperature to reach equilibrium.

10. Break equilibrium by transferring slides to racks and washing in 400 mL baths containing ice-cold 0.05 M Tris-HCl, pH 7.4, at 4°C (3×5 min).

11. Drain and wipe each section from the slide with a filter paper circle, transfer to a counting tube, and count in a gamma counter to measure DPM.

12. For autoradiography following **steps 1–10**, rinse sections once in deionized water to remove buffer salts, and dry rapidly in a stream of cold air prior to apposing to Radiation-sensitive film.

3.2.2. Analysis of Competition Binding Data: Running EBDA and LIGAND

1. Run the EBDA program, enter assay type (Competition), data type (DPM), specific activity of the label in dpm/pmol (typically 4.4×10^6 for a label with specific activity of ~2000 Ci/mmol), volume of incubation in mL (0.2 mL in above assay) and calculation type (specific bound).

Table 3
Competition Binding Assay

A	Label μL	Unlabeled ligand μL	Competing ligand μL	Buffer μL total
(×2)	225	–	–	25
NSB (×2)	225	25	–	–
Competing ligand (×21 Concentrations)	225	–	25	–

B	Series 1	Series 2	Series 3
Stock (1E-3 *M*) μL	10	20	50
Buffer μL	90	80	50
Target concentration	⇓	⇓	⇓
[M]	1E-4	2E-4	5E-4

	Series 1	Series 2	Series 3
C	1E-4	2E-4	5E-4
	1E-5	2E-5	5E-5
Serial Dilution	1E-6	2E-6	5E-6
10 μL + 90 μL Buffer	1E-7	2E-7	5E-7
	1E-8	2E-8	5E-8
	1E-9	2E-9	5E-9
		2E-10	5E-10

D Serial dilution 10 μL + 90 μL buffer	From serial dilutions	Final concentration
1	1E-3 (from stock)	1E-4
2	5E-4	5E-5
3	2E-4	2E-5
4	1E-4	1E-5
5	5E-5	5E-6
6	2E-5	2E-6
7	1E-5	1E-6
8	5E-6	5E-7
9	2E-6	2E-7
10	1E-6	1E-7
11	5E-7	5E-8
12	2E-7	2E-8
13	1E-7	1E-8
14	5E-8	5E-9
15	2E-8	2E-9
16	1E-8	1E-9
17	5E-9	5E-10
18	2E-9	2E-10
19	1E-9	1E-10
20	5E-10	5E-11
21	2E-10	2E-11

2. Enter total and NSB in DPM (common to all subsequent data points).
3. Enter each concentration (2×10^{-11} M is entered as 2E-11, etc.) and its corresponding counts in DPM from the gamma counter.
4. Check raw data input for accuracy and save data as an EBDA file to be used later by Ligand.
5. Select curve fitting and select the model to be fitted (one-site, two-site etc.), starting with a one-site model, and start curve fitting. In the above assay, unlabeled PD151242 is expected to compete for the binding of [^{125}I]-ET-1 biphasically with a high (nM) affinity for ET_A and low affinity (μM) at ET_B receptors. A one-site model is unlikely to be fitted and a two-site model should be chosen. Examine the initial estimates for a two-site model and if these are reasonable begin curve fitting. The program calculates initial estimates of the high and low affinity K_D values together with their corresponding receptor densities (B_{max}). Print these results to be used as initial estimates by the Ligand program and create a Ligand file.
6. Run the Ligand program and load the data file created in EBDA. Up to 10 files from separate assays can be loaded and co-analyzed. In this program the following notation is used:

   K—This is the association constant K_A, which is the reciprocal of the K_D value. LIGAND uses K_A instead of K_D.

   R—B_{max}, the maximum density of binding sites. This value is corrected using the amount of protein per section(s) mounted on the microscope slide in the incubation volume (*see* **Note 3**).

   N—B/F ratio at infinite free concentration and used to calculate NSB.

   C—This is a conversion factor used to adjust the amount of protein in different experiments if required, but not used in the following example.

3.2.2.1. ONE-SITE FIT

1. Start curve fitting by selecting a one-site fit.
2. Set the constant parameters: N2 C1 K11.
   N2—NSB of competing ligand (PD151242) set to 0.
   C1—Set to 1.
   K11—refers to the ligand binding to site 1, which for [^{125}I]-ET-1 is the reciprocal of the K_D.
3. Set the initial estimates of the floating parameters: K21 the estimate obtained from EBDA of the K_D for PD151242 (entered as the reciprocal of the K_D) and R1, the initial estimate from EBDA of the B_{max}.
4. The program iteratively refines the initial estimates and upon convergence displays the final estimates for the K_D (K21) and B_{max} (R1) together with the standard error.

3.2.2.2. TWO-SITE FIT

1. Start curve fitting by selecting a two-site fit.
2. Set the constant parameters: N1 C1 K11 K12 N2.
   K11—refers to the radioligand ([^{125}I]- ET-1) binding to site 1 (ET_A).

K12—refers to the radioligand ($[^{125}I]$-ET-1) binding to site 2 (ET_B).

Since $[^{125}I]$-ET-1 has equal affinity for both ET_A and ET_B receptors, these two values will be the same and for $[^{125}I]$-ET-1 the reciprocal of the K_D is entered.

N1—NSB for ligand 1 and is set to 0.

N2—NSB of competing ligand (PD151242) set to 0.

C1—is a conversion factor that can be applied but is not used in this example and is set to 1.

3. Set the initial estimates of the floating parameters: K21 and K22.

K21—refers to ligand 2 (unlabeled PD151242) binding to site 1 (ET_A).

K22—refers to ligand 2 (unlabeled PD151242) binding to site 2 (ET_B).

Both parameters are obtained from EBDA as initial estimates for the K_D for PD151242 (entered as the reciprocal of the K_D).

R1 and R2—are the initial estimates from EBDA of the B_{max} values for the two sites.

4. The program iteratively refines the initial estimates and upon convergence displays the final estimates for the K_D (K21) of PD151242 binding at the high affinity, ET_A site and K22, the low affinity, ET_B site. The density of ET_A (R1) and ET_B receptors (R2) is also given (*see* **Note 4**).

3.3. Binding Kinetics

Kinetic experiments determine the time course of ligand association and dissociation (**Fig. 5**). In association studies sections are labeled with a fixed concentration of radioligand for increasing time periods. Nonspecific binding is defined at each time point using a high concentration of unlabeled ligand. The plot of $\ln(B_{eq}/(B_{eq}-B_t))$ against time, where B_{eq} is the amount of ligand bound at equilibrium and B_t is the amount of ligand bound at time t, should yield a straight line through the points with slope equal to K_{obs}.

When equilibrium is reached, dissociation of the radioligand from the receptors is achieved either by incubation of tissue sections with a high concentration of unlabeled competitor or by infinite dilution of the labeled sections by immersion in a large volume of buffer. The plot of $\ln(B_t/B_0)$ against time, where B_0 is binding at time 0, should be linear with the slope equal to the dissociation rate constant (K-1, K21 or K_{off}). The association (K1, K12 or K_{on}) and dissociation rate constants are described by the following relationship: $K1 = (K_{obs}-K-1)/[L]$, where [L] is the concentration of free ligand. Kinetic experiments provide an additional means of calculating the equilibrium dissociation constant, $K_D = K-1/K1$, and this should be comparable to K_D values determined by saturation analysis (*see* **Subheading 3.1.**). While the above linear transformations give estimates of association and dissociation constants, the use of computer based nonlinear curve fitting, such as KINETIC in the KELL suite of programs (*see* **Subheading 3.1.3.**) are recommended for the analysis kinetic data.

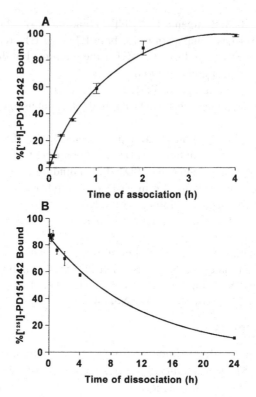

Fig. 5. **(A)** Association curve for a fixed concentration of [^{125}I]-PD151242 binding to sections of human ventricle. The curve plateaus after 2 h, indicating that equilibrium has been reached for this ligand. The calculated observed association rate constant (K_{obs}) was 0.0172 min^{-1}. **(B)** Time course for the dissociation of [^{125}I]-PD151242 initiated by washing the sections in a large volume of buffer. The calculated dissociation rate constant (K-1) was 0.00144 min^{-1}.

3.3.1. Association Binding Assays

1. Cut 16 consecutive cryostat sections (typically 10–30 μm) of fresh-frozen tissue per association assay. One section is used to measure total binding and one section for the NSB at each of eight time points.
2. Dilute the stock solution of radiolabeled [^{125}I]-PD151242 (5×10^{-8} *M*) to give a concentration of 1×10^{-10} *M* (corrected for decay, if any) in 4 mL of assay buffer (count a 200 μL aliquot in order to determine the total counts added, in DPM, to each slide for subsequent analysis). Remove 2 mL to define total binding and add unlabeled peptide to a final concentration of 1×10^{-6} *M*, to define the NSB. Vortex.
3. Preincubate 16 microscope slides bearing consecutive sections with 200 μL assay buffer for 15 min at room temperature.

4. Tip off preincubation buffer into tray and replace with 200 µL of total (8 slides) or NSB (8 slides). Transfer slides at intervals of 1, 2, 5 15, 30, 60, 120 and 240 min into racks, and wash in 400 mL baths containing ice-cold 0.05 M Tris-HCl, pH 7.4, at 4°C (3 × 5 min).
5. Drain and wipe each section from the slide with a filter paper circle, transfer to a counting tube, and count in a gamma counter to measure DPM.

3.3.2. Analysis of Association Binding Data

1. Run the Kinetic program, enter assay type (Association), data type (DPM), specific activity of the label in dpm/pmol (typically 4440000 for a label with specific activity of ~2000 Ci/mmol), volume of incubation in mL (0.2 mL in above assay), and calculation type (specific bound).
2. Enter time of sample, total, and NSB in DPM. Enter the amount of radioactivity added per 200 µL (DPM) which will be the same for each section.
3. Check raw data input for accuracy, view initial estimates, and save data as a Kinetic file.
4. Start curve fitting. Select the model to be fitted (one-site, two-site, etc.) starting with a one-site model. Commence curve fitting to refine the model estimates and if acceptable save the result in memory. The observed association rate constant (K_{obs}) is displayed as the exponent together with the error (units min^{-1}).
5. Repeat using a two-site model. In the above example, a second site could not be fitted indicating a one-site fit was an appropriate model for [^{125}I]-PD151242 binding (**Fig. 5A**).

3.3.3. Dissociation Binding Assays

1. Cut 16 consecutive cryostat sections (typically 10–30 µm) of fresh-frozen tissue per association assay. One section is used to measure total binding and one section for the NSB at each of eight time points.
2. Dilute the stock solution of radiolabel [^{125}I]-PD151242 (5×10^{-8} M) to give a concentration of 1×10^{-10} M (corrected for decay, if any) in 4 mL of assay buffer (count a 200 µL aliquot in order to determine the total counts added, in DPM, to each slide for subsequent analysis). Remove 2 mL to define total binding and add unlabeled peptide to a final concentration of 1×10^{-6} M, to define the NSB. Vortex.
3. Preincubate 16 microscope slides bearing consecutive sections with 200 µL assay buffer for 15 min at room temperature.
4. Tip off preincubation buffer into tray and replace with 200 µL of total (8 slides) or NSB (8 slides). Incubate for 2 h to reach equilibrium.
5. Starting with the last pair of slides, transfer slides at intervals of 1, 5, 60, 120, 240, and 1500 min into racks and wash in 400 mL baths containing ice-cold 0.05 M Tris-HCl, pH 7.4, at 4°C (3 × 5 min).
6. Drain and wipe each section from the slide with a filter paper circle, transfer to a counting tube, and count in a gamma counter to measure DPM (**Fig. 5B**).

3.3.4. Analysis of Dissociation Binding Data

The objective of the competition binding assay is to test whether the unlabeled ligand competes at one or two-sites for $[^{125}I]$-ET-1. Once the best model is fitted affinity constants (K_D) and B_{max} values for one or two-sites can be calculated by using KELL (*see* **Subheading 3.1.3.**).

1. Run the Kinetic program, enter assay type (Dissociation), data type (DPM), specific activity of the label in dpm/pmol (typically 4440000 for a label with specific activity of ~2000 Ci/mmol), volume of incubation in mL (0.2 mL in above assay), and calculation type (specific bound).
2. Enter time of sample, total, and NSB in DPM. Enter the amount of radioactivity added per 200 µL (DPM), which will be the same for each section.
3. Check raw data input for accuracy, view initial estimates, and save data as a Kinetic file.
4. Start curve fitting. Select the model to be fitted (one-site, two-site, etc.) starting with a one-site model. Commence curve fitting to refine the model estimates, and if acceptable, save the result in memory. The dissociation rate constant (K-1) is displayed as the exponent, together with the error.
5. Repeat using a two-site model. In the above example, a second site could not be fitted indicating a one-site fit was an appropriate model for $[^{125}I]$-PD151242 binding. Where a two-site model can be fitted, a partial F-test is used to determine which fit is preferred (**Fig. 5B**).

3.4. Autoradiography

Autoradiography can be used to visualize the localization of receptors in discrete regions of tissue and to confirm that the radioligand binds to cells that would be expected to express the target receptor. The principle of the technique is that the spatial distribution of radiolabeled ligands can be detected by the blackening of Radiation-sensitive film apposed directly to the section containing radiolabeled tissue. Slide mounted tissue sections or coverslips containing cultured cells are used. Sections are preincubated in buffer, labeled with the radioligand in the absence or presence of selective competing ligands, washed in buffer, dipped in water to remove buffer salts, and dried rapidly under a stream of cool dry air. The K_D (determined by saturation analysis) is used to calculate the concentration of the radioligand required to label a fixed proportion of receptors in the tissue. Using a concentration calculated to label 10% of the receptors results in a high ratio of total to NSB. At the end of the assay, sections are apposed to Radiation-sensitive film for macro-autoradiography and exposed in the dark for a period that will be determined by the type of isotope used, the density of binding sites in the tissue section and by the tissue section thickness. The films are then developed, fixed, and viewed. When higher resolution is required, sections can be apposed to coverslips coated in nuclear emulsion. Developed silver grains represent the location of the bound radioligand in the underlying tissue when viewed using a microscope equipped with darkfield illumination.

3.4.1. Quantitative Autoradiography Assays

Quantitative autoradiography can be used to analyze a number of different types of experiment. Sections can be apposed to Radiation-sensitive film following either saturation (*see* **Subheading 3.1.**) or competition (*see* **Subheading 3.2.**) binding assays. Sections can also be incubated with a fixed concentration of sub-type selective ligands under the same binding conditions (*see* **Subheading 3.2.**). [^{125}I]-PD151242 is used to measure the relative density of ET_A receptors and [^{125}I]-BQ3020 ET_B to determine the density of the ET_B sub-type. In both cases, nonspecific binding is defined in adjacent sections incubated with the radiolabel and 1 μM of the corresponding unlabeled peptide *(13)*. Alternatively, sections can be incubated with a fixed concentration of [^{125}I]-ET-1. Adjacent sections are incubated in the presence of a fixed concentration of an unlabeled ET_B ligand to block [^{125}I]-ET-1 binding to this sub-type thus delineating the ET_A receptors. A third section is incubated with a fixed concentration of an unlabeled ET_A ligand to define the ET_B receptors.

A fourth section is used to measure NSB ([^{125}I]-ET-1 + 1 μM unlabeled ET-1). For example, using human heart tissue, for BQ123, the K_D ET_A = 7 × 10^{-10} M and ET_B = 2.4 × 10^{-5} M. Using these K_D values, BQ123 at a concentration of 1 × 10^{-7} M is calculated to block >99% [^{125}I]-ET-1 binding to ET_A receptors but occupy <5% of the ET_B *(1,7)*. Similarly, for BQ3020, the K_D ET_B = 1.4 × 10^{-9} M and ET_A = 2 × 10^{-6} M. BQ3020 at a concentration of 2 × 10^{-7} M can be calculated to occupy >99% of ET_B but <9% ET_A. Once the appropriate binding assay has been completed and the tissue sections dried continue as follows.

1. Mount microscope slides bearing tissue sections onto card, together with a microscope slide bearing calibrated radioactive standards (^{125}I-Microscales, *5,45*) in an a light tight X-ray cassette. In a darkroom with a safelight, appose to a single coated Radiation-sensitive film (Kodak BioMax MR-1, Amersham Pharmacia Biotech, Little Chalfont, Bucks., UK) and leave for 2–5 d.
2. In a darkroom with a safelight, monitor the development of autoradiograms for up to 5 min in D19 developer; rinse for 30 s in deionized water to stop development. Fix for 30 min in Kodak Unifix (*see* **Note 6**).

3.4.2. Computer-Assisted Image Analysis

Analyze the resulting autoradiograms by measuring diffuse integrated optical density using a computer-assisted image analysis system (*see* **Note 7**).

1. Calibrate the image analyzer for densitometry. Autoradiograms are illuminated by reflected white light and the image captured by the videoscanner equipped with a zoom lens. Alter the zoom lens mounted on the videoscanner to produce a measuring field appropriate to the size of the autoradiographical image to be analyzed. Set the shading corrector to give an image, which appears uniformly white and compensate for any variation in illumination so that optical densities

can be measured accurately throughout the autoradiogram. Set the white level (100% transmission) and the scanner dark current (the current flowing in the scanner in the absence of a signal), which would otherwise contribute to the gray image. Finally calibrate the system against neutral density filters to convert gray levels into optical densities and the number of pixels per unit area are calculated by means of a measuring box (*see* **Note 8**).

2. Construct a standard curve from calibrated standards (*see* **Note 5**) for each film to relate optical densities to known amounts of radioactivity. Detect the autoradiographical image of each standard in turn using the cursor to draw around and isolate the image. Measure the integrated optical density for each standard together with the area. Enter the amount of radioactivity for each standard, measured by gamma counting in DPM (corrected for the efficiency of the counter and decay, if any), which is divided by the area to calculate radioactivity in dpm/mm^2. The specific activity of the label can be used to convert these values into amol/mm^2. Generate the natural log plot of optical density vs radioactivity to give a linear relationship.

3. Measure the density of ET receptors by digitizing each autoradiographical image of the tissue sections. Delineate regions of interest (or use other binary masks such as a circle) from the resulting gray image by using a cursor to draw around a defined anatomical region.

4. When all measurements have been made for a particular section, increase the threshold for detecting the autoradiogram to produce a template that can be used to align the autoradiographical image of the NSB section. Subtract the second image from the first to measure the amount of specific binding. Convert the resulting optical densities to the amount of specifically bound radioligand either in dpm/mm^2 for saturation/competition assays for analysis by EBDA and Ligand or in amol/mm^2 when comparing fixed concentration of ligand by interpolation from the standards curve.

4. Notes

1. In saturation experiments, the amount of radioligand added is increased while maintaining a constant specific activity of the radioligand. In practice, because of cost and hazards of handling high levels of radioactivity it is usually not possible to achieve concentrations of [^{125}I]-labeled ligand above 10 nM and saturation assays are limited to ligands with affinities in the sub-nanomolar range. An alternative is to use a constant concentration of radioligand and the specific activity of the radioligand is decreased by the addition of unlabeled ligand (*see* **Subheading 3.1.**).

2. The assay protocol can also be used for tissue homogenates *(13)*.

3. As a guide over the concentration range used in the above saturation assay, [^{125}I]-ET-1, [^{125}I]-ET-2, [^{125}I]-S6b would be expected to bind with similar sub-nanomolar affinity to ET_A/ET_B receptors and a one-site monophasic model is anticipated. Similarly [^{125}I]-PD1521242 binding to ET_A receptors and [^{125}I]-BQ3020 to ET_B would also be expected to bind monophasically. To check,

Ligand should be rerun by fitting a two-site model. In many cases, the program will be unable to do this, leading to an error message of overflow or ill-conditioning. Where a two-site fit is obtained, inspection of the resulting F-test which compares the two fits will show whether a one or two-site is statically a better fit.

4. The B_{max} value in the LIGAND printout is given in mol/L. To convert to pmoles of ligand bound/mg protein, divide R1 (if one-site or R1 and R2 if two-site fit, etc.) by the amount of protein measured in representative sections in mg/L.

5. Commercial standards (activity range 1.2–646 nCi/mg) consist of layers containing radioactivity incorporated at the molecular level in a methacrylate copolymer, separated by inert colored layers. Cut strips are expanded on water at 60°C and brushed flat onto gelatin-subbed slides to remove creases. Representative sections are sub-divided into the individual activity levels and counted in a gamma counter to measure the amount of radioactivity in DPM with correction for the efficiency of the counter. Since standards are designed to be used for up to a year, the amount of radioactivity should be corrected for decay from the time of counting the standards to the mid-time point between opposing and developing the film.

6. Optimum development can usually be assessed visually under safelight. However, if autoradiograms are too dark or too light, sections can be reopposed to film.

7. A range of image analyzers are available but in order to carry out accurate densitometry the machine should be equipped with a shading corrector and be able to digitize images into an array of at least 500 × 500 picture points with a minimum of 256 gray levels. The image-analyzer should also be able to subtract stored images. The details of operation of different commercial systems vary considerably, but the major procedures are similar.

8. This should be repeated each time the conditions are changed such as altering the magnification or using a different film.

Acknowledgments

Supported by grants from the British Heart Foundation, Royal Society, and Isaac Newton Trust.

References

1. Arai, H., Hori, S., Aramori, I., Ohkubo, H., and Nakanishi, S. (1990) Cloning and expression of a cDNA encoding an endothelin receptor. *Nature* **348,** 730–732.
2. Sakurai, T., Yanagisawa, M., Takuwa, Y., Miyazaki, H., Kimura, S., Goto, K., and Masaki, T. (1990) Cloning of a cDNA encoding a nonisopeptide-selective subtype of the endothelin receptor. *Nature* **348,** 732–735.
3. Davenport, A. P. (2000) Endothelin receptors. *Iuphar Compendium of Receptor Characterisation and Classification,* 2nd edition. Iuphar Media, London, UK. 182–188.
4. Davenport, A. P., O'Reilly, G., Molenaar, P., Maguire, J. J. Kuc, R. E., Sharkey, A., Bacon, C. R., and Ferro, A. (1993) Human endothelin receptors characterized using reverse transcriptase-polymerase chain reaction, *in situ* hybridization and sub-type selective ligands BQ123 and BQ3020: Evidence for expression of ET_B receptors in human vascular smooth muscle. *J. Cardiovasc. Pharmacol.* **22(S8),** 22–25.

5. Molenaar, P., O'Reilly, G., Sharkey, A., Kuc, R. E., Harding, D. P., Plumpton, P., Gresham, G. A., and Davenport, A. P. (1993) Characterization and localization of endothelin receptor sub-types in the human atrio-ventricular conducting system and myocardium. *Circ. Res.* **72**, 526–538.

6. Telemaque-Potts, S., Kuc, R. E., Yanagisawa, M., and Davenport A. P. (2000) Tissue-specific modulation of endothelin receptors in a rat model of hypertension. *J. Cardiovasc. Pharmacol.* **36(S1)**, 122–123.7.

7. Kuc, R. E. and Davenport A. P. (2000) Endothelin-A-receptors in human aorta and pulmonary arteries are down regulated in patients with cardiovascular disease: An adaptive response to increased levels of ET-1? *J. Cardiovasc. Pharmacol.* **36(S1)**, 377–379.

8. Keen, M. (ed.) (1999) *Receptor Binding Techniques.* Humana Press, Totowa, NJ.

9. Hulme, E. (1992) *Receptor-Ligand Interactions.* IRL, Oxford, UK.

10. Kenakin, T. (1993) *Pharmacologic Analysis of Drug-Receptor Interactions.* Raven Press, New York, USA.

11. Davenport, A. P. and Russell, F. D. (2001) Endothelin converting enzymes and endothelin receptor localisation in human tissues, in *Handbook of Experimental Pharmacology, vol. 152* (Warner, T. D. ed.), Springer-Verlag, Berlin, Germany, pp. 209–237.

12. Davenport, A. P. (1997) Distribution of endothelin receptors, in *Endothelins in Biology and Medicine* (Miller, R., Pelton, J. T., and Huggins, J., eds.), CRC Press Inc, Florida. pp. 45–68.

13. Davenport, A. P., O'Reilly, G., and Kuc, R. E. (1995) Endothelin ET_A and ET_B mRNA and receptors expressed by smooth muscle in the human vasculature: majority of the ET_A sub-type. *Br. J. Pharmacol.* **114**, 1110–1116.

14. Davenport, A. P. and Maguire, J. J. (1994) Endothelin-induced vasoconstriction is mediated by ET_A receptors in man. *Trends Pharmacol. Sci.* **15**, 136–137.

15. Gray, G. A. and Webb, D. J. (1996) The endothelin system and its potential as a therapeutic target in cardiovascular disease. *Pharmacol. Ther.* **72**, 109–148.

16. Douglas, S. A. and Ohlstein, E. H. (1997) Signal transduction mechanisms mediating the vascular actions of endothelin. *J. Vasc. Res.* **34**, 152–64.

17. Henry, P. J. and Goldie, R. G. (2001) Endothelin receptors, in *Handbook of Experimental Pharmacology, vol. 152* (Warner, T. D., ed), Springer-Verlag, Berlin, Germany, pp. 69–114.

18. Stanimirovic, D. B., Yamamoto, T., Uematsu, S., and Spatz, M. (1994) Endothelin-1 receptor binding and cellular signal transduction in cultured human brain endothelial cells. *J. Neurochem.* **62**, 592–601.

19. Zhang, Y. F., Jeffery, S., Burchill, S. A., Berry, P. A., Kaski, J. C. and Carter, N. D. (1998) Truncated human endothelin receptor A produced by alternative splicing and its expression in melanoma. *Br. J. Cancer* **78**, 1141–1146.

20. Shyamala, V., Moulthrop, T. H., Stratton Thomas, J., and Tekamp Olson, P. (1994) Two distinct human endothelin B receptors generated by alternative splicing from a single gene. *Cell Mol. Biol. Res.* **40**, 285–296.

21. Elshourbagy, N. A., Adamou, J. E., Gagnon, A. W., Wu, H. L., Pullen, M., and

Nambi, P. (1996) Molecular characterization of a novel human endothelin receptor splice variant. *J. Biol. Chem.* **271**, 25,300–25,307.

22. Mizuguchi, T., Nishiyama, M, Moroi, K., Tanaka, H., Saito, T., Masuda, Y., et al. (1997) Analysis of two pharmacologically predicted endothelin B receptor subtypes by using the endothelin B receptor gene knockout mouse. *Br. J. Pharmacol.* **120**, 1427–1430.

23. Molenaar, P., Kuc, R. E., and Davenport, A. P. (1992) Characterization of two new ET_B selective radioligands, [^{125}I]-BQ3020 and [^{125}I]-[Ala1,3,11,15]ET-1 in human heart. *Br. J. Pharmacol.* **107**, 637–639.

24. Davenport, A. P., Kuc, R. E., Hoskins, S. L., Karet, F. E., and Fitzgerald, F. (1994) [^{125}I]-PD151242: a selective ligand for endothelin ET_A receptors in human kidney which localizes to renal vasculature. *Brit. J. Pharmacol.* **113**, 1303–1310.

25. Peter, M. G. and Davenport A. P. (1996) Characterisation of endothelin receptor selective agonist BQ3020 and antagonists BQ123, FR139317, BQ788, 50235, Ro462005 and bosentan in the heart. *Brit. J. Pharmacol.* **117**, 455–462.

26. Russell, F. D. and Davenport, A. P. (1996) Characterisation of the binding of endothelin ET_B selective ligands in human and rat heart. *Brit. J. Pharmacol.* **119**, 631–636.

27. Flynn, M. A., Haleen, S. J., Welch, K. M., Cheng, X. M., and Reynolds, E. E. (1998) Endothelin B receptors on human endothelial and smooth-muscle cells show equivalent binding pharmacology. *J. Cardiovasc. Pharmacol.* **32**, 106–116.

28. Lecoin, L., Sakurai, T., Ngo, M. T., Abe, Y., Yanagisawa, M., and Le-Douarin, N. M. (1998) Cloning and characterization of a novel endothelin receptor subtype in the avian class. *Proc. Natl. Acad. Sci.* **95**, 3024–3029.

29. Karne, S., Jayawickreme, C. K., and Lerner, M. R. (1993) Cloning and characterization of an endothelin-3 specific receptor (ET_C receptor) from *Xenopus laevis* dermal melanophores. *J. Biol. Chem.* **268**, 19126–19133.

30. Davenport, A. P. and Morton, A. J. (1991) Binding sites for ^{125}I-^{125}I ET-1, ET-2, ET-3 and vasoactive intestinal contractor are present in adult rat brain and neurone-enriched primary cultures of embryonic brain cells. *Brain Res.* **554**, 278–285.

31. Bacon, C. R. and Davenport, A. P. (1996) Endothelin receptors in human coronary artery and aorta. *Brit. J. Pharmacol.* **117**, 986–992.

32. Maguire, J. J., Kuc, R. E., Rous, B. A., and Davenport A. P. (1996) Failure of BQ123, a more potent antagonist of sarafotoxin S6b than of endothelin-1, to distinguish between these agonists in binding experiments. *Brit. J. Pharmacol.* **118**, 355–342.

33. Davenport, A. P., Kuc, R. E., Fitzgerald, F., Maguire, J. J., Berryman, K., and Doherty, A. M. (1994) [^{125}I]-PD15242, a selective radioligand for human ET_A receptors. *Br. J. Pharmacol.* **111**, 4–6.

34. Davenport A. P., Kuc, R. E., Ashby, M. J., Patt, W. C., and Doherty, A. M. (1998) Characterisation of [^{125}I]-PD164333, an ET_A-selective nonpeptide radiolabeled antagonist, in normal and diseased human tissues. *Br. J. Pharmacol.* **123**, 223–230.

35. Ihara, M., Yamanaka, R., Ohwaki, K., Ozaki, S., Fukami, T., Ishikawa, K., et al. (1995) [^3H]-BQ-123, a highly specific and reversible radioligand for the endothelin ET_A receptor subtype. *Eur. J. Pharmacol.* **274**, 1–6.

36. Watakabe, T., Urade, Y., Takai, M., Umemura, I., and Okada, T. (1992) A reversible radioligand specific for the ET_B receptor, [^{125}I]-]Tyr13-Suc-[Glu9,Ala11,15]-endothelin-1(8–21), [^{125}I]-IRL1620. *Biochem. Biophys. Res. Commun.* **185,** 867–873.

37. Ihara, M., Noguchi, K., Saeki, T., Fukuroda, T., Tsuchida, S., Kimura, S., et al. (1992) Biological profiles of highly potent novel endothelin antagonists selective for the $ET_{(A)}$ receptor. *Life Sci.* **50,** 247–255.

38. Aramori, I., Nirei, H., Shoubo, M., Sogabe, K., Nakamura, K., Kojo, H., et al. (1993) Subtype selectivity of a novel endothelin antagonist, FR139317, for the two endothelin receptors in transfected Chinese hamster ovary cells. *Mol. Pharmacol.* **43,** 127–131.

39. William, D. L., Jr., Jones, K. L., Pettibone, D. J., Lis, E. V., and Clineschmidt, B. V. (1991) Sarafotoxin S6c, an agonist which distinguishes between endothelin receptor subtypes. *Biochem. Biophys. Res Commun.* **175,** 556–561.

40. Ishikawa, K., Ihara, M., Noguchi, K., Mase, T., Mino, N., Saeki, T., et al. (1994) Biochemical and pharmacological profile of a potent and selective endothelin B-receptor antagonist, BQ-788. *Proc. Natl. Acad. Sci. USA* **91,** 4892–4896.

41. Battistini, B. and Dussault, P. (1998) Blocking of the endothelin system: the development of receptor antagonists. *Pulm. Pharmacol. Ther.* **11,** 97–112.

42. Peter, M. G. and Davenport A. P. (1995) Selectivity of [^{125}I]-PD151242 for the human, rat and porcine endothelin ET_A receptors in the heart. *Brit. J. Pharmacol.* **114,** 297–302.

43. Munson, P. J. and Rodbard, D. (1980) Ligand: a versatile computerized approach for characterization of ligand-binding systems. *Anal. Biochem.* **107,** 220–239.

44. McPherson, G. A. (1985) Analysis of radioligand binding experiments. A collection of computer programs for the IBM PC. *J. Pharmacol. Meth.* **14,** 213–228.

45. Davenport, A. P. and Hall, M. D. (1988) Comparison between brain paste and polymer standards for quantitative receptor autoradiography. *J. Neurosci. Meth.* **25,** 75–82.

5

Using Receptor Antagonists in Binding Studies to Characterize a Mammalian Endothelin Receptor

J. Ruth Wu-Wong

1. Introduction

Endothelin (ET) is a peptide with 21-amino acid residues *(1)*. Three distinct members of the ET family, namely, ET-1, ET-2 and ET-3, have been identified in humans through cloning *(2)*. The effects of ETs on mammalian organs and cells are initiated by their binding to G-protein-linked receptors found in various tissues and cells *(3)*. Two types of mammalian ET receptors, ET_A and ET_B, have been characterized, purified *(4,5)*, and their cDNA have been cloned *(6,7)*. ET_A receptors are selective for ET-1 and ET-2, while ET_B receptors bind ET-1, ET-2 and ET-3 with equal affinity. In addition, an ET receptor specific for ET-3 (termed ETc receptor or ETcR) was cloned from *Xenopus laevis* dermal melanophores *(8)*. Although pharmacological studies suggest that there may be more endothelin receptor subtypes *(9)*, no additional homologous mammalian cDNAs other than ET_A and ET_B have been identified.

ET-1 is the most potent vasoconstrictor known. In addition to its potent effect on vasoconstriction, ETs play other biological roles. From both in vitro and in vivo studies, ETs are shown to be capable of eliciting a variety of physiological and pharmacological responses such as stimulating constriction in vascular and nonvascular tissues *(10,11)*, decreasing cardiac output *(12)*, decreasing glomerular filtration rate *(13)*, modulating cell proliferation and apoptosis *(14)*, and stimulating glucose uptake *(15,16)*. At the cellular level, binding of ETs initiates a complex signal transduction cascade *(17)*. ET-1 binding activates phospholipases C and D, causing increases in inositol 1,4,5-trisphosphate and neutral 1,2-diacylglycerol, which are associated with a biphasic increase in the intracellular Ca^{2+} concentration and

From: *Methods in Molecular Biology, vol. 206: Peptide Research Protocols: Endothelin*
Edited by: J. Maguire and A. Davenport © Humana Press Inc., Totowa, NJ

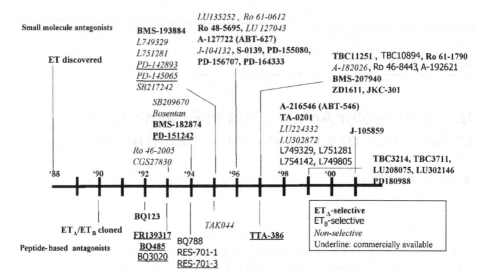

Fig. 1. Endothelin antagonists: a historical map. Antagonists that are commercially available are underlined. Adapted from **Fig. 1** in **ref. 44**.

activation of various kinase-mediated pathways involved in mitogenic responses *(18)*.

ETs have been shown to be involved in a wide range of pathological conditions such as atherosclerosis, pulmonary hypertension, cancer, congestive heart failure, coronary and cerebral vasospasm, restenosis, and so on. In most of these diseases, the ET-1 level is found to be elevated either in the plasma or in the tissue of interest. However, the elevation in the ET-1 level could be either the cause of the problem or the result of the condition. To differentiate between these two possibilities, it is important to employ ET receptor antagonists for further investigation.

Various antagonists and agonists for ET receptors have been developed. Although most of these ET receptor antagonists are intended for clinical development, they serve as useful tools for characterization of ET receptors. For discussion purposes, ET receptor antagonists developed during the past decade are shown in a chronicle order (**Fig. 1**). In **Fig. 1**, some of the commercially available ET receptor antagonists are marked for information purposes. It is worth noting that, although many ET receptor antagonists are not commercially available, requests sent to the appropriate companies for these compounds will usually be granted depending on the purpose of the request.

Since the discovery of ET in 1988, numerous papers have been published on the characterization of ET receptors in various cells and tissues. Although methods for characterizing an ET receptor seem well established, there are a number of factors that shall be considered when first venturing into the ET field. The goal of this chapter is to discuss these factors in order to provide information for researchers who need to characterize a new ET receptor employing known ET receptor agonists and antagonists in an in vitro binding study.

When using known agonists and antagonists to characterize a new ET receptor, the following factors shall be considered: (1) procedures for handling ET receptor agonists and antagonists, (2) tenacious binding characteristic of ETs, and (3) characteristics of different ET receptor agonists and antagonists.

1.1. Procedures for Handling ET Receptor Agonists and Antagonists

ET receptor agonists and antagonists are by nature very "sticky." The agents stick to the wall of a test tube or container easily. When we first started testing ET, we experienced a loss of >80% of ET-1 during a 60-min period when making a diluted 1 nM [^{125}I]ET-1 solution in a regular test tube. Not only are ET receptor agonists such as ET-1, -2, and -3 sticky, ET receptor antagonists also exhibit similar characteristics. Therefore, in order to obtain accurate concentrations for ET receptor agonists/antagonists, special care should be taken when making stock solutions or dilutions. The procedures followed in our laboratory for handling ET receptor ligands are described in **Subheading 3.1.**

1.2. Tenacious Binding Characteristic of ETs

To characterize a new ET receptor, one of the important steps is to determine the K_d value and the number of binding sites (B_{max}: maximal ET-1 or ET-3 binding) in a tissue/cell. The standard approach for obtaining these two pieces of information is to conduct a saturation binding study either using intact cells or membranes prepared from cells/tissues. The data are usually analyzed by Scatchard analysis. The procedure used in our laboratory to conduct a saturation binding study is described in **Subheadings 3.2.** and **3.3.**

Although most people, including ourselves, calculate the K_d values by Scatchard analysis out of convenience, the practice may not be appropriate for the ET system. The reason is that ET-1 binding to the receptor is tenacious and difficult to dissociate. Methods other than Scatchard analysis may be needed for the determination of binding parameters.

We have previously shown, in membranes prepared from a number of diverse tissues and cell types, that bound ET-1 and ET-3 are difficult to dissociate from the receptor *(19–24)*. For example, in membranes prepared from rat liver, [^{125}I]ET-1 binding reached a plateau after 120 min of incubation. Addition of ET-1 at 150 min dissociated <10% of bound [^{125}I]ET-1 after 240 min of incubation. Addition of guanosine 5'-O-3-thiotriphosphate (GTPγS), a nonhydrolyzable GTP analog which is known to interfere with ligand binding to G-protein-linked receptors, did not induce more dissociation *(24)*. We have shown in other studies that, even up to 20 h of incubation with a high concentration of unlabeled ET-1 or ET-3 plus GTPγS, very little dissociation of bound [^{125}I]ET-1 or [^{125}I]ET-3 was observed *(21)*. As a comparison, [^{3}H]ANG II (angiotensin II) binding to rat liver membranes reached a plateau after 30 min of incubation. Addition of unlabeled ANG II plus GTPγS dissociated ~60% of bound [^{3}H]ANG II within 20 min of incubation *(24)*. The irreversible binding characteristics of ETs have been reported by many different groups using membranes prepared from various tissues and cells *(25,26)*. The tenacious binding of ET may result from the formation of an unusually stable receptor-ligand complex.

Because of the tenacious receptor binding characteristics of ETs, a more accurate way to calculate K_d values is by kinetic analysis using the association and dissociation rate constants as shown below.

$$[L] + [R] \; \underset{k_{-1}}{\overset{k_1}{\rightleftarrows}} \; [LR] \tag{1}$$

L, ligand; R, receptor; and LR, ligand-receptor complex.

$$K_d = \frac{k^{-1}}{k^1} \tag{2}$$

k_1, association rate constant; k_{-1}, dissociation rate constant; K_d, equilibrium dissociation constant.

Discussion on how to calculate association and dissociation rate constants is beyond the scope of this chapter, and the information is available elsewhere *(24–27, see* Chapter 4). It is worth mentioning that Waggoner et al. *(25)* have suggested that the radioligand binding analysis program "Kinetic" (Biosoft, MO) can be modified to calculate kinetic data for ET binding. The K_d value for ET-1 binding to a given receptor calculated from kinetic analysis (e.g., $K_d = 0.075$ pM for ET-1 binding to rat liver membranes) can be about 1000-fold lower than that calculated from Scatchard analysis (e.g., $K_d = 0.1$ nM).

The tenacious binding characteristic of ETs and its impact on the determination of K_d may help to explain why sometimes a biological effect, e.g., an elevation in intracellular calcium concentration or an increase in the vascular tone, is induced by ET-1 at very low concentrations such as 1–20 pM *(28,29)*. Furthermore, the level of ET in circulation is usually in the range of 1–5 pM. Even under pathological conditions in which ET plays a role, the level of ET in circulation is seldom increased to the sub-nanomolar range. It is generally thought that ET in circulation is a "spillover" from a local synthesis site. However, if the K_d values for ET binding are in the sub-picomolar range as calculated from kinetic analysis, then perhaps the systemic level of ET does have physiological and/or pathological significance even though it seldom rises above 50 pM.

In conclusion, when determining the K_d and B_{max} values of a new ET receptor by Scatchard analysis, keep in mind that the K_d value may not reflect the true situation because of the tenacious binding characteristic of ETs.

1.3. Characteristics of Different Receptor Agonists and Antagonists

To characterize a new ET receptor, it is important to determine whether the receptor is ET_A, ET_B or a novel subtype. A common approach is to use known ET receptor agonists and antagonists for determining the subtype of a receptor. Before selecting agonists and antagonists for this purpose, it is important to know the characteristics of the various ET receptor ligands. **Table 1** shows the potency and selectivity of some ET receptor agonists and antagonists.

When comparing the potency and selectivity of ET receptor ligands, it is important to check whether data are generated from experiments using similar conditions, because the IC_{50} of an antagonist is very much dependent on the experimental conditions. This concern is based on the observation that (1) antagonists and agonists exhibit differences in the degree of tenacious binding, and (2) ET agonists/antagonists tend to interact with serum albumin.

1.3.1. Antagonists and Agonists Exhibit Differences in the Degree of Tenacious Binding

Ihara et al. have shown that [^{3}H]BQ123, an ET_A selective antagonist, bound to membranes prepared from human neuroblastoma cells can be readily dissociated by the addition of unlabeled BQ123 (10 μM) *(30)*. The binding of [^{3}H]SB209670, a nonpeptide ET receptor antagonist, to both human ET_A and ET_B receptors is shown to be reversible by the addition of unlabeled SB209670 at 1 μM *(31)*. The binding of [^{125}I]PD151242, another ET_A selective antagonist, is also reversible *(32)*.

Not only is antagonist binding much easier to dissociate than ET binding, but different antagonists may behave differently. For example, in a study comparing six ET receptor ligands, we found that the degree of reversibility of ligand binding to ET_A receptor is in the order of BQ123 > PD 156707 > Ro 47-0203 ≥ FR139317 > A-127722 ≥ ET-1. The details of the "bind-and-wash" procedure used to compare the "tenacity" of these ligands were reported previously *(20,21)*. In general, antagonist binding is more reversible than ET-1 binding, and the binding of different antagonists exhibit different degrees of tenacity.

The impact of different degrees of tenacious binding is reflected in the observation that the potency (IC_{50}) of an antagonist can change with incubation time.

Table 1
The IC_{50} Values of ET Receptor Ligands Against [^{125}I]ET-1
and [^{125}I]ET-3 Binding to Human ET_A and ET_B Receptors

	IC_{50} values, nM^a		
Ligand	ET_A	ET_B	Selectivity[d]
ET-1[b]	0.28	0.14	Nonselective
ET-3[b]	475	0.08	ET_B selective
IRL1620[b]	4263	14	ET_B selective
A-127722[c]	0.11	98.2	ET_A selective
ABT-627	0.055	85	ET_A selective
(Atrasentan)[c]			
ABT-546	0.49	15,400	ET_A selective
A-192621	8400	7.8	ET_B selective
A-182086	0.1	1.28	Nonselective
BMS-182874	307	67,320	ET_A selective
BQ123	7.6	34,405	ET_A selective
BQ788	390	2.8	ET_B selective
FR139317	0.99	10,311.9	ET_A selective
L-749329	44.59	1878.9	Nonselective
L-754142	**0.35**	**26**	Nonselective
PD 142893	91	228	Nonselective
PD 156707	0.23	2457.7	ET_A selective
RES-701-1	**>5000**	**10**	ET_B selective
Ro 46-2005	230	1101	Nonselective
Ro 46-8443	**6800**	**69**	ET_B selective
Ro 47-0203	7.13	474.8	Nonselective
(Bosentan)			
SB209670	0.32	35	Nonselective
TAK-044	**6.4**	**60**	Nonselective
TBC-10894	**3300**	**36**	ET_B selective

[a]The IC_{50} values in bold are obtained from the literature. Other IC_{50} values are obtained from our lab using the competition binding protocol described in **Subheading 3.3.2.** with membranes (10 µg of protein) from CHO cells stably transfected with human ET_A or ET_B receptors.

[b]ET-1, -3, and IRL1620 are agonists. The rest are antagonists.

[c]ABT-627 is the active enantiomer of A-127722, a chiral molecule. For references on these antagonists, please *see* the review article by Wu-Wong *(24)*.

[d]The determination of selectivity is somewhat arbitrary. For discussion of how the selectivity of a ligand is determined, please *see* Chapter 11.

Because ET-1 binding is less reversible than antagonist binding, the potency of an antagonist in inhibiting ET-1 binding to the receptor will decrease when the incubation time is increased. For example, in a competition binding study using MMQ cell membranes comparing three incubation time points of 1 h, 3 h, or

24 h, the IC_{50} values of ET-1 against $[^{125}I]$ET-1 binding remained in the sub-nanomolar range at the three different time points (0.35, 0.64, and 0.90 nM at 1, 3, and 24 h, respectively). As a comparison, the IC_{50} values of Ro 47-0203 changed from 2.7 nM at 1 h to 5.8 nM at 3 h, and to 56.7 nM at 24 h of incubation. These results suggest that the potency of an ET receptor antagonist is critically dependent on the incubation time because antagonist binding is more reversible than ET binding. Also, different antagonists exhibit different reversible characteristics and are affected differently by the length of incubation time.

1.3.2. ET Agonists/Antagonists Interact with Serum Albumin

We have previously shown that ET-1, ET-3 and ET receptor antagonists such PD 156707, L-749329, Ro 47-0203, and A-127722, exhibit a high degree of binding to plasma proteins, especially serum albumin, because of the lipophilic nature of many of these compounds *(33)*. We have also shown that addition of bovine and human serum albumin (BSA or HSA) into the binding buffer has impacts on ET-1 binding and the potency of antagonists *(33)*. For example, in the absence of HSA, the IC_{50} values for A-127722 and L-749329 were 0.22 nM and 0.29 nM, respectively. When the amount of HSA was increased to 1%, the IC_{50} values of both compounds increased to 2.75 nM and 13.1 nM, respectively, with L-749329 being affected more than A-127722. These studies suggest that serum albumin can decrease the potency of an ET receptor antagonist. In addition, some antagonists are affected to a greater degree than others.

In vitro binding studies are usually conducted using buffers that contain serum albumin and different labs often use different concentrations of serum albumin. For example, HSA or BSA at 0.01% was used in the binding assays by Williams et al. *(34)* and Sogabe et al. *(35)*. BSA at 0.1% was used in the assays by Webb et al. *(36)* and Reynolds et al. *(37)*, while 0.5% BSA was used by Clozel et al. *(38)*. In our own laboratory, 0.2% BSA is routinely included in the buffer system for binding studies using membranes as described in **Subheading 2.2.**

In conclusion, it is important to keep the experimental conditions such as incubation time and temperature, the ingredients used in the binding buffer, the final incubation volume, the tools and instruments employed, etc., as constant as possible when conducting receptor binding studies. When comparing binding data from different labs, it is advisable to take into consideration whether the difference observed in the data is from different conditions employed. Furthermore, when reporting the characteristics of a new ET receptor, the amount of serum albumin used in the binding studies should be clearly defined.

Regarding subtype determination, in competition binding studies, if $[^{125}I]$ET-1 binding can be replaced by ET-1 and ET-3 with very similar IC_{50} values, likely the receptor belongs to the ET_B subtype. If ET-1 is more potent than ET-3 in replacing $[^{125}I]$ET-1, then the situation becomes more complicated because two possibilities exist: (1) The receptor is ET_A, and (2) both receptor subtypes co-exist in the same cell or tissue type of interest. When this happens, it is necessary to enlist antagonists in order to differentiate between these two possibilities. Because of the difference in binding characteristics of antagonists, it may be necessary to use several antagonists with different selectivity profiles simultaneously in order to gain a better understanding of the receptor of interest. For example, in characterizing the ET receptors in human pericardial smooth muscle cells, we found that ET-1 was more potent than ET-3 in inhibiting $[^{125}I]$ET-1 binding. When comparing four different antagonists, BQ123, FR139317, Ro 46-2005 and PD 142893, BQ123 and FR139317 (ET_A-selective) inhibited $[^{125}I]$ET-1 binding by ~70% with IC_{50} values in the 1–5 nM range, while Ro 46-2005 and PD 142893 (nonselective) inhibited $[^{125}I]$ET-1 binding completely, but were less potent (IC_{50} values > 5 nM). The results suggest that the receptors in these cells are heterogeneous, and likely both ET_A and ET_B receptors co-exist. To further confirm the observation, we tested the combined effect of two ligands by first blocking $[^{125}I]$ET-1 binding to ET_A using an ET_A selective antagonist at a fixed concentration, and then determining the effect of an ET_B selective antagonist in a concentration dependent manner (39). Usually when nonselective antagonists or a combination of both ET_A and ET_B receptor antagonists are needed to completely block $[^{125}I]$ET-1 binding, it is an indication that both ET_A and ET_B subtypes are present.

If both ET_A and ET_B subtypes are present, to determine the ratio between ET_A and ET_B in a particular tissue or cell type, saturation binding studies can be conducted for $[^{125}I]$ET-1 and $[^{125}I]$ET -3. Since ET_A receptors are selective for ET-1 and ET_B receptors bind ET-1 and ET-3 with equal affinity, the B_{max} obtained from the $[^{125}I]$ET-1 saturation binding indicates the combined binding sites of ET_A and ET_B, and the B_{max} obtained from the $[^{125}I]$ET-3 saturation binding determines the density of ET_B. Thus, the distribution ratio between ET_A and ET_B can be calculated.

Occasionally, a portion of $[^{125}I]$ET -1 binding may be resistant to inhibition by various ET ligands, or may exhibit unusual characteristics. It raises the question of whether there are novel ET receptor subtypes that are yet to be defined. For example, in canine spleen membranes, Nambi et al. (40) reported the presence of an ET_B receptor subtype that was sensitive to BQ123, an antagonist thought to be highly ET_A-selective. The same group also reported that, in human bronchus, a combination of BQ123 and Sarafotoxin 6C (an ET_B receptor agonist) or BQ788 (an ET_B receptor antagonist) failed to completely inhibit $[^{125}I]$ET-1 binding (41). It is plausible that there are several mammalian ET_B subtypes – ET_{B1} which is sensitive to RES-701 and BQ788, but insensitive to BQ123 (42), ET_{B2} which is insensitive to RES-701 and BQ123, but can be inhibited by BQ788 and

Ro 47-0203 (a nonselective antagonist), a third one that is sensitive to BQ123, and a fourth one that is resistant to various antagonists. Although pharmacological studies suggest the presence of more than two mammalian ET receptor subtypes *(9)*, no additional homologous mammalian cDNAs other than ET_A and ET_B have been identified. Until the molecular cloning evidence becomes available, the true identity of these different ET_B subtypes remains a mystery.

2. Materials
2.1. ET Receptor Ligands

ET-1 and ET-3 and radiolabeled [^{125}I]ET-1 and [^{125}I]ET-3 are commercially available (*see* **Note 1**). Some of the commercially available antagonists are shown in **Fig. 1** (*see* **Note 2**).

2.2. Binding Studies

1. Thermostatically controlled incubator or cold box.
2. Microtiter plates: 96-well plates when using membranes, 48-well plates when using intact cells.
3. A device to separate bound ligands from unbound (*see* **Note 3**).
4. Gamma counter.
5. Binding buffer for intact cells: 140 mM NaCl, 5 mM KCl, 1.8 mM CaCl$_2$, 0.8 mM MgSO$_4$, 5 mM glucose, 25 mM HEPES, 0.1 % bovine serum albumin, 5 μg/mL pepstatin A, 0.1 mM phosphoramidon, 0.01 mM PMSF, and 0.025% bacitracin, pH 7.4.
6. Binding buffer for membranes: 20 mM Tris, 100 mM NaCl, 10 mM MgCl$_2$, 3 mM EDTA, 0.1 mM phenylmethylsulfonyl fluoride, and 5 μg/mL pepstatin A, 0.025% bacitracin and 0.2% bovine serum albumin, pH 7.4.
7. Hemocytometer or Coulter cell counter.

2.3. Preparation of Membranes

1. Centrifuge and ultracentrifuge.
2. Tissue homogenizer: polytron.
3. Cell homogenizer: micro-ultrasonic cell disruptor (Kontes, Vineland, NJ).
4. Homogenization buffer: 10 mM HEPES, pH 7.4, containing 0.25 M sucrose and protease inhibitors (3 mM EDTA, 0.1 mM. phenylmethylsulfonyl fluoride, and 5 μg/mL pepstatin A).
5. Membrane resuspending buffer: 20 mM Tris-HCl, 100 mM NaCl, 10 mM MgCl$_2$, 3 mM EDTA, 0.1 mM phenylmethylsulfonyl fluoride, and 5 μg/mL pepstatin A, 0.025% bacitracin, pH 7.4.

3. Methods
3.1. Handling ET Receptor Agonists and Antagonists

1. To make a stock solution, dissolve ET-1 (or ET-3) in distilled water to a final concentration of 200 μM (*see* **Note 4**). Immediately, aliquot the peptides, 100 μL per

tube, into prelubricated microcentrifuge tubes (*see* **Note 5**) and store at −20°C. Use each tube with no more than 5 cycles of freezing and thawing (*see* **Note 6**).

2. On the day of conducting the receptor binding experiment, thaw a tube of the ET-1 stock solution. To make dilutions from the ET stock solution, it is advisable to use containers that are either siliconized or precoated with BSA. We routinely make dilutions using a microtiter plate (the dilution preparation plate) precoated with 0.1% BSA (*see* **Note 7**).

3. To prepare the [^{125}I]ET-1 solution for experiments, if only one concentration is needed (e.g., in a competition binding study), prepare the solution in a prelubricated or BSA-coated microcentrifuge tube by diluting the [^{125}I]ET-1 solution from the vendor in binding buffer to make a 10-fold stock solution, and then transfer 20 µL to a well in the incubation microtiter plate (precoated with 0.1% BSA) to mix with other ingredients (membranes and test ligands, etc.) to a final volume of 200 µL (*see* **Note 8**). When multiple [^{125}I]ET-1 concentrations are needed (e.g., in a saturation binding study), first make a stock solution in a prelubricated or BSA-coated tube by mixing unlabeled ET-1 with [^{125}I]ET-1 in binding buffer to a desired twofold ET-1 concentration with ≥300,000 cpm of radioactivity. Make a series of dilutions from the stock solution using prelubricated or BSA-coated tubes (*see* **Note 9**). Transfer 100 µL of each concentration to a well in the incubation microtiter plate to mix with other ingredients (membranes and test ligands, etc.) to a final volume of 200 µL. While making the dilutions, carry out all the pipeting rapidly to minimize the amount of ETs that may stick to the pipet tips. If a large scale receptor binding assay is conducted and more time and steps are required for liquid handling, then the pipet tips may need to be precoated with BSA (*see* **Note 10**).

4. Dissolve ET receptor antagonists in DMSO to make a stock solution of 10 mM. As before, dilutions of the antagonist stock solution should also be made using containers that are either siliconized or precoated with BSA (*see* **Note 11**). Again, we use a microtiter plate (the dilution preparation plate) precoated with 0.1% BSA for making dilutions.

3.2. Radioligand Binding to Intact Cells (see Note 12)

1. Incubate cells (~80 % confluency, *see* **Note 13**) in 48-well culture plates with 0.2 mL/well binding buffer containing [^{125}I]ET-1 (or [^{125}I]ET-3) for 4 h at 4°C (*see* **Note 14**). In a saturation binding study, increasing concentrations of [^{125}I]ET-1 are tested. In a competition binding study, increasing concentrations of a ligand are tested against 0.1 nM of [^{125}I]ET-1.

2. Determine nonspecific binding in the presence of 1 µM ET-1.

3. After the incubation, remove the incubation buffer by gentle suction, wash the cells twice with 0.5 mL/well of ice-cold phosphate-buffered saline (PBS), and solubilize with 0.2 mL of 0.1 N NaOH.

4. In order to analyze data, determine the cell number (*see* **Note 15**).

5. For saturation binding studies, calculate the radioactivity added to wells at each ET-1 concentration (*see* **Note 15**). An example for the layout of wells and plates in a saturation binding study with each concentration tested in triplicate is shown in **Fig. 2**.

Plate #1   Plate #2

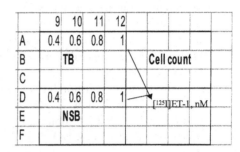

	1	2	3	4	5	6	7	8
A	0.01	0.02	0.04	0.06	0.08	0.1	0.15	0.2
B	TB							
C								
D	0.01	0.02	0.04	0.06	0.08	0.1	0.15	0.2
E	NSB (+1 μM ET-1)							
F								

TB: total binding; NSB: non-specific binding

Fig. 2. An example of the plate and well layout for a saturation binding study using intact cells in a 48-well plate.

6. Once all the data are gathered, analyze binding results manually (*see* **Subheading 3.3.2.**) or using the radioligand binding analysis program "EBDA & LIGAND" (Biosoft, MO) to calculate B_{max}, K_d and IC_{50} values (*see* Chapter 4).

3.3. Radioligand Binding to Membranes

3.3.1. Preparation of Membranes

Membranes can be prepared from either tissues or cells. The protocols are similar with only minor differences.

1. Homogenize tissues or cells (*see* **Note 16**) in 25 vol (w/v) of homogenization buffer, using a polytron for 10 s at 13,500 rpm for 3× with 10 s intervals for tissues, and using a micro-ultrasonic cell disruptor (Kontes) for cells.
2. Centrifuge the mixture at 1000*g* for 10 min. Collect the supernatant and centrifuge at 30,000*g* for 30 min for tissue or at 60,000*g* for 60 min for cells. Resuspend the precipitate in membrane resuspending buffer, and centrifuge again using the same parameters. Resuspend the final pellet in the same buffer to a protein content of 5–10 mg/mL, and then store at −80°C until use. Determine protein content using the Bio-Rad dye-binding protein assay.

3.3.2. Radioligand Binding Assay

1. Perform binding assays in 96-well microtiter plates precoated with 0.1% bovine serum albumin. Dilute membranes in binding buffer to a final concentration of 0.05 mg/mL of protein per well (*see* **Note 17**).
2. For competition binding studies, incubate membranes with 0.1 n*M* of [125I]ET-1 or [125I]ET-3 in binding buffer (final volume: 0.2 mL) in the presence of increasing concentrations of unlabeled test ligands for 4 h at 25°C.
3. For saturation binding studies, incubate membranes with increasing concentrations of [125I]ET-1 or [125I]ET-3 in binding buffer (final volume 0.2 mL) in the presence or absence of unlabeled test ligands for 4 h at 25°C (*see* **Note 18**).

4. Determine nonspecific binding using 1 μM ET-1 or 1 μM ET-3.

5. After incubation, separate unbound ligands from bound ligands by vacuum filtration using glass-fiber filter strips in a PHD cell harvester, followed by washing the filter strips with saline (1 mL), 3×.

6. Analyze the data manually or using the radioligand binding analysis program "EBDA & LIGAND" to calculate B_{max}, K_d and IC_{50} values. To calculate IC_{50} manually from competition binding data, *see* **Subheading 3.1.3.** in Chapter 11. **Table 2** and **Fig. 3** show an example of how to analyze data from a saturation binding study in order to obtain B_{max} and K_d values for ET-1 binding to membranes prepared from CHO cells transfected with human ET_A receptor. An example of the layout of wells and plates in a saturation binding study with each concentration tested in duplicates can be found in **Fig. 3** in Chapter 11.

7. As described in **Subheading 3.2.**, the amount of radioactivity added to wells at each ET-1 concentration has to be determined (*see* **Note 15**, **Table 2**: columns 10–13, lower portion). From the highest [^{125}I]ET-1 concentration (1 nM final concentration in this example), which is also the stock solution used to make the other diluted concentrations, use the cpm per pmol to calculate the actual ET-1 concentration at each dilution. In this particular case, the actual ET-1 concentrations (column 2, **Table 2**) are very close to the planned ET-1 concentrations (column 1, **Table 2**), indicating that the dilution and handling were done accurately. Because the final volume is 0.2 mL/well, the ET-1 molality in pmol can be calculated (column 3, **Table 2**). Radioactivity bound to membranes (cpm/well, $n = 2$) is shown in column 4 and the average is shown in column 5 of **Table 2**. The bound radioactivity in cpm is divided by the cpm in the ET-1 standard (304,022 cpm at 0.2 pmol ET-1 in this case) to calculate total ET-1 bound in pmol (column 7, **Table 2**), which is then converted into pmol/mg (TB: total binding) by using the protein content (0.015 mg/well) as the normalization basis (column 9, **Table 2**). To calculate free ET-1 (column 8, **Table 2**), use the following equation:

$$\text{Free ET-1 (n}M) = (\text{column 3} - \text{column 7})/0.2 \text{ mL}$$

In **Fig. 3A**, the ET-1 bound in pmol/mg (TB from column 9, **Table 2**) is plotted against free ET-1 (column 8, **Table 2**) for both sets of data in the absence (TB) and presence (NSB: nonspecific binding) of 1 μM ET-1. In this particular case, the free ET-1 concentrations for both sets of data points are similar, which may not be so in other studies. Therefore, to calculate the true NSB for a particular free concentration in the TB curve, an equation is derived from the linear NSB curve in **Fig. 3A** (in this case $y = 0.11608x$). Each free ET-1 concentration is plugged into the equation to calculate y, the NSB to be subtracted at that ET-1 concentration (column 11, **Table 2**). Afterwards, SB (specific binding, column 12, **Table 2**) can be calculated by subtracting NSB from TB. Then, SB (column 12, **Table 2**) is divided by free ET (column 8, **Table 2**) to calculate SB/F (column 13, **Table 2**).

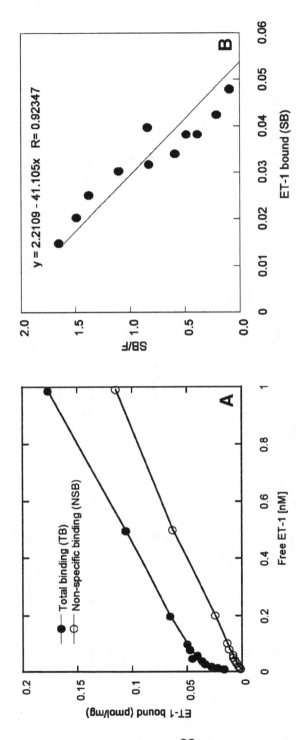

Fig. 3. Scatchard analysis. (A) Membranes (0.015 mg/well) from CHO cells transfected with human ET_A receptor were incubated for 3 h at 25°C with increasing concentrations of [^{125}I]ET-1 in the absence of presence of 1 μM unlabeled ET-1. Data were calculated as in **Table 2**. (B) Scatchard analysis of data from (A).

Table 2
Analysis of Radiolabeled ET-1 Saturation Binding Data

1	2	3	4	5	6	7	8	9	10	11	12	13
Planned [ET-1], nM	Actual [ET-1], nM	Actual ET-1, pmol	Bound ET, cpm/well	Bound ET, cpm/well (mean)	STDEV, CPM	Bound ET, pmol	Free ET, nM	TB, pmol/mg	Stdev of TB, pmol/mg	NSB to be subtracted	SB, pmol/mb	SB/F
0.01	0.0101	0.00202	374 346	360	only applicable when $n=3$	0.0002369	0.0089	0.0158	only applicable when $n=3$	0.0010	0.0148	1.6553
0.015	0.0152	0.00304	554 441	498		0.0003274	0.0136	0.0218		0.0016	0.0203	1.4932
0.02	0.0202	0.00404	644 595	619		0.0004075	0.0182	0.0272		0.0021	0.0251	1.3797
0.03	0.0298	0.00596	807 716	761		0.0005007	0.0273	0.0334		0.0032	0.0302	1.1068
0.04	0.0405	0.0081	787 853	820		0.0005394	0.0378	0.0360		0.0044	0.0316	0.8352
0.05	0.0503	0.01006	1047 1010	1029		0.0006767	0.0469	0.0451		0.0054	0.0397	0.8455
0.06	0.0599	0.01198	961 886	924		0.0006076	0.0569	0.0405		0.0066	0.0339	0.5963
0.08	0.081	0.0162	1138 1011	1074		0.0007067	0.0775	0.0471		0.0090	0.0381	0.4921
0.1	0.102	0.0204	1150 1109	1130		0.0007433	0.0983	0.0496		0.0114	0.0381	0.3881
0.2	0.203	0.0406	1529 1452	1490		0.0009804	0.1981	0.0654		0.0230	0.0424	0.2139
0.5	0.505	0.101	2541 2275	2408		0.0015841	0.4971	0.1056		0.0577	0.0479	0.0964
1	1	0.2	3991 4048	4020		0.0026444	0.9868	0.1763		0.1158	0.0605	0.0613

(Continued)

+1 μM ET-1 (NSB)

0.01	0.0101	0.00202	32 / 25	28	0.0000186	0.0100	0.0012
0.015	0.0152	0.00304	45 / 47	46	0.0000304	0.0150	0.0020
0.02	0.0202	0.00404	80 / 67	73	0.0000482	0.0200	0.0032
0.03	0.0298	0.00596	109 / 102	106	0.0000696	0.0295	0.0046
0.04	0.0405	0.0081	156 / 119	137	0.0000904	0.0400	0.0060
0.05	0.0503	0.01006	189 / 161	175	0.0001151	0.0497	0.0077
0.06	0.0599	0.01198	189 / 163	176	0.0001158	0.0593	0.0077
0.08	0.081	0.0162	269 / 245	257	0.0001690	0.0802	0.0113
0.1	0.102	0.0204	316 / 273	294	0.0001936	0.1010	0.0129
0.2	0.203	0.0406	594 / 491	543	0.0003570	0.2012	0.0238
0.5	0.505	0.101	1550 / 1325	1437	0.0009455	0.5003	0.0630
1	1	0.2	2600 / 2622	2611	0.0017177	0.9914	0.1145

Volume = 0.2 mL/well (final)
protein = 0.015 mg/well

[125I]ET-1 added to each well:

Planned [ET-1], nM (Final concentration)	Radioactivity cpm/well	Actual [ET-1] nM (Final)
0.01	3080	0.0101
0.015	4631	0.0152
0.02	6131	0.0202
0.03	9059	0.0298
0.04	12310	0.0405
0.05	15291	0.0503
0.06	18201	0.0599
0.08	24740	0.0814
0.1	31116	0.1023
0.2	61776	0.2032
0.5	153537	0.505
1	304022	1

[125I]ET-1 Standard: 0.2 pmol = 304,022 cpm
Note: 100 μL of [125I]ET-1 (2 nM) was added to the well

Note: (1) The study was conducted using membranes prepared from CHO cells transfected with human ET_A receptor. (2) TB, total binding; SB: specific binding; NSB, nonspecific binding; Stdev, standard deviation; F, free ET-1.

In **Fig. 3B**, SB/F is plotted against SB and an equation of $y = 2.2109 - 41.105x$ is derived. When $y = 0$, $x = 0.054$ pmol/mg, which is the B_{max} for the CHO cells (Clone #2) transfected with human ET_A receptor (*see* **Note 19**). The K_d value is 0.024 nM, calculated from $K_d = -1/slope$.

4. Notes

1. Many different companies sell ET-1 and ET-3. We purchase ET-1 and -3 from American Peptide Co. (Santa Clara, CA). Both DuPont New England Nuclear (NEN, Boston, MA) and Amersham (Little Chalfont, Bucks, UK) sell [^{125}I]ET-1 and [^{125}I]ET-3. We purchase [^{125}I]ET-1 and [^{125}I]ET-3 from NEN. The specific activity for [^{125}I]ET-1 or [^{125}I]ET-3 is ~2200 Ci/mmol. The concentration is ~36 nM. All these materials are stored at $-20°C$.
2. We have never tried commercially available antagonists. All the antagonists used in our studies were made by Abbott chemists.
3. If the binding study is conducted using intact cells that form a monolayer in culture, a vacuum line to remove liquid from the microtiter plate is adequate. If the binding study is conducted using membranes prepared from cells or tissues, it is necessary to employ a device that separates the bound radiolabeled ligand from the unbound before the bound radioactivity in the membranes can be determined. Usually, the membranes with bound radioactivity can be separated from the incubation buffer containing unbound ligands by either centrifugation or filtration. In our laboratory, we use the filtration method by employing glass-fiber filter strips (Cambridge Technology, Inc., Watertown, MA, presoaked in saline just before use) together with a PHD cell harvester (a vacuum filtration device from Cambridge Technology, Inc.).
4. We calculate the amount of water needed to make the stock solution and add water directly into the vial that contains the ET-1 (or ET-3) powder. Since ETs are very sticky, we advise against trying to weigh out a certain amount. If there is a doubt about the amount of ET-1 listed on the vial, one can weigh the vial before and after handling. From our experience, the amount listed on the vial is usually accurate. If the powder does not dissolve, it may be necessary to add a small amount of acetic acid into water to make it slightly acidic.
5. We purchase prelubricated microcentrifuge tubes from Costar (Corning, NY).
6. We mark directly on the tube each time it is taken out for use.
7. To coat microtiter plates with BSA: fill wells of a microtiter plate (96-well or other sizes dependent on the need). with 0.1% BSA for at least 3 h at room temperature. After the incubation, shake off the BSA solution and blot the plate on paper towel. Make sure that the plate is dry before use.
8. In a competition binding study, we use [^{125}I]ET-1 or [^{125}I]ET-3 at a fixed final concentration of either 0.05 or 0.1 nM, depending on the receptor density. If the receptor density is high, use 0.1 nM with a smaller amount of membranes (*see* **Note 17**) to avoid ligand depletion.
9. In a saturation binding study, we usually make the [^{125}I]ET-1 concentration in the range of 0.02–2 nM. Thus, the final ET-1 concentrations will be 0.01–1 nM

after 100 μL of [^{125}I]ET-1 is mixed with other ingredients to a final volume of 200 μL. To save radiolabeled materials, we make the stock solution by mixing unlabeled ET-1 with [^{125}I]ET-1 to a concentration of 2 nM with ≥300,000 cpm of radioactivity. Thus, the radioactivity is adequate to allow a series of dilutions so that even the lowest concentration gets good counts.

10. When a lot of liquid handling is required for a large scale receptor binding study, we use a Hamilton liquid handling station with tips precoated with 0.1% BSA.

11. In a competition binding study, we usually prepare the test ligand solutions at 10-fold concentrations. For example, if the desired final concentrations are in the range of 10^{-11} to 10^{-4} M, we prepare the dilutions in the range of 10^{-10} to 10^{-3} M. Then, 20 μL is transferred to a well in the incubation microtiter plate to mix with other ingredients to a final volume of 200 μL.

12. The method is for cells that form a monolayer in culture. When intact cells are used in the binding study, agonist-induced receptor internalization and recycling is always a concern. The experiment can be done at 4°C to minimize receptor internalization.

13. The microtiter plate and the number of cells used are dependent on the cell type. For a new cell type, it may be necessary to first test one concentration of [^{125}I]ET-1 (e.g., 0.1 nM) in the presence or absence of 1 μM ET-1 to estimate the number of binding sites. If very little specific binding is detected, then it is necessary to increase the well size and also increase the cell number in order to obtain enough counts. If the receptor density is very high, e.g., in CHO cells transfected with ET$_A$ or ET$_B$ receptor, then the cell number has to be reduced to avoid ligand depletion.

14. The culture medium is removed by gentle suction, and each well rinsed with 500 μL of ice-cold binding buffer. The order of adding the various ingredients is as follows: add binding buffer first, followed by the test ligand, and finally add the radiolabeled ET-1. The plate is then sealed and shaken gently to ensure homogeneous mixing of the ingredients.

15. To have an accurate cell number determination, it is advisable to treat the wells designated for cell number determination with the same binding process except addition of radiolabeled ligands. Also, in saturation binding studies, we routinely determine the radioactivity added into wells at each concentration of [^{125}I]ET-1. We advise against determining only the radioactivity at the highest concentration of [^{125}I]ET-1, and then using that number as the basis for calculating the counts at lower concentrations. From our experience, when making a series of dilutions, the dilution process will result in some loss of radioactivity at the lower concentrations because [^{125}I]ET-1 is very sticky. Therefore, we count the radioactivity at each concentration in order to determine the actual amount of radioactivity added to the wells. It is also a good practice to have some counting vials prepared in advance so that when 100 μL of [^{125}I]ET-1 at a certain concentration is transferred to a well in the incubation plate, a portion is transferred at the same time to a vial for counting. Never wait until the end of an experiment to count [^{125}I]ET-1 out of a tube containing the diluted [^{125}I]ET-1 solution. No matter how much precaution is taken, it is difficult to completely prevent [^{125}I]ET-1 from binding to the wall of a tube.

16. We usually start with 15–20 g of tissues or cells from 10 roller bottles. The tissues are dissected and immediately frozen in liquid nitrogen before stored at −80°C. On the day of membrane preparation, tissues are taken out of the freezer and processed in the frozen state. Never thaw tissues! We break the tissues into smaller pieces by hammering the frozen tissues wrapped in several layers of plastic storage bags. Afterwards, it can be weighed. For cells, we try to collect cells on the day of membrane preparation. If it cannot be done on the same day, cells can be collected in advance with the weight determined at the end of collection, and then stored at −80°C until use. If only a small piece of tissue is available, then it will not be possible to prepare membranes, but it is possible to use tissue sections for autoradiographic studies. [^{125}I]ET-1 autoradiographic studies using tissue sections have been reported before *(43)* and *see* Chapter 4.

17. Depending on the density of binding sites on membranes, the protein content used in each study will vary. We have experienced using 10 μg/well for some membranes that have a large number of binding sites to 350 μg/well for membranes that contain a low receptor density. For membranes prepared from a cell or tissue type for which the ET receptors have not been characterized before, it may be necessary to first test the membranes at different concentrations (e.g., 10–500 μg per well) using one concentration of [^{125}I]ET-1 (e.g., 0.1 n*M*) in the presence or absence of 1 μ*M* ET-1. The procedure for doing such a testing is described in **Subheading 3.1.2.** in Chapter 11.

18. In a binding study using membranes, the order of addition of the various ingredients is as follows: add binding buffer first, followed by radiolabeled ET-1 and the test ligand, and finally add membranes. The plate is then sealed and shaken gently to ensure homogeneous mixing of the ingredients.

19. When intact cells are used in the saturation binding study, replace the protein content with the cell number per well and calculate TB and SB into pmol per million cells. Once the B_{max} is obtained, the number of binding site per cell can be determined by the following equation:

Binding sites per cell = B_{max} (pmol per million cells) × 6.02 × 10^{23} sites/mol

For example, if the B_{max} is 0.02 pmol per million cells,
then binding sites per cell is 12,040 sites per cell.

References

1. Yanagisawa, M., Kurihara, H., Kimura, S., Tomobe, Y., Kobayashi, Y., Mitsui, M., et al. (1988) A novel potent vasoconstrictor peptide produced by vascular endothelial cells. *Nature* **332,** 411–415.
2. Inoue, A., Yanagisawa, M., Kimura, S., Kasuya, Y., Miyachi, T., Goto, K., and Masaki, T. (1989) The human endothelin family: Three structurally and pharmacologically distinct isopeptides predicted by three separate genes. *Proc. Natl. Acad. Sci. USA* **86,** 2863–2867.
3. Sokolovsky, M. (1992) Structure-function relationships of endothelins, sarafotoxins, and their receptor subtypes. *J. Neurochem.* **59,** 809–821.

4. Kozuka, M., Ito, T., Hirose, S., Lodhi, K. M., and Hagiwara, H. (1991) Purification and characterization of bovine lung endothelin receptor. *J. Biol. Chem.* **266,** 16,892–16,896.

5. Wada, K., Tabuchi, H., Ohba, R., Satoh, M., Tachibana, Y., Akiyama, N., et al. (1990) Purification of an endothelin receptor from human placenta. *Biochem. Biophys. Res. Commun.* **167,** 251–257.

6. Arai, H., Hori, S., Aramori, I., Ohkubo, H., and Nakanishi, S. (1990) Cloning and expression of a cDNA encoding an endothelin receptor. *Nature* **348,** 730–732.

7. Sakurai, T., Yanagisawa, M., Takuwa, Y., Miyazaki, H., Kimura, S., Goto, K., and Masaki, T. (1990) Cloning of a cDNA encoding a nonisopeptide selective subtype of the endothelin receptor. *Nature* **348,** 732–735.

8. Karne, S., Jayawickreme, C. K., and Lerner, M. R. (1993) Cloning and characterization of an endothelin-3 specific receptor (ET$_C$ receptor) from Xenopus laevis dermal melanophores. *J. Biol. Chem.* **268,** 19,126–19,133.

9. Bax, W. and Saxena, P. (1994) The current endothelin receptor classification: time for reconsideration? *Trends Pharmacol. Sci.* **15,** 379–386.

10. Haynes, W. G. and Webb, D. J. (1994) Contribution of endogenous generation of endothelin-1 to basal vascular tone. *Lancet* **344,** 952–854.

11. Salamoussa, A., Lau, W. A., Pennefather, J. N., and Ventura, S. (2000) The contractile effects of endothelins on the smooth muscle of the rat prostate gland. *Eur. J. Pharmacol.* **403,** 139–145.

12. Wagner, O. F., Vierhapper, H., Gasic, S., Nowotny, P., and Waldhausl, W. (1992) Regional effects and clearance of endothelin-1 across pulmonary and splanchnic circulation. *Eur. J. Clin. Invest.* **22,** 277–282.

13. Benigni, A. and Remuzzi, G. (1995) Endothelin in the progressive renal disease of glomerulopathies. *Miner Electrolyte Metab.* **21,** 283–291.

14. Wu-Wong, J. R. (2002) Endothelins in cellular proliferation and apoptosis: biological roles and clinical application. *Analytical Pharmacology*, in press.

15. Wu-Wong, J. R., Berg, C. E., Wang, J., Chiou, W. J., and Fissel, B. (1999) Endothelin stimulates glucose uptake and GLUT4 translocation via activation of endothelin ET$_A$ receptor in 3T3-L1 adipocytes. *J. Biol. Chem.* **274,** 8103–8110.

16. Wu-Wong, J. R., Berg, C. E., and Kramer, D. (2000) Endothelin stimulates glucose uptake via activation of endothelin ET$_A$ receptor in neonatal rat cardiomyocytes , *J. Cardiovasc. Pharmacol.* **36,** S179–S183.

17. Simonson, M. S. (1993) Endothelins: Multifunctional renal peptides. *Physiol. Rev.* **73,** 375–411.

18. Wu-Wong, J. R. and Opgenorth, T. J. (1998) Endothelin and isoproterenol counter-regulate cAMP and mitogen-activated protein kinases. *J. Cardiovasc. Pharmacol.* **31,** S185–S191.

19. Chiou, W., Magnuson, S. R., Dixon, D. B., Sundy, S., Opgenorth, T. J., and Wu-Wong, J. R. (1997) Dissociation characteristics of endothelin receptor ago-

nists and antagonists in cloned human type-B endothelin receptor, *Endothelium: J. Endothelial Cell Res.* **5,** 179–189.

20. Wu-Wong, J. R., Chiou, W., Naugles, Jr., K. E., and Opgenorth, T. J. (1994) Endothelin receptor antagonists exhibit diminishing potency following incubation with agonist. *Life Sci.* **54,** 1727–1734.

21. Wu-Wong, J. R., Chiou, W., Magnuson, S. R., and Opgenorth, T. J. (1994) Endothelin receptor agonists and antagonists exhibit different dissociation characteristics. *Biochim. Biophys. Acta* **224,** 288–294.

22. Wu-Wong, J. R., Chiou, W., Magnuson, S. R., and Opgenorth, T. J. (1995) Endothelin receptor in human astrocytoma U373MG cells: binding, dissociation, receptor internalization. *J. Pharm. Exp. Ther.* **274,** 499–507.

23. Wu-Wong, J. R., Chiou, W., Dixon, D. B., and Opgenorth, T. J. (1995) Dissociation characteristics of endothelin ET_A receptor agonist and antagonists. *J. Cardiovasc. Pharmacol.* **26,** S380–S384.

24. Wu-Wong, J. R. (1998) "Sticky" conundrums in the endothelin system: Unique binding characteristics of receptor agonists and antagonists. In *Endothelin Receptors and Signaling Mechanisms,* (Pollock, D., ed.), R. G. Landes Company Biomedical Publishers, pp. 23–40.

25. Waggoner, W. G., Genova, S. L. and Rash, V. A. (1992) Kinetic analyses demonstrate that the equilibrium assumption does not apply to [^{125}I]endothelin-1 binding data. *Life Sci.* **51,** 1869–1876.

26. Takasuka, T., Horii, I., Furuichi, Y., and Watanabe, T. (1991) Detection of an endothelin-1-binding protein complex by low temperature SDS-PAGE. *Biochem. Biophys. Res. Commun.* **176,** 392–400.

27. Keen, M. and MacDermot, J. (1993) Analysis of receptor by radioligand binding. In *Receptor Autoradiography* (Wharton, J. and Polak, J. M., eds.), Oxford University Press, pp. 22–55.

28. Sokolovsky, M., Shraga-Levine, Z., and Galron, R. (1994) Ligand-specific stimulation/inhibition of cAMP formation by a novel endothelin receptor subtype. *Biochemistry* **33,** 11,417–11,419.

29. Bkaily, G., Wang, S., Bui, M., and Menard, D. (1995) ET-1 stimulates Ca^{2+} currents in cardiac cells. *J. Cardiovasc. Pharmacol.* **26,** S293–S296.

30. Ihara, M., Yamanaka, R., Ohwaki, K., Ozaki, S., Fukami, T., Ishikawa, K., et al. (1995) [^{3}H]BQ-123, a highly specific and reversible radioligand for the endothelin ET_A receptor subtype. *Eur. J. Pharmacol.* **274,** 1–6.

31. Nambi, P., Pullen, M., Wu, H.-L., Lee, D., Saunders, D., Heys, R., et al. (1996) Nonpeptide endothelin receptor antagonists. VII: Binding characteristics of [^{3}H]SB 209670, a novel nonpeptide antagonist of endothelin receptors. *J. Pharm. Exp. Ther.* **277,** 1567–1571.

32. Peter, M. G. and Davenport, A. P. (1995) Selectivity of [^{125}I]-PD151242 for human, rat and porcine endothelin ET_A receptors in the heart. *Br. J. Pharmacol.* **114,** 297–302.

33. Wu-Wong, J. R., Chiou, W., Hoffman, D. J., Winn, M., von Geldern, T. W., and Opgenorth, T. J. (1996) Endothelins and endothelin receptor antagonists: binding to plasma proteins. *Life Sci.* **58**, 1839–1847.

34. Williams, Jr., D. L., Murphy, K. L., Nolan, N. A., O'Brien, J. A., Pettibone, D. J., Kivlighn, S. D., et al. (1995) Pharmacology of L-754,142, a highly potent, orally active nonpeptidyl endothelin antagonist. *J. Pharm. Exp. Ther.* **275**, 1518–1526.

35. Sogabe, K., Nirei, H., Shoubo, M., Nomoto, A., Ao, S., Notsu, Y., and Ono, T. (1993) Pharmacological profile of FR139317, a novel, potent endothelin ET_A receptor antagonist. *J. Pharm. Exp. Ther.* **264**, 1040–1046.

36. Webb, M. L., Bird, J. E., Liu, E. C. K., Rose, P. M., Serafino, R., Stein, P. D., and Moreland, S. (1995) BMS-182874 is a selective, nonpeptide endothelin ET_A receptor antagonist. *J. Pharm. Exp. Ther.* **272**, 1124–1134.

37. Reynolds, E. E., Keiser, J. A., Haleen, S. J., Walker, D. M., Olszewski, B., Schroeder, R. L., et al. (1995) Pharmacological Characterization of PD 156707, an orally active ET_A receptor antagonist. *J. Pharm. Exp. Ther.* **273**, 1410–1417.

38. Clozel, M., Breu, V., Gray, G.A., Kalina, B., Loffler, B.M., Burri, K., et al. (1994) Pharmacological characterization of bosentan, a new potent orally active nonpeptide endothelin receptor antagonist. *J. Pharm. Exp. Ther.* **270**, 228–235.

39. Wu-Wong, J. R., Chiou, W., Huang, Z.-J., Vidal, M. J., and Opgenorth, T. J. (1994) Endothelin receptor in human pericardium smooth muscle cells: antagonist potency differs on agonist-evoked responses, *Am. J. Physiol.* **267**, C1185–C1195.

40. Nambi, P., Pullen, M., Kincaid, J., Nuthulaganti, P., Aiyar, N., Brooks, D. P., et al. (1997) Identification and characterization of a novel endothelin receptor that binds both ET_A- and ET_B-selective ligands. *Mol. Pharmacol.* **52**, 582–589.

41. Douglas, W. P., Hay, D. W., Luttmann, M. A., Pullen, M. A., and Nambi, P. (1998) Functional and binding characterization of endothelin receptors in human bronchus: evidence for a novel endothelin B receptor subtype? *J. Pharmacol. Exp. Ther.* **284**, 669–677.

42. Douglas, S. A., Beck, G. R., Jr., Elliott, J. D., and Ohlstein, E. H. (1995) Pharmacologic evidence for the presence of three functional endothelin receptor subtypes in rabbit saphenous vein. *J. Cardiovasc. Pharmacol.* **26**, S163–S168.

43. Kobayashi, S., Tang, R., Wang, B., Opgenorth, T., Stein, E., Shapiro, E., and Lepor, H. (1994) Localization of endothelin receptors in the human prostate. *J. Urol.* **151**, 763–766.

44. Wu-Wong, J. R. (1999) Endothelin receptor antagonists: past, present, and future. In *Current Opinion in Cardiovascular, Pulmonarys and Renal Investigational Drugs* (Ripka, W. C. and Doherty, A. M., eds.), Pharma Press, London, UK, 346–351.

6

Quantification of Endothelin Receptor mRNA by Competitive RT-PCR

Paula J. W. Smith and Juan Carlos Monge

1. Introduction

The potent effects of the endothelins (ETs), including their vasoconstrictor, positive inotropic and co-mitogenic actions, are mediated by at least two distinct ET receptor subtypes, ET_A *(1)* and ET_B *(2)*. The ET_A receptor is selective for ET-1, with binding affinity ET-1>ET-2>>ET-3, while the ET_B receptor is nonisoform selective. Both subtypes are structurally similar, having seven transmembrane domains characteristic of the G-protein-coupled superfamily *(1,2)*. In several pathophysiological conditions, including myocardial infarction *(3)*, congestive heart failure *(4)*, and renal failure *(5)*, there is altered expression of ET receptors. These changes further implicate ET in the pathogenesis of such conditions and provide additional characterization of the disease process. It is, therefore, essential to have an accurate and reliable means of measuring ET receptor expression. Traditional Northern analysis has the disadvantage of low sensitivity, and while the reverse transcription-polymerase chain reaction (RT-PCR) offers 1000–10,000-fold greater sensitivity, the exponential nature of its amplification kinetics makes it difficult to obtain truly quantitative information. Competitive RT-PCR obviates this problem by co-amplifying the gene of interest with a known concentration of mutant cDNA, which as the name suggests, competes for primer binding and PCR substrates. The subsequent PCR products from wild-type and mutant are distinguished by size or the presence or absence of a restriction enzyme site. By constructing plots of the ratio of wild-type to competitor densities vs molar concentration of competitor cRNA, the starting concentration of the wild-type RNA can be calculated.

From: *Methods in Molecular Biology, vol. 206: Peptide Research Protocols: Endothelin*
Edited by: J. Maguire and A. Davenport © Humana Press Inc., Totowa, NJ

This chapter describes a competitive RT-PCR approach for the accurate quantification of ET_A and ET_B receptor mRNA from whole tissue and cell-culture extracts, and provides a more detailed account of our previously published report *(6)*. The mutants for the ET_A and ET_B receptor have been designed to amplify with equal efficiency to the respective wild-type cDNA, hence the ratio of products remains constant throughout the reaction. For the ET_A receptor mutant, site-directed mutagenesis was used to introduce a novel EcoRV site, while, for the ET_B receptor mutant, a 105-bp deletion was made through restriction enzyme digests. As mentioned, the application of the competitive RT-PCR technique for quantitative analysis of ET receptors is of particular importance in pathophysiological conditions in which the ET system has been implicated. We have used this technique to characterize changes in ET_A and ET_B receptor expression in rat models of heart failure *(7,8)* and following balloon injury of the rat carotid artery *(9)*. Given that tissue samples can be small, such as the carotid artery, and ET receptor mRNA is found in low abundance, competitive RT-PCR is an ideal method for quantitative analysis of limited amounts of RNA by virtue of its extreme sensitivity. Similarly, this feature overcomes the difficulty in examining gene expression in human tissue, where patient biopsies are usually small. Furthermore, the primer sequences for both ET_A and ET_B are chosen to be within regions of maximum homology between species and make this method applicable to RNA isolated from human, rat, mouse, rabbit, dog, bovine and porcine sources.

2. Materials

1. Total RNA extracted from tissue and cell-culture samples (*see* **Note 1**).
2. DEPC (RNase-free) water: add 1 mL diethylpyrocarbonate (DEPC) to 1 L of double-distilled, deionized H_2O (i.e., final concentration 0.1%); shake well, incubate overnight at 37°C, and then autoclave for at least 45 min, or until DEPC scent has disappeared.
3. RT-PCR reagents: Moloney Murine Leukemia Virus (M-MLV) reverse transcriptase (Gibco-BRL, Burlington, ON, Canada); *Taq* DNA polymerase (Boehringer Mannheim, Laval, QC, Canada); deoxynucleotide triphosphates (dNTPs) (Gibco-BRL, Burlington, ON, Canada); Random Primer oligodeoxyribonucleotides (Gibco-BRL, Burlington, ON, Canada).
4. First strand buffer: final concentration, 50 mM Tris-HCl, pH 8.3, at 37°C, 75 mM KCl, 3 mM $MgCl_2$ (Gibco-BRL, Burlington, ON, Canada).
5. PCR reaction buffer: final concentration, 10 mM Tris-HCl, pH 9.0, at 25°C, 50 mM KCl and 1.5 mM $MgCl_2$ (Boehringer Mannheim, ON, Canada).
6. Restriction enzymes: *Eco*RV, *Sac*I, and *Sal*I (Pharmacia Biotech, Canada); *Nhe*I and *Bal*I (Promega Corporation, Madison, WI).
7. Cloning vectors and reagents: Original TA cloning kit (Invitrogen, San Diego, CA); pGEM-T Vector system (Promega Corporation, Madison, WI); T4 DNA

Table 1
GenBank Accession Numbers and Primer Sequence Locations for ET$_A$ and ET$_B$ Receptors in the Species Tested

Species	ET$_A$ GenBank ref. no.	ET$_A$ sense primer location	ET$_A$ anti-sense primer location	ET$_B$ Gen-Bank ref. no.	ET$_B$ sense primer location	ET$_B$ anti-sense primer location
Mouse	AF039892	–	207–186	U32329	847–867	1399–1377
Rat	M60786	312–333	543–522	X57764	844–864	1396–1374
Rabbit	AF311974	218–239	449–428	–	–	–
Dog	–	–	–	AF034530	818–838	1370–1348
Bovine	X57765	736–757	967–946	D90456	788–808	1340–1318
Porcine	S80652	329–350	560–539	–	–	–
Human	L06622	275–296	506–485	L06623	877–897	1429–1408

–, denotes no data currently available.

ligase (Gibco-BRL, Burlington, ON, Canada); Klenow Fragment of DNA Polymerase I (Pharmacia Biotech, Canada).

8. In vitro transcription kit: RiboMAX Large scale RNA production system–T7 (Promega Corporation, Madison, WI) (*see* **Note 2**).

9. Thermal cycler (e.g., PTC-200 Peltier Thermal Cycler, MJ Research Inc., Watertown, MA), gel electrophoresis system (e.g., Mupid-21 mini-gel electrophoresis system, Helixx Technologies Inc., Scarborough, ON, Canada), gel extraction kit (e.g., QIAquick gel extraction kit, QIAGEN Inc., Chatsworth, CA), gel documentation system (e.g., GS-700, Bio-Rad, Mississauga, ON, Canada).

3. Methods

3.1. Oligonucleotide Primer Design

1. Obtain available nucleotide sequences for ET$_A$ and ET$_B$ receptors from the GenBank database and compare homology between species using the BLAST program *(10)*.

2. Choose PCR primer sequences to be within regions of complete homology between all species included in the database and optimize using the computer software program OLIGO (National Biosciences).

3. Synthesize primer sequences using, e.g., a PerSeptive Expedite nucleic acid synthesizer (Millipore, Canada Ltd., Mississauga, ON, Canada).

4. Design the primer pair for each receptor to span one or more introns such that they will not give rise to genomic DNA templated PCR products.

5. For the ET$_A$ receptor, the sense and antisense primers are 5'-TTTTCATC-GTGGGAATGGTGGG-3' and 5'-GACTTCTGCAAAAAGGGGAACA-3' respectively. For the ET$_B$ receptor, the sense and antisense primers are 5'-CAAAATGGACAGCAGTAGAAA-3' and 5'-GACTTAAAGCAGTTTTTGA-ATCT-3' respectively (*see* **Table 1**).

3.2. RT-PCR

The ability of the homologous primers to work in multiple species has been tested using RNA isolated from human placenta, rat left ventricle (LV), mouse lung, rabbit LV, dog LV, bovine lung, and pig LV for both ET receptors.

1. Carry out cDNA synthesis at 37°C for 90 min by incubating total RNA (2 μg per sample) (*see* **Note 3**) with 200 U of M-MLV reverse transcriptase, 0.5 mM dNTPs, 1.5 nM Random Primer oligodeoxyribonucleotides in first strand buffer to a final volume of 20 μL (*see* **Note 4**).
2. Inactivate the reverse transcriptase by heating at 95°C for 4 min before proceeding to the PCR step.
3. Use 10 μL of the cDNA from the RT reaction for PCR amplification using the PTC-200 Peltier Thermal Cycler. To the cDNA add 5 U *Taq* DNA polymerase, 200 μM dNTPs, 100 pM specific primers for ET_A or ET_B in PCR reaction buffer to a final volume of 50 μL (*see* **Note 4**). We routinely use a "hot start" of 95°C for 2 min to reduce nonspecific amplification.
4. Use the following amplification profile for ET_A: 95°C for 1 min, 59°C for 1 min, 72°C for 2 min for 30 cycles, followed by strand extension at 72°C for 10 min. Use the following amplification profile for ET_B: 95°C for 1 min, 62°C for 1 min, 72°C for 2 min for 35 cycles, followed by 10 min at 72°C (*see* **Note 5**).
5. Load the reaction products on to a 2% agarose gel and electrophorese for 45 min at 100 V, before visualizing using ethidium bromide staining.

The primer pair works in all of the seven species studied for both the ET_A and ET_B receptor, including species for which the cDNA sequences of the receptors has not been described previously (*see* **Table 1**), generating cDNA bands of the predicted size of 232 and 553 bp respectively (**Fig. 1**).

3.3. Design and Synthesis of ET_A Receptor cDNA Mutant

The ET_A receptor cDNA mutant is engineered to contain a single-base mutation, thus introducing a novel EcoRV restriction enzyme site that is not present in the wild-type fragment (**Fig. 2**). The "megaprimer" method of site-directed mutagenesis was chosen to make the single nucleotide change *(11)*. This approach uses only 3 primers in two rounds of PCR. The first round uses either the sense or antisense primer originally designed (*see* **Subheading 3.1.**), together with a primer containing the desired mutation.

1. For the ET_A receptor, the original sense primer is used in conjunction with a mutant primer designed to introduce an EcoRV site in to a rat cDNA fragment (a PCR product generated with the original ET_A receptor primer pair), by replacing a guanine base for a thymine base at 101 bp of the reverse and complement sequence (GAGATC→GAT!ATC). The sequence of the mutant primer is as follows: 5'-GGG**GATATC**AATGACCACGTAG-3'. This mutant primer is designed so that its first 5' nucleotide follows a thymine residue in the template

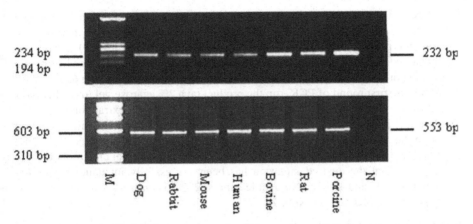

Fig. 1. RT-PCR 2% agarose gel electrophoresis. RT-PCR was performed with 2 μg total RNA isolated from seven species for ET_A (upper gel) and ET_B (lower gel) respectively. Bands of the expected size were generated for ET_A (232 bp) and ET_B (553 bp). M = φX174 RF DNA/HaeIII fragments marker, N = negative control (i.e., minus template).

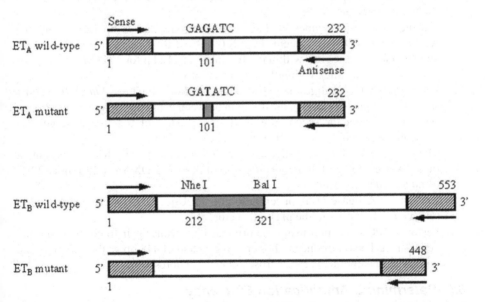

Fig. 2. Diagram of competitive PCR fragments. Site-directed mutagenesis was used to introduce an EcoRV site into the ET_A receptor cDNA mutant by replacing a guanine residue for a thymine residue at 101 bp. For the ET_B receptor, a double restriction enzyme digest using NheI and BalI created a 105-bp deletion mutant. The primer pairs for both the ET_A and ET_B receptors are identical for the wild-type and mutant fragments, which allows equal amplification efficiencies.

cDNA in order to obviate the nonspecific, nontemplate addition of a single adenine residue at the 3' end of the megaprimer by *Taq* DNA polymerase *(12)*, and thus prevent any unwanted mutations. Landt and colleagues *(13)* also recommend reducing the dNTP concentration in the first round of PCR, which although results in lower product yield, reduces random mutations (*see* **Note 6**).

2. After the first round of PCR, run the product on a 2% agarose gel to confirm it is of the expected size, and then purify using a QIAquick gel extraction kit.

3. Use this product as a megaprimer for the second round of PCR in conjunction with the original antisense primer. Digest the PCR product with EcoRV (12 U) for 3 h at 37°C, and subsequently separate by 2% agarose gel electrophoresis to confirm that the desired mutation has been successfully introduced, yielding bands of 101 and 131 bp. No visible band at 232 bp confirms that the digest has gone to completion (*see* **Note 7**).

3.4. Design and Synthesis of ET_B Receptor cDNA Mutant

The ET_B receptor cDNA mutant is created as a deletion mutant in order to distinguish it from the wild-type fragment of 553 bp.

1. Firstly, generate a rat ET_B cDNA fragment using the PCR described with the original ET_B receptor primer pair (*see* **Subheading 3.2.**), and then clone it into the plasmid vector pGEM-T.

2. Use the restriction enzymes *Nhe*I and *Bal*I to introduce a 105-bp deletion into the wild-type ET_B cDNA fragment (**Fig. 2**) (*see* **Note 8**). These enzymes have only single endonuclease sites within the fragment, at 212 bp for *Nhe*I and 321 bp for *Bal*I, and have no sites within the plasmid vector.

3. Carry out the double digest in two separate reactions. First use *Nhe*I followed by *Bal*I (1 U enzyme/µg DNA), purifying in between using the QIAquick PCR purification kit. After the second digest, run the product on a 1% agarose gel and subsequently purify using a QIAquick gel extraction kit.

4. The sticky-ends of the post-digestion product are removed by Klenow Fragment of DNA Polymerase I at a concentration of 0.5 U/µg DNA for 20 min at 22°C (4 nucleotides filled in).

5. Use T4 DNA ligase at a concentration of 0.5 U/µg DNA overnight at 4°C to religate the fragment in the plasmid vector.

6. Perform a PCR reaction using the original ET_B primer pair to confirm that the deletion has been introduced, thus creating a band of 448 bp vs the 553 bp of the wild-type in subsequent 2% agarose gel electrophoresis.

3.5. Determining Amplification Efficiency

1. In order for competitive PCR to be effective, there has to be equal amplification efficiency between the wild-type and mutant fragments. To determine the amplification efficiency, perform PCR as described above (*see* **Subheading 3.2.**) using mixed samples of wild-type and mutant cDNA, each at a starting concentration = 1 fmol (obtain by diluting known concentrations of RT-PCR products that have been determined by spectrophotometry) for each receptor.

2. Remove samples (5% of reaction vol) every 2 cycles between 20 and 40 cycles by pausing the thermal cycler just prior to the end of the 72°C extension phase (*see* **Note 9**). Run PCR products on a 2% agarose gel (following EcoRV digestion, for ET_A) and stain with ethidium bromide, before quantifying the intensity of the bands by densitometry. Amplification efficiency is primarily determined by the sequence of primers *(14,15)*.

In the competitive RT-PCR approach described here, we use the same primer pair for the mutant competitor and wild-type cDNA, for both ET_A and ET_B, and achieve identical amplification efficiencies for wild-type and competitor cDNA fragments (**Fig. 3**), despite a single nucleotide difference and a 105-bp difference between the fragments for the ET_A and ET_B receptor respectively. Although sequence data is not available for every species we tested, the primer sequences were chosen from regions with 100% homology, and it is very likely that the homology is present in the other species. Thus, the technique is unequivocally quantitative for those species for which the sequence is known, and has the potential to be quantitative for the other species tested.

3.6. DNA Cloning and Sequencing

1. Clone the PCR product of the ET_A receptor mutant into the vector pCR 2.1 using the Original TA cloning kit. Clone the ET_B receptor mutant into the pGEM-T vector.
2. Carry out large-scale isolation of plasmid DNA s with a Plasmid Maxi kit. Confirm that only the desired mutations are present by sequencing the insert for both the ET_A and ET_B constructs.

3.7. In Vitro Transcription

To obtain an absolute measurement of the ET receptor mRNA present in tissue samples, we use competitor cRNA fragments (*see* **Note 10**).

1. The DNA templates for the ET_A and ET_B mutants are linearized prior to in vitro transcription to produce RNA of defined length. For the ET_A mutant, use *Sac*I (1 U/μg DNA) to digest 100 μg of DNA template; use *Sal*I (1 U/μg DNA) for the same quantity of ET_B mutant.
2. After digestion, run the mutants on a 1% agarose gel with undigested template to confirm complete linearization. Follow by excision and purification using a QIAquick gel extraction kit.
3. Blunt the resulting 3' overhangs in the ET_A template using Klenow Fragment of DNA Polymerase I at a concentration of 5 U/μg DNA for 15 min at 22°C.
4. Carry out in vitro transcription using a RiboMAX Large Scale RNA Production System–T7. Determine the concentration of cRNA (suspended in DEPC-treated water) by spectrophotometric analysis, and its integrity by denaturing gel electrophoresis.
5. Store 8-μL aliquots of the cRNA, each sufficient for one experiment, at −80°C in order to prevent freeze-thaw steps.

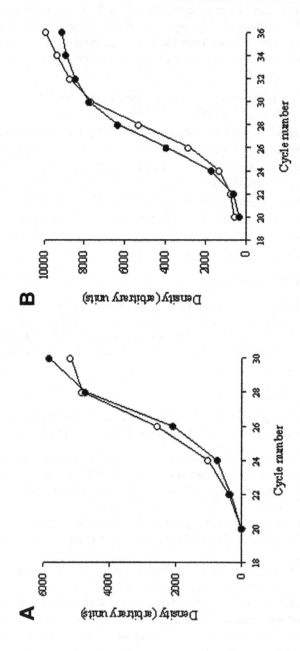

Fig. 3. Amplification kinetics of the wild-type and mutant cDNA templates for ET_A and ET_B receptors. 1 fmol each of the respective receptor wild-type and mutant cDNA were combined and PCR was performed as described (*see* **Subheadings 3.2.** and **3.5.**). After 20 cycles, 5% aliquots were removed from the reaction every 2 cycles up to 40 cycles. Following 2% agarose gel electrophoresis, densitometric analysis of the bands was carried out, and the values within the linear range were plotted vs cycle number. The open and closed circles denote wild-type and mutant cDNA respectively for (**A**) ET_A and (**B**) ET_B.

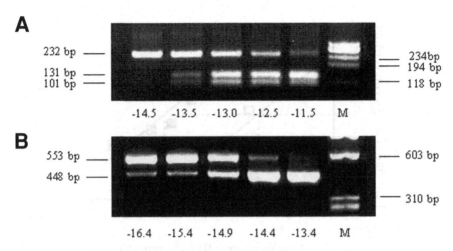

Fig. 4. Co-amplification competitive RT-PCR analysis of ET_A and ET_B mRNA levels in rat left ventricle. (**A**) Five serial dilutions of the ET_A mutant ($10^{-11.5} - 10^{-14.5}$ M) were used to compete 2 μg of total RNA extracted from the rat left ventricle. PCR products were digested with EcoRV for 3 h to distinguish wild-type (232 bp) from mutant (131 and 101 bp). (**B**) Five serial dilutions of the ET_B mutant ($10^{-13.4} - 10^{-16.4}$ M) were used to compete 2 μg of total RNA extracted from the rat left ventricle. Since the templates differed by 105 bp, the wild-type fragment (553 bp) could be distinguished from the mutant (448 bp) immediately post-PCR. M = φX174 RF DNA/*Hae*III fragments marker.

3.8. Competitive RT-PCR

1. Prepare a dilution series in logarithmic increments for the ET_A and ET_B receptor mutant cRNA. RT-PCR is performed as described above (*see* **Subheading 3.2.**) by combining the total RNA (2 μg per sample) extracted from tissue with 1 μL vol of mutant cRNA in increasing concentrations, giving a total of six vials (including negative control) (*see* **Note 11**).
2. Carry out gel electrophoresis and stain with ethidium bromide.
3. Quantify the intensity of the bands by densitometry, normalize relative to the density of competitor and then plot as log (wild-type /competitor) ratio vs log (competitor cRNA). The exact amount of ET_A and ET_B receptor mRNA present in each sample is then calculated by intrapolating from the intersection of the curves at the point of molar equivalence, i.e., where the ratio of wild-type/competitor = 1, the log of one being equal to zero. **Figure 4** shows representative competitive RT-PCR experiments for (A) ET_A and (B) ET_B receptors in rat LV. As predicted for competitive templates, **Fig. 5** illustrates the linear nature of the log-log plots of the ratio of wild-type to competitor density vs concentration of competitor cRNA. At the point of molar equivalence, the starting concentration of target RNA is equal to the known starting concentration of mutant competitor. In the examples shown, the concentration of ET_A mRNA isolated from rat LV is 89 fmol/μg total RNA, and that of ET_B is 2.50 fmol/μg total RNA (**Fig. 5**). The

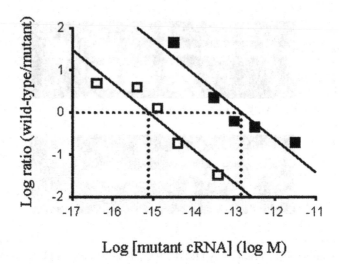

Log [mutant cRNA] (log M)

Fig. 5. Quantitative analysis of ET_A and ET_B mRNA levels in rat left ventricle. The intensity of the bands shown in **Fig. 4** was measured by densitometry and a logarithmic plot of the ratio of wild-type to mutant density vs molar concentration of mutant was constructed. The solid lines were drawn from a linear regression analysis of each of the five data points, and the dotted lines indicate the point of molar equivalence between the wild-type and mutant. The closed and open squares denote data derived from ET_A and ET_B, respectively.

inter-/intra- coefficients of variation are 9%/10% and 10%/12% for ET_A and ET_B respectively ($n = 4$ experiments).

Although the initial development of the mutant RNA fragments for the ET receptors may appear somewhat laborious, once they are synthesized on a large scale, the technique described offers a relatively fast, inexpensive and extremely sensitive method to quantify ET_A and ET_B receptor mRNA in most of the species commonly used in research.

4. Notes

1. We generally use the method described by Chomczynski and Sacchi *(16)* to extract total RNA from tissue, but have also used commercially available kits (e.g., RNeasy Mini kit from QIAGEN Inc.), which reduce extraction times but are obviously more expensive. For isolation of RNA from cell culture samples we recommend using Trizol reagent (Gibco-BRL).
2. For consistency, we recommend preparing a sufficiently large quantity of cRNA to allow the same batch to be used to analyze a complete study's samples. The RiboMAX Large Scale RNA production kit produces milligram amounts of RNA, which are stable for at least 6 mo when stored at $\leq -70°C$.

3. We routinely use lower starting concentrations of RNA, e.g., 200 ng, particularly if the yield following extraction from small tissue samples is low.

4. We recommend preparing a master mix for reactions when multiple samples are to be analyzed. A master mix should contain all the components except the RNA or DNA source, and should be made up to a vol (× the number of samples + 10%) that allows for loss during pipeting. If nonspecific background appears to be a problem (despite the "hot start" procedure), the use of 2 PCR master mixes is recommended. (1) All nucleic acids: dNTPs + primer + template + half of the water, (2) all other components: buffer + enzyme + half of the water. Bring mixes together on ice immediately before aliquoting to cDNA tubes and transferring to the thermal cycler.

5. Cycling conditions may have to be adjusted depending on the particular thermal cycler used.

6. We used the same mix as listed for normal PCR but with half-concentrations of dNTPs, i.e., 100 μM final concentration.

7. It is essential to confirm in preliminary experiments the conditions that are required for the digest to go to completion. Undigested mutant will obviously affect the density of wild-type bands and lead to erroneous quantification.

8. Gilliland and co-workers *(17)* have demonstrated that competitor fragments differing by ~100 bp from wild type are able to give identical quantitative results to competitors that contain a single base pair substitution, emphasizing that the major determinant of amplification is the sequence of the primer pair.

9. We found that this cycle window generates bands ranging from barely visible to plateau, allowing plots of the linear range of amplification to be constructed. This window may have to be altered depending on the thermal cycler being used.

10. Although quantification can be made when using mutant cDNA *(17)*, this approach does not control for the efficiency of the RT-step and negates the ability to express the concentration of mRNA in absolute units. By performing in vitro transcription to generate cRNA mutants, we are able to calculate ET receptor expression in moles of RNA.

11. In initial reactions, logarithmic increments of molar concentrations of specific competitor are used to obtain a rough estimate of the amount of cDNA present. After appropriate concentrations have been determined for a particular source of sample mRNA, competitive RT-PCR is carried out using half-log increments to more accurately quantify the concentration of ET receptor mRNA in each sample.

References

1. Arai, H., Hori S., Aramori, I., Ohkubo, H., and Nakanishi, S. (1990) Cloning and expression of a cDNA encoding an endothelin receptor. *Nature* **348,** 730–732.

2. Sakurai, T., Yanagisawa, M., Takuwa, Y., Miyazaki, H., Kimura, S., Goto, K., and Masaki, T. (1990) Cloning of a cDNA encoding a nonisopeptide-selective subtype of the endothelin receptor. *Nature* **348,** 732–735.

3. Nambi, P., Pullen, M., Egan, J. W., and Smith, E. F. (1991) Identification of cardiac endothelin binding sites in rats: downregulation of left atrial endothelin binding sites in response to myocardial infarction. *Pharmacology* **53**, 84–89.

4. Morawietz, H., Szibor, M., Goettsch, W., Bartling, B., Barton, M., Shaw, S., et al. (2000) Deloading of the left ventricle by ventricular assist device normalizes increased expression of entothelin ET(A) receptors but not endothelin-converting enzyme-1 in patients with end-stage heart failure. *Circulation* **102(19 Suppl. 3)**, III188–193.

5. Shimizu, T., Hata, S., Kuroda, T., Mihara, S., and Fujimoto, M. (1999) Different roles of two types of endothelin receptors in partial ablation-induced chronic renal failure in rats. *Eur. J. Pharmacol.* **381**, 39–49.

6. Smith, P. J., Brooks, J. I., Stewart, D. J., and Monge, J. C. (1999) Quantification of endothelin ETA and ETB receptor mRNA by competitive reverse transcription-polymerase chain reaction: development of amultispecies assay. *Anal. Biochem.* **271**, 93–96.

7. Picard, P., Smith, P. J. W., Monge, J. C., Rouleau, J. L., Nguyen, Q. T., Calderone, A., and Stewart, D. J. (1998) Coordinated upregulation of the cardiac endothelin system in a rat model of heart failure. *J. Cardiovasc. Pharmacol.* **31(Suppl. 1)**, S294–S297.

8. Smith, P. J. W., Ornatsky, O., Stewart, D. J., Picard, P., Dawood, F., Wen, W. H., et al. (2000) Effects of estrogen replacement on infarct size, cardiac remodeling, and the endothelin system after myocardial infarction in ovariectomized rats. *Circulation* **102**, 2983–2989.

9. Picard, P., Smith, P. J. W., Monge, J. C., and Stewart, D. J. (1998) Expression of endothelial factors after arterial injury in the rat. *J. Cardiovasc. Pharmacol.* **31(Suppl. 1)**, S323–S327.

10. Altschul, S. F., Gish, W., Miller, W., Myers, E. W., and Lipman, D. J. (1990) Basic local alignment search tool. *J. Mol. Biol.* **215**, 403–410.

11. Sarkar, G. and Sommer, S. S. (1990) The "megaprimer" method of site-directed mutagenesis. *BioTechniques* **8**, 404–407.

12. Clark, J. M. (1988) Novel nontemplated nucleotide addition reactions catalyzed by procaryotic and eucaryotic DNA polymerases. *Nucl. Acid Res.* **16**, 9677–9686.

13. Landt, O., Grunert, H.-P., and Hahn, U. (1990) A general method for rapid site-directed mutagenesis using the polymerase chain reaction. *Gene* **96**, 125–128.

14. Wang, A. M., Doyle, M. V., and Mark, D. F. (1989) Quantitation of mRNA by the polymerase chain reaction. *Proc. Natl. Acad. Sci. USA* **86**, 9717–9721.

15. Siebert, P. D. and Larrick, J. W. (1992) Competitive PCR. *Nature* **359**, 557–558.

16. Chomczynski, P. and Sacchi, E. (1987) Single-step method of RNA isolation by acid guanidinium thiocyanate-phenol-chloroform extraction. *Anal. Biochem.* **162**, 156–159.

17. Gilliland, G., Perrin, S., Blanchard, K., and Bunn, H. F. (1990) Analysis of cytokine mRNA and DNA: detection and quantitation by competitive polymerase chain reaction. *Proc. Natl. Acad. Sci. USA* **87**, 2725–2729.

III

Endothelin-Converting Enzyme Protocols

7

Detection and Assessment of Endothelin-Converting Enzyme Activity

Carolyn D. Jackson and Anthony J. Turner

1. Introduction

The biologically active vasoconstrictor peptide endothelin (ET-1) is produced from its inactive precursor big endothelin (big ET-1) in a process catalyzed by an endothelin-converting enzyme (ECE). Two potential human endothelin-converting enzymes, ECE-1 and ECE-2, have been cloned (*1–3*) and a third ECE activity, designated ECE-3, has been described in bovine iris (*4*). ECE-1 is a member of the M13 family of zinc metalloproteases that includes the well-characterized neprilysin, or NEP, to which ECE-1 has 37% identity (*5*). Like NEP, ECE-1 is a type II integral membrane protein with a short N-terminal cytoplasmic region, a single transmembrane domain and a large C-terminal region containing the active site, the zinc-binding domain and a number of potential glycosylation sites (**Fig. 1**). Significant differences exist between NEP and ECE-1. ECE-1 is a disulfide-linked dimer whereas NEP is a monomer, and they also exhibit different inhibitor profiles. The zinc metallopeptidase inhibitors phosphoramidon and thiorphan both inhibit NEP at nanomolar concentrations whereas micromolar levels of phosphoramidon are required to inhibit ECE-1, which is also relatively insensitive to thiorphan ($I_{50} > 200\ \mu M$). There are also marked differences in substrate specificity, NEP having a much broader profile of substrates. ECE-1 cleaves big ET-1 and big ET-2 at the Trp^{21}-Val^{22} bond and big ET-3 at the Trp^{21}-Ile^{22} to produce ET-1, -2 and -3 respectively (**Fig. 2**). Originally thought to be specific for these big ET substrates, it has since been shown that ECE-1 efficiently cleaves some other substrates including bradykinin and substance P, and even hydrolyzes insulin B chain at multiple sites (*6,7*). ECE-1 is expressed predominantly in endothelial cells but it has also been shown to be expressed in smooth muscle

From: *Methods in Molecular Biology, vol. 206: Peptide Research Protocols: Endothelin*
Edited by: J. Maguire and A. Davenport © Humana Press Inc., Totowa, NJ

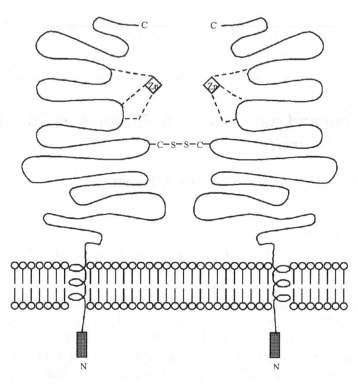

Fig. 1. The topology of ECE-1 as a dimeric type II integral membrane protein. The subunits are linked by disulfide bonds as illustrated. Each subunit has a zinc ion coordinated by three zinc ligands that form the catalytic centre. The hatched areas at the N-termini represent the regions that differ between the different isoforms of ECE-1.

cells and neurones and glia in the brain *(8)*. The subcellular localization of the enzyme has been the subject of much debate, with both intracellular and cell surface localization being reported, and is further complicated by the presence of four known isoforms of ECE-1, designated ECE-1a, -1b, -1c and -1d in the human, produced from distinct promoters within the same gene *(9,10)*. These isoforms are identical in their C-terminal and transmembrane domains but differ significantly in their N-terminal domains (*see* **Table 1**). Potential tyrosine and dileucine based localization sequences in these short regions have been suggested to be responsible for different subcellular localizations of the isoforms *(11–14)*.

Finally, it should be borne in mind that, although ECE-1 is widely viewed as the major activity cleaving big ET-1, other proteases can catalyze this reaction. However, several reports, such as that which illustrates only a 40% reduction in ET-1 levels in ECE-1 null mice with no increase in big ET-1 levels *(15)*,

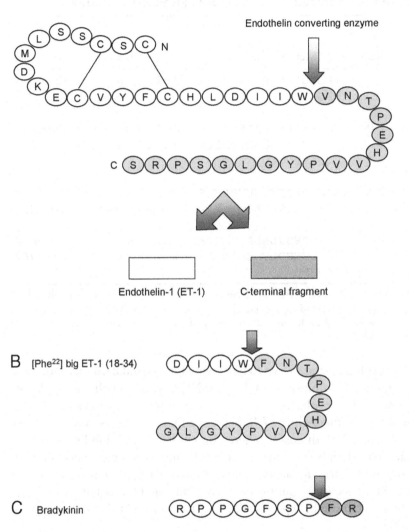

Fig. 2. Schematic representation of the cleavage of some substrates of ECE-1. (**A**) Cleavage of big ET-1 to produce ET-1 and the C-terminal fragment, (**B**) the synthetic peptide [Phe^{22}] big ET-1, and (**C**) bradykinin. Cleavage sites are indicated by arrows.

suggest that the enzymes identified thus far are not solely responsible for this cleavage. In particular, antisense experiments suggest that ECE-1 is not primarily involved in big ET-1 conversion in bovine pulmonary artery smooth muscle cells *(16)*.

Table 1
Summary of the Characteristics of the Human ECE-1 Isoforms

ECE-1 Isoform	Number of residues	N-terminal sequence	Localization	Reference
a (β)	758	MPLQGLGLQRNPFLQGKR GPGLTSSPPLLPPSLQ–	Predominantly plasma membrane	Shimada et al. *(2)*
b	770	MRGVWPPPVSALLSALGM STYKRATLDEEDLVDSLS EGDAYPNGLQ–	Exclusively intracellular	Schweizer et al. *(9)*
c (α)	754	MMSTYKRATLDEEDLVDS LSEGDAYPNGLQ–	Plasma membrane and intracellular	Schmidt et al. *(1)*
d	767	MEALRESVLHLALQMTYK RATLDEEDLVDSLSEGDA YPMGLQ-	Intermediate between a and c	Valdenaire et al. *(10)*

Two isoforms of ECE-1 were originally identified in the rat and designated a and b. Subsequently, the human forms were identified and given Roman rather than Greek symbols for identification. It is now established that the rat isoforms a and b correspond to human ECE-1c and ECE-1a, respectively.

ECE-1 levels have been shown to be elevated in several cardiovascular diseases and combined inhibition of ECE-1 and NEP, which is believed to elevate ANP and lower ET-1 levels, has shown positive effects in several animal models of vascular pathophysiology *(17)*. Selective ECE inhibitors may also prove effective in respiratory diseases, where compounds which inhibit both ECE and NEP are likely to have detrimental effects by increasing the levels of bradykinin, a bronchoconstrictor, substance P and endothelin, thereby exacerbating the disease. Studies carried out thus far have indicated the potential of selective ECE inhibitors both in experimental investigation and therapeutic applications *(18–21)*.

Since the discovery of endothelin in 1988 *(22)*, the involvement of ECE-1 in both nonpathological and disease states has become apparent, illustrating the potential of the biosynthetic pathway for ET-1, in particular ECE-1, as drug targets for the treatment and control of disease states. The measurement and assessment of ECE-1 expression, in particular isoform expression, and the use of cultured cells to assess the effectiveness of ECE inhibitors is, therefore, increasingly relevant.

This chapter will focus on ECE-1 and will describe methods that can be used in the detection and assessment of ECE-1 expression and activity. In particular the production of ECE-1 isoform-specific antibodies, their uses and HPLC assay methodology will be discussed. Direct cellular assays of ET-1 production by immunological methods are described in Chapters 1 and 2.

2. Materials

2.1. Production of Isoform-Specific Antibodies

1. Purified peptides (many suppliers, e.g., Genosys Biotechnologies Ltd., Cambs, UK). Store desiccated and refrigerated.
2. Ovalbumin.
3. Dialysis tubing.
4. 10 mM Sodium phosphate buffer: 10 mM NaH$_2$PO$_4$, pH 7.4, stored, as all buffers, at 4°C.
5. 50 mM N-ethylmaleimide. Freshly prepared for each use.
6. m-Maleimidobenzoyl-N-hydroxysulfosuccinimide ester (Sulfo MBS, Pierce, IL) solution (20 mg/mL) freshly prepared for each use.
7. Sephadex G50 and G10.
8. 50 mM Sodium phosphate buffer: 50 mM NaH$_2$PO$_4$, pH 6.0.
9. 0.5 M Dithiothreitol (DTT). Freshly prepared for each use.
10. 5 mM 5,5'-Dithiobis(2-nitrobenzoic acid) (DTNB) in 100 mM NaH$_2$PO$_4$, pH 7.4.
11. 96-Well plates and plate-reader.
12. 0.1 M NaOH.
13. 10 mM NaH$_2$PO$_4$, 145 mM NaCl, pH 7.2.
14. Phosphate-buffered saline (PBS): 150 mM NaCl, 20 mM NaH$_2$PO$_4$, 200 mM Na$_2$PO$_4$, pH 7.4.
15. Complete and Incomplete Freund's adjuvant.
16. Low-fat milk powder.
17. Coating buffer: 50 mM NaHCO$_3$, 10 mM NaOH, pH 9.6.
18. Antibody buffer: PBS containing 1% low-fat milk powder.
19. Tween-20.
20. Goat anti-rabbit horseradish peroxidase IgG.
21. Substrate solution: 5.5 mg 2,2'-azino-bis(3-ethylbenzthiazoline-6-sulphonic acid) (ABTS) in 5.72 mL 0.1 M citric acid, 4.27 mL 0.2 M Na$_2$HPO$_4$, 1 μL 30% H$_2$O$_2$, pH 4.3.
22. 1 M Citric acid.
23. Tris buffer: 50 mM Tris-HCl, 5 mM EDTA, pH 8.5.
24. Sulfolink coupling gel (Pierce, IL).
25. 50 mM Cysteine in Tris buffer.
26. 1 M NaCl.
27. 10 mM NaH$_2$PO$_4$, 800 mM NaCl, pH 7.2.
28. 0.2 M glycine/HCl, pH 2.4.
29. Polyethylene glycol (PEG) (M$_r$ 10,000).
30. Sodium azide (2%).
31. Tris-buffered saline (TBS): 25 mM Tris-HCl, 137 mM NaCl, pH 7.6.
32. Triton X-100.

33. TBST: TBS containing 1% Tween-20.
34. Bicinchoninic acid solution (BCA).
35. Copper (II) sulphate solution (4% w/v).
36. Pump, e.g., Microperpex S peristaltic pump (LKB Bromma).
37. Spectrophotometer, e.g., Ultrospec 2000 (Pharmacia Biotech).
38. Fraction collector, e.g., Frac100 (Pharmacia).
39. Sterile 19 gauge needles.
40. Teflon tubing.
41. Syringes.
42. Falcon tubes.
43. Rotor/mixer, e.g., Spiramix 5 (Denley).

2.2. Immunoprecipitation

1. TBS-TX: TBS containing 1% Triton X-100.
2. Protein A immobilized on sepharose CL-4B. Store in PBS/azide (2%) at 4°C (Sigma).

2.3. SDS-PAGE and Western Blotting

1. 5X Sample buffer: 0.065 M Tris-HCl, pH 6.8, 2% SDS, 5% sucrose, 0.02% bromophenol blue.
2. 2-Mercaptoethanol.
3. Acetone.
4. 30% Acrylamide/Bis solution (37.5:1).
5. 1.5 M Tris-HCl, pH 8.8.
6. 1 M Tris-HCl, pH 6.8.
7. Sodium dodecyl sulfate (SDS).
8. 10% Ammonium persulfate, freshly prepared for each use.
9. $N,N,N'N'$-Tetramethylethylene diamine (TEMED).
10. Running buffer (5X: 14.5 g Tris, 72.4 g glycine, 5 g SDS made up to 1 L with dH$_2$O.
11. Whatman 3mm paper.
12. Immobilon-P polyvinylidene difluoride (PVDF) membrane (Millipore UK Ltd., Herts, UK).
13. Methanol.
14. CAPS buffer, pH 11: 1.1 g CAPS, 10% methanol, freshly prepared for each use.
15. ECL kit (Amersham Pharmacia Biotech, UK).
16. Western blotting apparatus, e.g., Trans-blot-SD, semi-dry transfer cell (Bio-Rad).

2.4. Immunocytochemistry

1. Dulbecco's phosphate-buffered saline (DPBS).
2. Methanol/acetone (1:1).
3. Normal goat serum.
4. Gelatin.
5. Species-specific FITC- or TRITC-conjugated whole antibody.
6. Species-specific biotinylated whole antibody.
7. Streptavidin-fluorescein.

Table 2
Fluorogenic ECE Substrates S_1, S_2, and S_3

S_1	Ac-Ile-Ile-**Pya-Nop**-Asn-Thr-Pro-Glu-His-Val-Val-Pro-Tyr-Gly-Leu-Gly-Ser-COOH
S_2	Ac-Ser-Gly-**Pya**-Lys-Ala-Phe-Ala-**Nop**-Gly-Lys-NH$_2$
S_3	(7-methoxycoumarin-4-yl)acetyl-Arg-Pro-Pro-Gly-Phe-Ser-Ala-Phe-Lys(2,4 dinitrophenyl)

The fluorescent chromophore, pyrenylalanine (Pya), and the quencher, p-nitrophenylalanine (Nop) in S_1 and S_2, are indicated in bold.

8. Vectashield mounting medium (Vector Laboratories Inc.).
9. Ethanol.
10. 1% H_2O_2 in methanol.
11. 0.1% Phenylhydrazine chloride in TBS.
12. Acetone.
13. 3,3'-Diaminobenzidine (DAB) tablets.
14. DPX mounting medium.

2.5. ECE Assays

2.5.1. HPLC Assay

1. 100 mM Tris-HCl buffer, pH 7.0.
2. Captopril (100 µM, stored at $-20°C$).
3. Thiorphan (5 mM in ethanol, stored at $-20°C$ for 1 mo).
4. Phosphoramidon stored as 5 mM stock at $-20°C$.
5. Bradykinin stored as 5 mM stock at $-20°C$.
6. Reverse-phase µBondapak C_{18} column.
7. Acetonitrile (9–91%) in 0.02% (v/v) trifluoroacetic acid, pH 2.5.

2.5.2. Fluorescence-Based Assay

1. Synthetic substrates: *see* **Table 2**.
2. 50 mM Tris-maleate buffer, pH 6.8.
3. Solvent A: 0.05% (v/v) trifluoroacetic acid in water.
4. Solvent B: 0.038% (v/v) trifluoroacetic acid in CH_3CN/H_2O 90:10 (v/v).

3. Methods

3.1. Production of Isoform-Specific Antibodies

3.1.1. Peptide Design

There are several criteria when designing peptides for raising polyclonal antibodies against any protein including hydrophilicity, surface accessibility, and secondary structure (for discussion, *see* **ref. 23**). However, in the particular

Table 3
Peptide Sequences, Based on the Human ECE-1 Isoforms,
to Which the Antibodies Are Raised

Isoform	Peptides used for antibody production	Isoform detected
ECE-1a	CQGKRGPGLTSPNH$_2$	ECE-1a
ECE-1b	RGVWPPPVSALLSALGCNH$_2$	ECE-1b
ECE-1c	SYKRATLDEEDLCNH$_2$	ECE-1b and ECE-1c
ECE-1d	EALRESVLHLALQCNH$_2$	ECE-1d

Because the N-terminal sequence of ECE-1c is contained within ECE-1b, apart from a single extra methionine residue at the N-terminus of ECE-1c, a unique sequence for ECE-1c is not available for anti-peptide antibody production. NH$_2$ represents C-terminal amidation.

case of the ECE-1 isoforms, peptides based on the sequences of their N-terminal domains are necessary to distinguish between them (**Table 3**). A minimum purity of 70% of the peptides is confirmed by mass spectrometry. C-terminal amidation of the peptides minimizes desulfurization of cysteine residues.

3.1.2. Conjugation

1. Dialyze ovalbumin (10 mg) in 625 µL 10 mM NaH$_2$PO$_4$ buffer, pH 7.4, overnight at 4°C against 2 L of the same buffer.
2. Transfer to an Eppendorf and centrifuge at 10,000g to remove precipitated material. Transfer 500 µL (80 µg ovalbumin) to a fresh Eppendorf, add 10 µL of 50 mM NEM and incubate at 25°C for 10 min (*see* **Note 1**).
3. Slowly add Sulfo MBS (4 mg in 200 µL H$_2$O) to the mixture and incubate at 25°C for 30 min. Remove excess NEM and Sulfo MBS by chromatography using a 1 × 20 cm column of Sephadex G50 equilibrated with 50 mM NaH$_2$PO$_4$, pH 6.0, at a flow rate of 20 mL/h. Measure the absorbance of 1-mL fractions at 280 nm, collect the peak void volume fractions and store on ice.
4. Add 40 µL 0.5 M DTT to 8 mg of the synthetic peptide and incubate for 1 h at 25°C under nitrogen.
5. Separate the reduced peptide from excess DTT by chromatography on a 1 × 20 cm column of Sephadex G10 equilibrated in 50 mM NaH$_2$PO$_4$, pH 6.0 at a flow rate of 15 mL/h at 4°C. Collect 1 mL fractions and measure their absorbance at 230 nm. Pool the peak fractions containing the peptide and store on ice.
6. To ensure the complete separation of excess DTT from the reduced protein, assay the fraction using the DTNB assay: on a 96-well plate, add 13 µL 5 mM DTNB, 60 µL 100 mM NaH$_2$PO$_4$, pH 7.4 and 17 µL H$_2$O to 10 µL of each fraction. Incubate the samples at room temp for 10 min and measure the absorbance at 405 nm using a plate reader.

7. To couple the activated peptide and carrier, mix the pooled fractions of the activated ovalbumin from **step 3** and reduced peptide from **step 5** and adjust the pH to 7.4 with 0.1 M NaOH.

8. Incubate at 25°C for 4 h then dialyze the fractions against 2 L of 10 mM NaH$_2$PO$_4$, 145 mM NaCl, pH 7.2, at 4°C overnight.

9. Determine the protein concentration by BCA assay *(24)*.

3.1.3. Immunization

1. Ensure that a preimmune bleed is taken from each rabbit prior to immunization. Allow the blood to clot then centrifuge and remove the serum. Divide the serum into aliquots and store at −70°C.

2. Dilute approx 200 µg of the conjugated protein from **Subheading 3.1.2.** in 0.5 mL PBS. For the initial injection mix the conjugate with 0.5 mL Complete Freund's Adjuvant. To do this, connect two sterile 19 gauge needles via a short length of Teflon tubing. With the required amount of adjuvant or conjugated protein in separate syringes, attach the syringes to the needles and mix the contents by forcing the emulsion through the tubing several times. Once thoroughly mixed, draw the emulsion into one of the syringes for immunization.

3. Inject each peptide into two New Zealand white rabbits subcutaneously in the back.

4. Administer the first booster injection 4 wk after the initial injection. The booster injections should consist of 100 µg of protein in Incomplete Freund's Adjuvant, prepared as described in **step 2**. Subsequent booster injections may be given at minimum intervals of 4 wk.

5. Obtain the first test bleed (20–40 mL) 7–10 d after the first booster injection, and subsequent test bleeds 7–10 d after each booster injection.

6. Allow the blood from each test bleed to clot, centrifuge to remove cellular material, aliquot the serum and store at −70°C.

7. Determine the sensitivity and specificity of the response by ELISA.

3.1.4. ELISA

1. Each assay is carried out in triplicate. Blank wells, binding of preimmune serum, and binding to an alternative peptide are used as controls in each case.

2. Coat the wells of a 96-well plate with 80 µL (0.25 µg/mL) of the peptide to which the antiserum was raised, or an opposing peptide, in coating buffer overnight at 4°C.

3. Remove the antigen and wash the plate 3× with PBS, 0.05% v/v Tween-20.

4. Add 200 µL PBS containing 5% (w/v) low-fat milk powder to each well and incubate for 2 h at 37°C, then repeat the washes as described in **step 2**.

5. Add 100 µL of serially diluted antiserum in antibody buffer to each well and incubate for 2 h at 37°C. Repeat the washes as described in **step 2**.

6. Add 100 µL of anti-rabbit horseradish peroxidase IgG (1/1000 in antibody buffer) to each well and incubate for 2 h at 37°C. Repeat the washes as described in **step 2**.

7. Add 100 μL of substrate solution to each well and incubate in the dark for 30 min at room temp. Stop the reaction by adding 100 μL of 1 *M* citric acid to each well.

8. Measure the absorbance at 405 nm.

3.1.5. Purification

1. Purification is carried out by affinity chromatography, attaching the cysteine-containing peptides, to which the antisera are raised, to iodoacetyl-agarose.

2. Pour a 1 × 20 cm column of Sephadex G10 and equilibrate by pumping through several column volumes of Tris buffer at a flow rate of 12 mL/h.

3. Reduce 3 mg of synthetic peptide in 500 μL Tris buffer by incubating with 25 μL of 1 *M* DTT under nitrogen at room temp for 1 h, then apply to the G10 column at a flow rate of 12 mL/h.

4. Collect 1-mL fractions, measure their absorbance at 230 nm and carry out DTNB assays (as described in **Subheading 3.1.2.**) to confirm the separation of the excess DTT from the reduced peptide. Pool the peak peptide fractions and store on ice.

5. Wash 3 mL of Sulfolink coupling gel (6 mL of slurry) at room temp with 6 volumes of Tris buffer to remove the storage buffer. Transfer the gel into a 10-mL Falcon tube, centrifuge for 1 min at 100*g* and discard the supernatant.

6. Add the pooled fractions from **step 4** to the gel and incubate at room temperature, slowly rotating the tube for 25 min in the dark. Continue the incubation for a further 30 min without rotation.

7. Centrifuge the gel for 1 min at 100*g* and discard the supernatant, retaining samples to assay for thiol content to determine the efficiency of coupling if required.

8. Remove excess peptide by washing 3× with Tris buffer.

9. Add 5 mL 50 m*M* cysteine in Tris buffer and incubate at room temp in the dark for 25 min with rotation, then 30 min without. Centrifuge for 1 min at 100*g* and discard the supernatant.

10. Wash the gel with 50 mL of 1 *M* NaCl, then equilibrate by washing with PBS. Pour the gel into a 5 mL column and pump through several volumes of PBS at a flow rate of 12 mL/h.

11. Thaw the antiserum on ice and filter through a sterile 0.45 μm filter before loading onto the column.

12. Collect 2-mL fractions and measure their absorbance at 280 nm.

13. Elute with 10 m*M* NaH_2PO_4, 800 m*M* NaCl, pH 7.2, until the A_{280} falls to zero, retaining fractions for protein assay.

14. Elute with 0.2 *M* glycine/HCl, pH 2.4, pool peak fractions, as indicated by A_{280}, and rapidly neutralize with NaOH.

15. Dialyze the pooled fractions against 2 L PBS overnight at 4°C. Concentrate the antiserum in the dialysis tubing using PEG 10,000, then add sodium azide at a final concentration of 0.02% for storage at 4°C.

3.2. Immunoprecipitation

1. Wash the protein A beads 3×, by centrifuging in TBS-TX at 100*g* for 1 min then discarding the supernatant to remove the storage buffer.

2. Dilute the protein preparation from which the ECE-1 isoform is to be immuno-precipitated to 1 mg/mL in TBS-TX and incubate with 10% w/v protein A for 1 h at 4°C with shaking.
3. Centrifuge the sample to remove the beads then divide the supernatant into 2 aliquots. Add 0.5 μL of preimmune serum to one aliquot and 0.5 μL of purified antiserum to the other then incubate the samples on ice for 1 h.
4. Add 10% w/v protein A to each sample and incubate for 1 h at 4°C with rocking.
5. Collect the beads by centrifugation and remove and retain the supernatant.
6. Wash the beads 3× with TBS-TX, removing as much of the supernatant as possible in the final wash.
7. Add 20 μL of 5X sample buffer to each sample and heat at 85°C for 10 min.
8. Centrifuge at 10,000g, remove the supernatant and store at −20°C. The beads may be discarded.
9. For SDS-PAGE and Western blotting, add 1 μL of 2-mercaptoethanol to each sample and heat at 100°C for 4 min. Analyze the supernatants from **steps 5** and **8** to illustrate binding efficiency.

3.3. SDS-PAGE and Western Blotting

1. Analyze samples by SDS-PAGE according to the methods of Laemmli *(25)* using a 7.5% gel.
2. Set up Western blotting apparatus. Prior to assembly, soak the PVDF membrane in methanol for a few seconds then rinse in water. Soak the SDS gel, Whatman 3mm chromatography paper and PVDF membrane in CAPS buffer for 10 min, then assemble. Probe with specific antibodies and anti-rabbit or anti-mouse HRP conjugated antibody. A band of 120 kDa is visualized using the ECL kit (**Fig. 3**).

3.4. Immunocytochemistry

3.4.1. Cultured Cells (*Fig. 4*)

1. Fix and stain cells (e.g., CHO) grown on coverslips 24–48 h post-transfection as follows.
2. Remove normal growth medium from the cells and wash them 3× with DPBS.
3. Fix the cells by adding methanol:acetone (1:1) for 10 min then wash 3× with TBS.
4. Block the cells with TBS containing 1% normal goat serum and 0.2% gelatin for 30 min at room temperature.
5. Incubate in primary antibody at room temp for 2 h.
6. Wash the cells 3× with TBS.
7. For transfected cells, incubate with the secondary, FITC-conjugated antibody (1/100) for 30 min at room temperature.
   For cell lines and stably transfected cells, incubate with species-specific biotinylated whole antibody (1/100) for 1 h followed by streptavidin-fluorescin (1/400) for 30 min.
8. Wash the cells 3× in TBS and mount on glass slides in Vectashield.

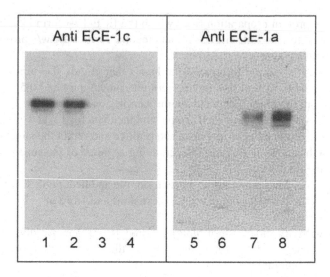

Fig. 3. Western blotting using antipeptide antibodies to ECE-1c and ECE-1a. Solubilised membranes from CHO cells expressing ECE-1c (lanes 1, 2, 5, and 6) or ECE-1a (lanes 3, 4, 7, and 8) were probed with isoform-specific antipeptide antibodies to ECE-1c and ECE-1a.

3.4.2. Tissue Samples

1. Deparaffinize sections from tissue samples in xylene for 10 min.
2. Rinse in 100% ethanol for 5 min.
3. Block endogenous peroxidase activity by incubating in 1% H_2O_2 in methanol for 20 min then 0.1% phenylhydrazine hydrochloride in TBS for 20 min.
4. Rinse twice in water then place the slides in ice-cold acetone for 10 min.
5. Rinse in TBS for 10 min.
6. Block for 30 min in TBS containing 0.2% gelatin and 1% normal goat serum.
7. Add primary antibody diluted in block solution and incubate overnight at 4°C.
8. Wash slides 3× with TBS.
9. Add species-specific biotinylated whole antibody (1/50) and incubate for 1 h at room temperature.
10. Wash slides 3× with TBS.
11. Add streptavidin-horseradish peroxidase conjugate (1/100) for 30 min at room temperature.
12. Wash slides 3× with TBS.
13. Add DAB substrate and incubate for 15 min.
14. Dehydrate slides in 75%, 95%, then 100% ethanol, dry, then mount in DPX.

3.5. ECE Assays

To aid the investigation of potential ECE-selective inhibitors, several types of ECE assay have been developed (*see* **Note 2**). These can be immunological,

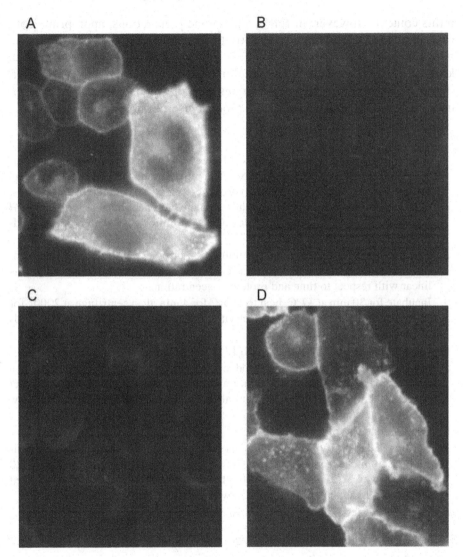

Fig. 4. Immunofluorescence studies of expressed ECE-1 in CHO cells using the isoform-specific antibodies. CHO cells transfected with ECE-1c (**A** and **B**) or ECE-1a (**C** and **D**) were stained with antibodies to ECE-1c (**A** and **C**) or ECE-1a (**B** and **D**).

HPLC-based or fluorometric. Since separation of big ET-1 from ET-1 is difficult to achieve efficiently by HPLC, ET-1 based immunoassays are the preferred methodology for directly measuring ET-1 production in cell culture (*see* Chapter 2). For HPLC-based assays, other substrates of ECE-1 are more convenient, either natural or synthetic. Bradykinin has a similar k_{cat}/K_m as big ET-1 with ECE-1 *(6,7)*, is readily available commercially and is hence valuable in this context. However, in cell or membrane preparations, appropriate controls are needed to eliminate other activities hydrolysing the chosen substrate. In addition, synthetic peptides, such as [Phe^{22}] big ET-1 (**Fig. 2**) have been developed which are hydrolyzed much more efficiently than big ET-1 itself. The discovery of further ECE-1 substrates may allow more efficient assay techniques to be developed or adapted to produce useful fluorogenic substrates.

3.5.1. HPLC Assay

1. Add 10 µg of total protein from solubilized membranes in a total volume of 100 µL 100 mM Tris-HCl buffer, pH 7.0, with captopril (1 µM) and thiorphan (10 µM) to block angiotensin-converting enzyme (ACE) and NEP activities, respectively. Assays should be conducted in the presence and absence of 100 µM phosphoramidon (or other suitable ECE-1 inhibitor), the difference providing the ECE-1 activity.
2. Start the reaction by adding bradykinin (BK), or other substrate, to a final concentration of 0.1–2.0 mM. Maintain reaction conditions such that hydrolysis is linear with respect to time and protein concentration.
3. Incubate for 30 min at 37°C, heat to 100°C for 4 min, then centrifuge at 2000g for 20 min at 4°C. Depending on the activity in the preparation, longer time periods of incubation may be necessary.
4. Analyze the reaction products by HPLC.
5. Separate BK from its hydrolysis products, BK(1-7) and BK(8-9) (Phe-Arg), on a reverse-phase µBondapak C$_{18}$ column, using trifluoroacetic acid/acetonitrile/water as the mobile phase. Carry out all the separations at room temp at a flow rate of 1.5 mL/min.
6. Filter and degas solvents before use.
7. Resolve and quantify BK, BK(1–7) and BK(8–9) by HPLC using a linear gradient of acetonitrile from 9–91% in 0.02% (v/v) trifluoroacetic acid, pH 2.5, for 20 min, followed by a 5-min wash at final conditions. Product detection is carried out at 214 nm and quantification achieved by use of an appropriate standard.
8. Other substrates and their products can be analyzed using similar procedures.

3.5.2. Fluorescence-Based Assays

An alternative type of assay is the fluorescence-based assay utilizing a fluorogenic substrate. This generally has advantages of sensitivity and speed, allowing continuous monitoring of enzyme activity. In this method, two new ECE substrates are described below (S$_1$ and S$_2$), based on the concept of intramolecularly-quenched fluorescence, whose cleavage generates intense fluorescence emission *(26)*. An additional internally-quenched fluorescent substrate (S$_3$), derived from bradykinin, has been developed *(27)*, which is suitable for rapid continuous assay of the enzyme using a microplate format in a fluorescent plate reader (**Table 2**). As with HPLC-based assays, appropriate controls are needed to eliminate other protease activities in the preparation under study.

1. ECE substrates S_1, which is the (19–35) fragment of big ET-1, and S_2 from a biased substrate peptide library (**Table 2**), and their corresponding fluorescent metabolites were synthesized as described *(26)*.

2. To determine the fluorescence increase with substrate degradation, establish calibration curves by adding increasing quantities of the fluorescent metabolites and decreasing quantities of substrate to 100 µL in 50 m*M* Tris-maleate buffer (pH 6.8).

3. The ECE assays can be carried out in 96-well plates in a final volume of 100 µL. Incubate reactions for 1 h at 37°C. Stop the reaction by immediately cooling to 4°C for 10 min and measure the fluorescence (λ_{ex} = 340 nm, λ_{em} = 400 nm).

4. Reaction products formed by the hydrolysis of S_1 and S_2 can also be characterized by HPLC. Inject 50 µL of the reaction mixture onto a C_{18} column. Elute using a gradient of 0–100% Solvent B over 30 min with a flow rate of 1 mL/min.

4. Notes

1. NEM blocks free SH groups on the protein. The succinimide ester end of the Sulfo MBS will react with the protein amino groups, yielding a protein covered with maleimide groups. Incubation with DTT ensures that all the peptide thiol groups are reduced. DTNB reacts with sulphydryl compounds to yield a mixed disulfide and the bright yellow thionitrobenzoate anion at alkaline pH.

2. Early assay developments included using the scintillation proximity assay principle and [125I] big ET-1 as the substrate *(28)*; a rapid bioassay for ET-1 together with ELISA *(29)* and a radioassay based on the quantitative determination of [125I] ET-1 released from (3-[125I] iodo-tyrosyl(13))big ET-1 by binding to the ET receptor *(30)*. Further developments include: a procedure for individual measurement of big ET-1 and the two products, ET-1 and the C-terminal fragment, using selective solid phase extraction and specific immunoassays *(31)* and a live-cell assay for studying extracellular and intracellular ECE activity using a luciferase reporter cell line that permanently expresses the ET_A receptor *(32)*. More recently, the identification of bradykinin as a suitable substrate in ECE assays and the development of fluorescence assays have increased the ease and efficiency of assaying ECE activity. Big ET-1 itself is not necessarily the best substrate to use in such ECE assays. The N-terminal disulfide-loop structure in big ET-1 appears to hinder conversion since truncated forms have substantially higher specific activity *(33)*. However, [Phe[22]]big ET-1 (18–34) exhibits 12-fold higher specific activity than big ET-1 itself and is a useful synthetic substrate for assay of ECE.

Acknowledgments

We thank the National Research Fund (UK) for financial support.

References

1. Schmidt, M., Kroger, B., Jacob, E., Seulberger, H., Subkowski, T., Otter, R., et al. (1994) Molecular characterization of human and bovine endothelin converting enzyme (ECE-1). *FEBS Lett.* **356**, 238–243.

2. Shimada, K., Matsushita, Y., Wakabayashi, K., Takahashi, M., Matsubara, A., Iijima, Y., and Tanzawa, K. (1995) Cloning and functional expression of human endothelin-converting enzyme cDNA. *Biochem. Biophys. Res. Comm.* **207,** 807–812.
3. Emoto, N. and Yanagisawa, M. (1995) Endothelin-converting enzyme-2 is a membrane-bound, phosphoramidon-sensitive metalloprotease with acidic pH optimum. *J. Biol. Chem.* **270,** 15,262–15,268.
4. Hasegawa, H., Hiki, K., Sawamura, T., Aoyama, T., Okamoto, Y., Miwa, S., et al. (1998) Purification of a novel endothelin-converting enzyme specific for big endothelin-3. *FEBS Lett.* **428,** 304–308.
5. Turner, A. J., Isaac, R. E., and Coates D. (2001) The neprilysin (NEP) family of zinc metalloendopeptidases: genomics and function. *Bioessays* **23,** 261–269.
6. Hoang, M. V. and Turner, A. J. (1997) Novel activity of endothelin-converting enzyme: hydrolysis of bradykinin. *Biochem. J.* **327,** 23–26.
7. Johnson, G. D., Stevenson, T., and Ahn, K. (1999) Hydrolysis of peptide hormones by endothelin-converting enzyme-1 *J. Biol. Chem.* **274,** 4053–4058.
8. Barnes, K., Walkden, B. J., Wilkinson, T. C., and Turner, A. J. (1997) Expression of endothelin-converting enzyme in both neuroblastoma and glial cell lines and its localization in rat hippocampus. *J. Neurochem.* **68,** 570–577.
9. Schweizer, A., Valdenaire, O., Nelbock, P., Deuschle, U., Dumas Milne Edwards, J. B., Stumpf, J. G., and Loffler, B. M. (1997) Human endothelin-converting enzyme (ECE-1): three isoforms with distinct subcellular localizations. *Biochem. J.* **328,** 871–877.
10. Valdenaire, O., Lepailleur-Enouf, D., Egidy, G., Thouard, A., Barret, A., Vranckx, R., et al. (1999) A fourth isoform of endothelin-converting enzyme (ECE-1) is generated from an additional promoter. *Eur. J. Biochem.* **264,** 341–349.
11. Barnes, K., Brown, C., and Turner, A. J. (1998) Endothelin-converting enzyme: ultrastructural localization and its recycling from the cell surface. *Hypertension* **31,** 3–9.
12. Emoto, N., Nurhantari, Y., Alimsardjono,H., Xie, J., Yamada, T., Yanagisawa, M., and Matsuo, M. (1999) Constitutive lysosomal targeting and degradation of bovine endothelin-converting enzyme-1a mediated by novel signals in its alternatively spliced cytoplasmic tail. *J. Biol. Chem.* **274,** 1509–1518.
13. Valdenaire, O., Barret, A., Schweizer, A., Rohrbacher, E., Mongiat, F., Pinet, F., et al. (1999b) Two di-leucine-based motifs account for the different subcellular localizations of the human endothelin-converting enzyme (ECE-1) isoforms. *J. Cell Sci.* **112,** 3115–3125.
14. Cailler, F., Zappulla, J. P., Boileau, G., and Crine, P. (1999) The N-terminal segment of endothelin-converting enzyme (ECE)-1b contains a di-leucine motif that can redirect neprilysin to an intracellular compartment in Madin-Darby canine kidney (MDCK) cells. *Biochem. J.* **341,** 119–126.
15. Yanagisawa, H., Yanagisawa, M., Kapur, R. P., Richardson, J. A., Williams, S. C., Clouthier, D. E., et al. (1998) Dual genetic pathways of endothelin-mediated intercellular signalling revealed by targeted disruption of endothelin-converting enzyme-1 gene. *Development* **125,** 825–836.

16. Barker, S., Khan, N. Q., Wood, E. G., and Corder, R. (2001) Effect of an antisense oligodeoxynucleotide to endothelin-converting enzyme-1c (ECE-1c) on ECE-1c mRNA, ECE-1 protein and endothelin-1 synthesis in bovine pulmonary artery smooth muscle cells. *Mol. Pharmacol.* **59,** 163–169.
17. DeLombaert, S., Ghai, R. D., Jeng, A. Y., Trapani, A. J., and Webb, R. L. (1994) *Biochem. Biophys. Res. Comm.* **204,** 407–412.
18. Wallace, E. M., Moliterni, J. A., Moskal, M. A., Neubert, A. D., Marcopulos, N., Stamford, L. B., et al. (1998) Design and synthesis of potent, selective inhibitors of endothelin-converting enzyme. *J. Med. Chem.* **41,** 1513–1523.
19. Ahn, K., Sisneros, A. M., Herman, S. B., Pan, S. M., Hupe, D., Lee, C., et al. (1998) Novel quinazoline inhibitors of endothelin-converting enyme-1. *Biochem. Biophys. Res. Comm.* **243,** 184–190.
20. Russell, F. D. and Davenport, A. P. (1999) Evidence for intracellular endothelin-converting enzyme-2 expression in cultured human vascular endothelial cells. *Circ. Res.* **84,** 891–896.
21. Wada, A., Tsutamoto, T., Ohnishi, M., Sawaki, M., Fukai, D., Maeda, Y., and Kinoshita, M. (1999) Effects of a specific endothelin-converting enzyme inhibitor on cardiac, renal, and neurohumoral functions in congestive heart failure: comparison of effects with those of endothelin A receptor antagonism. *Circulation* **99,** 570–577.
22. Yanagisawa, M., Kurihara, H., Kimura, S., Tomobe, Y., Kobayashi, M., Mitsui, Y., et al. (1988) A novel potent vasoconstrictor peptide produced by vascular endothelial cells. *Nature* **332,** 411–415.
23. Baldwin, S. A. (1994) *Methods in Molecular Biology, vol 27: Biomembrane Protocols: II, Architecture and Function.* (Graham, J. M., ed.) Humana, Totowa, NJ.
24. Smith, P. K., Krohn, R. I., Hermanson, G. T., Mallia, A. K., Gartner, F. H., Provenzano, M. D., et al. (1985) Measurement of protein using bicinchoninic acid. *Anal. Biochem.* **150,** 76–85.
25. Laemmli, U. K. (1970) Cleavage of structural proteins during the assembly of the head of bacteriophage T4. *Nature* **227,** 680–685.
26. Luciani, N., De Rocquigny, H., Turcaud, S., Romieu, A., and Roques, B. P. (2001) Highly sensitive and selective fluorescence assays for rapid screening of endothelin-converting enzyme inhibitors. *Biochem. J.* **356,** 813–819.
27. Johnson, G. D. and Ahn, K. (2000) Development of an internally quenched fluorescent substrate selective for endothelin-converting enzyme-1. *Anal. Biochem.* **286,** 112–118.
28. Matsumura, Y., Umekawa, T., Kawamura, H., Takaoka, M., Robinson, P. S., Cook, N. D., and Morimoto, S. (1992) A simple method for measurement of phosphoramidon-sensitive endothelin-converting enzyme activity *Life Sci.* **51,** 1603–1611.
29. Warner, T. D., Budzik, G. P., Mitchell, J. A., Huang, Z. J., and Murad, F. (1992) Detection by bioassay and specific enzyme-linked-immunosorbent assay of phosphoramidon-inhibitable endothelin-converting enzyme activity in brain and endothelium. *J. Cardiovasc. Pharmacol.* **20(Suppl. 12),** S19–S21.

30. Fawzi, A. B., Cleven, R. M., and Wright, D. L. (1994) A rapid and selective endothelin-converting enzyme assay - characterization of a phosphoramidon-sensitive enzyme from guinea-pig membrane. *Anal. Biochem.* **222,** 342–350.

31. Plumpton, C., Haynes, W. G., Webb, D. J., and Davenport, A. P. (1995) Measurement of C-terminal fragment of big endothelin-1 in humans *J. Cardiovasc. Pharmacol.* **26(Suppl. 3),** S34–S36.

32. Parnot, C., LeMoullec, J. M., Cousin, M. A., Guedin, D. Corvol, P., and Pinet, F. (1997) A live cell assay for studying extracellular and intracellular endothelin-converting enzyme activity. *Hypertension* **30,** 837–844.

33. Turner, A. J. and Murphy, L. J. (1996) Molecular pharmacology of endothelin-converting enzymes *Biochem. Pharmacol.* **51,** 91–102.

8

Quantitative Measurement of mRNA Levels by RT-PCR

Studies of ECE-1 Isoforms

Delphine M. Lees, Noorafza Q. Khan, Stewart Barker, and Roger Corder

1. Introduction

The original description of endothelin-1 (ET-1) included the concept that a novel processing enzyme, referred to as endothelin-converting enzyme (ECE), was required for cleavage of the Trp^{21}-Val^{22} bond in the biosynthetic intermediate big ET-1 (1). Initially it was thought that ECE could be a chymotrypsin-like enzyme because of the nature of the peptide bond being cleaved (1). The challenge of identifying ECE was soon taken up by many groups and a variety of different proteolytic activities were proposed as potential ECEs (2). By 1990, studies of endogenous ET-1 synthesis by cultured endothelial cells and investigations of the systemic pressor effect of intravenously administered big ET-1 indicated that the physiological ECE was a phosphoramidon-sensitive enzyme (3–5). Phosphoramidon was also shown to inhibit hydrolysis of exogenous big ET-1 by cultured vascular smooth muscle and endothelial cells (6). The pursuit of an ECE that could selectively hydrolyze big ET-1 and was inhibited by phosphoramidon led quickly to the purification and cloning of a metallopeptidase called endothelin-converting enzyme-1 (ECE-1) (7–9). Shortly after this, a second phosphoramidon-sensitive peptidase, with ~59% structural homology to ECE-1, was cloned and called ECE-2 (10). ECE-1 and ECE-2 are members of a family of type II integral membrane peptidases that also includes neutral endopeptidase 24.11 and the KELL and PEX proteins (11).

Four isoforms of ECE-1 have now been identified—namely, ECE-1a, ECE-1b, ECE-1c and ECE-1d (12–15). The four isoforms are synthesized from the same

From: *Methods in Molecular Biology, vol. 206: Peptide Research Protocols: Endothelin*
Edited by: J. Maguire and A. Davenport © Humana Press Inc., Totowa, NJ

gene by differential splicing of the first four exons in the 5' gene sequence *(12,13)*, with the result that the four isoforms differ only in their N-terminal amino acid sequences. From the transmembraneous sequence through to the C-terminus, the four ECE-1 proteins have identical amino acid sequences. The identification of ECE-1 in endothelial cells led to it being proposed as the physiologically relevant ECE for ET-1 biosynthesis *(7–9)*. Subsequent studies have shown all four ECE-1 isoforms are expressed in endothelial cells, but only ECE-1b and ECE-1c are expressed to any extent in vascular smooth muscle cells *(13,15)*. A widespread cell and tissue distribution of ECE-1 mRNA has been described *(16,17)*, but neither the factors regulating cell specific expression of ECE-1 isoforms nor the relationship of specific isoforms to ET-1 synthesis have been fully investigated. Our studies of endothelial cells did not reveal any link between the up- or down- regulation of ET-1 synthesis and the level of ECE-1 expression *(18)*. In blood vessels ECE-1 is more abundant in endothelial cells than vascular smooth muscle cells *(16,19)*. However, the synthesis of ECE-1 increases in the vascular smooth muscle of diseased vessels *(20,21)* and following balloon injury *(21,22)*. This suggests that ECE-1 plays a role in the processes of vascular remodeling irrespective of whether this is linked to changes in ET-1 synthesis.

Ultrastructural studies have shown ET-1 processing in endothelial cells occurs intracellularly *(23)*. Hence, the relationship between particular ECE-1 isoforms and ET-1 synthesis may be a function of their intracellular location. In this respect, ECE-1a and ECE-1c have been localized mainly to the luminal surface of endothelial cells with the characteristics of a classical ectoenzyme *(24–26)*. But ECE-1 immunoreactivity has also been found at intracellular sites sometimes co-localized with ET-1 *(19,26)*. When the four isoforms of ECE-1 are expressed in CHO cells or Madin-Darby canine kidney (MDCK) cells there is a tendency for each isoform to have a specific intracellular distribution *(26–28)*. ECE-1a localizes to the cell surface, ECE-1b is found mainly at intracellular sites such as the *trans*-Golgi network (TGN), and ECE-1c and ECE-1d accumulate both on the cell surface and intracellularly. However, the role played by ECE-1 protein at different cellular sites is uncertain. Indeed, ECE-1 protein associated with the TGN may be newly synthesized protein in transit to other cellular locations where it plays its physiological function. The results from these localization studies should not be overinterpreted because the cellular distribution of ECE-1 isoforms in CHO or MDCK cells may not be consistent with that occurring in cells where there is physiological expression of the respective ECE-1 isoforms.

Although it has been widely assumed that ECE-1 plays a physiological role in ET-1 synthesis, *ECE-1* gene deletion studies failed to confirm this. The phenotype of *ECE-1*$^{-/-}$ mice displays features that are compatible with a combined

ET-1/ET-3 knockout *(29)*. However, evidence that ET-1 or ET-3 synthesis was perturbed as a result of disruption of the physiological ECE was largely inconclusive. Thus, tissue levels of ET-1 in the nonviable $ECE\text{-}1^{-/-}$ fetuses were reduced, but by only 48% compared with control levels *(29)*. As big ET-1 content was not increased, it seems likely that the decreased amount of ET-1 was a result of reduced ET-1 gene expression in ECE-1$^{-/-}$ mice. Work carried out in our laboratory has cast further doubts on the role of ECE-1 in ET-1 biosynthesis *(15)*. Bovine pulmonary artery smooth muscle cells express mainly ECE-1c and some ECE-1b, with negligible amounts of ECE-1a and ECE-1d *(15*; **Fig. 1)** (*see* **Subheading 3.4.2.4.**). Treatment of these cells with an antisense oligonucleotide to ECE-1c depleted *ECE-1* protein levels by ≈70% but was virtually free of any effect on ET-1 synthesis *(15)*. This suggests that an ECE distinct from ECE-1 is the physiologically-relevant processing enzyme.

The physiological function of ECE-1 and its relationship to the actions of the endothelin family of peptides remains to be elucidated. The observation that ET-1 synthesis is not prevented in $ECE\text{-}1^{-/-}$ mice, even though the phenotype has parallels with combined ET-1/ET-3 knockout, suggests a role in receptor mediated events rather than peptide biosynthesis. Indeed, interference with ET_A and ET_B receptor function would be expected to have a similar effect as ET-1 and ET-3 gene deletion *(29)*. Therefore, sensitive methods for quantifying the expression of specific ECE-1 isoforms can play an important part in studying the pattern of ECE-1 expression under different conditions.

In recent years, reverse transcription-polymerase chain reaction (RT-PCR) has become one of the most widely used methods for studying gene expression *(30)*. Compared to other methods to evaluate mRNA levels it has the advantages of being both nonradioactive and highly sensitive because it allows the exponential amplification of very low levels of specific mRNA to produce a measurable level of product. The polymerase chain reaction cannot be performed with mRNA as the template, so the first step in RT-PCR based measurements of mRNA levels is the reverse transcription to synthesize a cDNA template suitable for amplification using gene-specific primers. This is followed by the PCR reaction, gel electrophoresis of the products, and quantification by densitometry. Judicious choice of reaction conditions for RT-PCR can provide a semi-quantitative procedure where the yield of product is proportional to the quantity of RNA template *(15,18,31)*. In addition, careful choice of primers can allow the selective measurement of closely related mRNA sequences such as the isoforms of ECE-1 described here. The protocols described below show how readily available commercial reagents can be applied to the quantification of mRNA levels by semi-quantitative RT-PCR *(15,18,31)*. In addition, we describe how the same primer pairs can be applied to quantitative measurements of mRNA levels using the technique of real-time RT-PCR *(30)*.

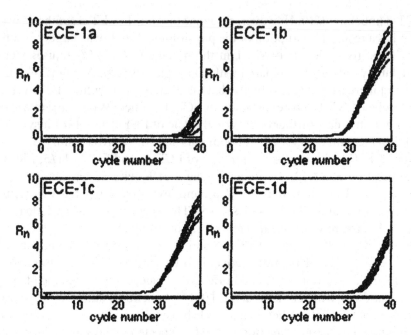

Fig. 1. Amplification plots showing the relative basal levels of ECE-1a, ECE-1b, ECE-1c, and ECE-1d mRNA in total RNA extracted from cultured bovine pulmonary artery smooth muscle cells. The calculated mean Ct values were 34.9 (ECE-1a), 27.8 (ECE-1b), 26.5 (ECE-1c), and 31.6 (ECE-1d). Using the Ct values for the reaction with primers for measuring total ECE-1 isoforms as the internal reference, these samples were found to contain the following relative amounts of each isoform 0.03 % ECE-1a, 22.77% ECE-1b, 76.68% ECE-1c, and 0.53% ECE-1d. This is consistent with previous comparisons made by semi-quantitative RT-PCR *(15)*.

2. Materials

2.1. Chemicals and Solutions

1. Strataprep total RNA miniprep kit (400711, Stratagene, La Jolla, CA).
2. 70% Ethanol: in a sterile tube, mix 7 mL of absolute ethanol with 3 mL of DEPC-treated water, store at room temperature.
3. DEPC-treated water: in a fume hood, add 2–3 drops of DEPC (diethyl pyrocarbonate, Sigma; DEPC stock is stored at +4°C; it is very toxic, therefore, manipulate in a fume hood wearing gloves, eye protection, and a labcoat) to ~200 mL UHQ-water in a 250-mL Duran bottle. Autoclave the solution (*see* **Note 1**).
4. RiboGreen RNA quantitation reagent (R-11491, Molecular Probes, Eugene, OR); store at –20°C, note that this reagent is light-sensitive (caution–potential mutagen).
5. TE buffer: 10 mM Tris-HCl, pH 8.0, 1 mM EDTA, molecular grade, e.g., V2631 Promega, Madison, WI.

6. Access RT-PCR system (A1280, Promega); store at –20°C.
7. Oligo(dT)$_{15}$ primers (e.g., C1101, Promega); store at –20°C.
8. Agarose gel running buffer: in a 1 L cylinder, mix 100 mL 10X TBE buffer (10X TBE: 89 mM Tris base, 89 mM boric acid, 2 mM EDTA) (e.g., T4415, Sigma) and 900 mL UHQ-water. Add 25 µL of a 10 mg/mL solution of ethidium bromide (toxic, carcinogen) (e.g., 161-0433, Bio-Rad, Hercules, CA).
9. Agarose, molecular biology grade.
10. 3X Glycerol loading buffer: in a 50 mL sterile conical tube mix 20 mg bromophenol blue (e.g., B5525, Sigma), 2 mL 10X TBE and 14 mL UHQ-water. Add 4 mL glycerol (e.g., G7757, Sigma), mix by vortexing and store at +4°C.
11. DNA size markers (e.g., ΦX174/HaeIII fragments, 15611-015, Gibco-BRL, Paisley, UK). To the stock solution, add 990 µL of nuclease-free water and 530 µL of 3X glycerol loading buffer. Prepare 200 µL aliquots and store at –20°C.
12. Nuclease-free water (e.g., P1193, Promega).
13. Reverse Transcription System (A3500, Promega); store at –20°C.
14. SYBR® Green PCR Master Mix (SYBR Green 1 dye, AmpliTaq Gold™ DNA polymerase, dNTPs with dUTP, passive reference 1 and optimized reaction buffer; 4309155, Applied Biosystems, Foster City, CA); store at +4°C.
15. Specific custom synthesized oligodeoxynucleotide primers (*see* **Table 1**; e.g., from Oswel, Southampton, UK); store at –20°C.
16. TaqMan® universal PCR Master Mix (AmpliTaq Gold™ DNA polymerase, AmpErase® uracyl-*N*-glycosylase, dNTPs with dUTP, passive reference 1 and optimized reaction buffer; 4304437, Applied Biosystems); store at +4°C.
17. TaqMan® ribosomal RNA control reagents, VIC™ probe (4308329, Applied Biosystems). Prepare aliquots of the primers and probe upon delivery, and avoid multiple freeze/thaw cycles, particularly of the probe. Store the probe overnight at +4°C if you are going to use it again the following day rather than refreezing it.
18. Random hexamers (e.g., C1181, Promega).

2.2. Equipment

1. Autoclaved nuclease-free 1.5-mL microtubes and tips.
2. Microtubes heating block or 60°C water bath.
3. Programmable thermal cycler (e.g., Perkin-Elmer GeneAmp PCR system 2400; Cambridge, UK).
4. Sterile flat-bottom, clear 96-well plates.
5. Fluorescence plate reader.
6. Thin-walled PCR tubes (0.5 mL), nuclease-free.
7. Flat-bed gel electrophoresis apparatus and power pack.
8. UV transilluminator for capturing in real-time fluorescent gel images for computer acquisition and subsequent quantification or analysis (e.g., Gel Doc 1000 system, Bio-Rad, with PowerMac computer).
9. Densitometry software for band analysis and quantification (e.g., Molecular Analyst software, Bio-Rad).
10. Equipment for real-time PCR (e.g., Applied Biosystems, 5700 GeneAmp Sequence Detection System).

Table 1
Oligonucleotide Primers and Cycling Conditions Used for Semi-Quantitative and Real-Time RT-PCR of ECE-1 Isoforms (15,18,31)

Gene	Amplicon size (nt)	Sequence	Sense or antisense	Annealing time/temp	Extension time/temp	Number of cycles
hECE-1a	734	CTGAGACAGGAGGCAGC	S	60/65	120/72	40
hECE-1b/c/d	699	GATGTCGACGTACAAGC	S	60/60	120/68	25
hECE-1b	715	TGCTGTCGGCGCTGGGGATG	S	60/62	120/68	24
hECE-1c	715	GGAGCACGCGAGCTATGATG	S	60/62	120/68	24
hECE-1	n/a	CTGTTGGAGTTCTTGGAATC	AS			
hGAPDH	859	TGAAGGTCGGAGTCAACGGA	S	60/65	120/72	20
		GTGTCGCTGTTGAAGTCAGA	AS			
bECE-1a	767	GGTGGCCGTTCCTCCTCCTGGATTAG	S	60/60	120/68	23
bECE-1b	253	CGCTGTCGGCGCTGGGGATG	S	30/60	60/72	25
bECE-1c	253	GGAGCGCGCGAGCGATGATG	S	30/60	60/72	25
bECE-1d	269	CTTAAGGAGTCCGTGCTGCA	S	30/60	60/72	25
bECE-1a/b/c/d	n/a	GGCGTTCTTGTCTGGTATTGGA	AS			
bECE-1 total	461	TACCAGACAAGAACGCCCTC	S	60/60	120/68	23
		TCGGCACTGACGTAGACGGA	AS			
bGAPDH	556	CGAGATCCTGCCAACATCAA	S	60/60	120/68	20
		GCCTGCTTCACCACCTTCTT	AS			

When performing real-time PCR with the GeneAmp 5700 Sequence Detection System, all reactions are performed using the default conditions of 50°C for 2 min, 95°C for 10 min and (95°C for 15 s, 60°C for 1 min) for 40 cycles.

11. MicroAmp® optical 96-well reaction plates and optical caps (403012, Applied Biosystems).
12. Centrifuge with adapter for 96-well plates.

3. Methods

3.1. Total RNA Isolation

Total RNA is isolated using the Strataprep total RNA miniprep kit (*see* **Note 2**).

1. Aspirate the growth medium from confluent cells grown on 12 × 22 mm-well plates.
2. Prepare the lysis solution by adding 7 μL of β-mercaptoethanol to the lysis buffer for each milliliter of lysis solution needed.
3. Lyse the cells by addition of 350 μL of lysis buffer per well.
4. Reduce the viscosity of the lysate by repeated pipeting and transfer the solution to a sterile 1.5 mL microtube (*see* **Note 3**).
5. Vigorously vortex the tube to homogenize the lysate.
6. Transfer the homogenate to a Prefilter Spin Cup (blue) seated in a 2 mL receptacle tube and close the cap.
7. Centrifuge the tube in a microcentrifuge at maximum speed for 5 min (*see* **Note 4**), remove the Prefilter Spin Cup from the tube and discard it.
8. Retain the filtrate and add 350 μL of 70% ethanol to it. Mix the solution by repeated pipeting.
9. Transfer the solution to a Fibre-Matrix Spin Cup (white) seated in a clean 2 mL receptacle tube and cap it.
10. Centrifuge the tube for 1 min at maximum speed in a microcentrifuge. Open the tube, lift the spin cup with forceps, and discard the filtrate, replace the spin cup in the tube.
11. Add 600 μL of low salt wash buffer, cap the tube and centrifuge for 1 min at maximum speed in a microcentrifuge.
12. Discard the filtrate, replace the spin cup in the receptacle tube, close it, and centrifuge for 2 min at maximum speed in a microcentrifuge.
13. Mix gently in a sterile microtube 50 μL of DNase digestion buffer with 5 μL of RNAse-free DNase I.
14. Add 50 μL of the DNase solution directly onto the fiber matrix and cap the tube, incubate for 15 min at 37°C in an air incubator.
15. Add 600 μL of high salt wash buffer to the spin cup, cap the tube, and centrifuge for 1 min at maximum speed in a microcentrifuge. Discard the filtrate and replace the spin cup in its receptacle tube.
16. Add 600 μL of low salt wash buffer, cap the tube, and centrifuge for 1 min at maximum speed in a microcentrifuge. Discard the filtrate and replace the spin cup in its receptacle tube.
17. Add 300 μL of low salt wash buffer, cap the tube and spin for 2 min at maximum speed in a microcentrifuge to dry the fiber matrix.
18. Transfer the spin cup to a fresh 1.5 mL microtube and discard the 2 mL receptacle tube.
19. Add 30 μL of elution buffer prewarmed to 60°C directly onto the fiber matrix.

20. Cap the tube, incubate for 2 min at room temperature and centrifuge it for 1 min at maximum speed in a microcentrifuge.
21. Repeat **steps 19** and **20** to maximize the yield of RNA.
22. Store the RNA stock solution at –80°C.

3.2. RNA Quantification

The concentration of RNA in each sample is measured using the RiboGreen dye, a sensitive fluorescent nucleic acid stain for quantification of RNA in solution.

1. In one well of a sterile 96-well plate mix by repeated pipeting 105 μL sterile TE with 5 μL of RNA sample solution (dilution factor = 22).
2. From this first well, transfer 10 μL of RNA solution to another well containing 90 μL of TE (dilution from stock = 220).
3. Prepare a 2 μg/mL RNA standard solution in TE (*see* **Note 5**). Dilute the 2 μg/mL RNA solution in the wells, as follows:

Volume (μL) of TE	Volume (μL) of 2 μg/mL RNA standard solution	Final RNA concentration
100	0	0
98	2	20 ng/mL
90	10	100 ng/mL
50	50	500 ng/mL
0	100	1 μg/mL

4. Dilute the stock RiboGreen solution 1/200 in TE, add 100 μL per well, mix by gently tapping the plate, and incubate 2–5 min at room temperature, protected from light.
5. Measure the fluorescence of the samples and standards using a microplate fluorescence reader that is set to the fluorescein wavelengths (excitation ~ 480 nm, emission ~ 520 nm).
6. Generate a standard curve of fluorescence vs RNA concentration, and use this standard curve to calculate the RNA concentration of each sample.

3.3. Semi-Quantitative RT-PCR

3.3.1. Reverse Transcription and Amplification of Sample RNA

The reverse transcription (RT) and polymerase chain reaction (PCR) are performed using the Access RT-PCR system, which is a one-step/two-enzymes system, allowing both reactions to be performed in the same tube.

1. To an autoclaved thin-walled 0.5 mL PCR reaction tube, add the following components, on ice:

Reagent	Amount	Final concentration
Nuclease-free water	to a final volume of 50 μL	
AMV/*Tfl* 5X reaction buffer	10 μL	1X
10 m*M* dNTP mix	1 μL	0.2 m*M*
50 μ*M* sense primer (*see* **Note 6**)	1 μL	1 μ*M*
50 μ*M* antisense primer (*see* **Note 6**)	1 μL	1 μ*M*
50 μ*M* oligo(dT)$_{15}$	1 μL	1 μ*M*
25 m*M* MgSO$_4$	2 μL	1 m*M*
AMV RT (5 U/μL)	1 μL	0.1 U/μL
Tfl DNA polymerase (5 μ/μL)	1 μL	0.1 U/μL
RNA template (*see* **Notes 7** and **8**)	100 ng	

2. Cap the tube and vortex gently to mix the solution.
3. Place the tubes in a microcentrifuge and centrifuge for ~10 s to bring all the liquid to the bottom of the tube.
4. Place the tubes in the thermal cycler heating block and incubate for 45 min at 48°C to perform the reverse transcription step to synthesize the cDNA template for PCR amplification.
5. Denature the RNA/cDNA hybrid and inactivate the reverse transcriptase by incubating the samples for 2 min at 94°C.
6. Amplify the cDNA by incubating for the indicated number of cycles using a programmable thermal cycler (denaturation: 30 s at 94°C; annealing as indicated; extension as indicated [*see* **Table 1**]), followed by a final extension step of 7 min.

3.3.2. Agarose Gel Electrophoresis

1. Prepare a 1.2% (w/v) agarose gel solution: in a 500 mL conical flask pour 150 mL of agarose gel running buffer, add 1.8 g agarose and swirl gently to mix the solution.
2. Swell the agarose by boiling the solution in a microwave on full power (~4–5 min), remove from the microwave after ~2 min and swirl gently to mix the solution. (*Caution*–do not seal flask. Use heat protecting gloves and face shield when handling hot agarose solutions. *See* **Note 1**.)
3. Allow the solution to cool down sufficiently to be able to handle the flask without heat protection (this usually takes about 15 min), and pour the solution in a 10 × 15 cm gel tray containing a thin comb (well size 1 × 5 mm width).
4. Leave the gel to set at room temperature for 30 min.
5. Mix by vortexing 16 μL of the PCR reaction with 8 μL of 3X glycerol loading buffer.
6. Centrifuge for 10 s in a microcentrifuge to bring all the liquid to the bottom of the tube.
7. Place the gel in the tank and cover it with agarose gel running buffer.
8. Carefully remove the comb.
9. In each well load 20 μL of sample diluted in gel loading buffer.
10. Load 10 μL DNA size markers in one lane.

11. Set the gel electrophoresis apparatus to run for 15 min at 50 V to allow the samples to enter the gel, then increase the voltage to 120 V and leave to run for an additional 45–60 min.
12. Turn off the electrophoresis power supply and analyze the gel.

3.3.3. Results Analysis (see *Note 9*)

3.3.3.1. DIGITIZED IMAGE ACQUISITION

1. Place the gel, without its tray, on the UV transilluminator and close the cabinet door.
2. Switch on the UV light.
3. On the camera, adjust the zoom so that the region of interest on the gel fills the window.
4. Click on "Show saturated pixels" to activate this option and avoid over exposure of the images.
5. By modifying the camera aperture and the integration time, optimize the image illumination so that it is just below saturation (*see* **Note 10**).
6. Capture the image and save it to disk for later analysis.

3.3.3.2. IMAGE ANALYSIS

1. Select the rectangle in the volume integration tools.
2. Draw a rectangle around the band representing your PCR product in the first sample lane (*see* **Note 9**).
3. Copy the rectangle and place it around the next lane's band, repeat this until all the bands you want to quantify are included.
4. Click on "Analysis," select the "Local background" option.
5. Click on "Analysis" again, select the "Autointegrate" option.
6. Print the results window.

3.3.3.3. CALCULATIONS

All the calculations are done using the "% volume" values. The results are expressed as percentage of controls, relative to a reference gene (or so-called housekeeping gene) such as GAPDH.

1. For each sample, divide the value for the target gene by the value obtained for GAPDH with the same RNA sample.
2. Mean the value for the controls.
3. Divide each value by the mean value for the controls, and multiply by 100 to yield values as a % of control.
4. Mean the values obtained for each treatment and perform statistical comparisons using standard methods used for other biological variables *(15,18,31)*.

3.4. Quantitative Real Time PCR

Because of the very high sensitivity of real-time PCR quantification, it is advisable to perform the reverse transcription step separately from the amplification reaction.

3.4.1. Reverse Transcription

A stock solution of cDNA is prepared for each sample that will be used for all the different PCR reactions including the measurement of mRNA for the reference gene. The first strand cDNA synthesis is performed using the Reverse Transcription System kit from Promega.

1. Prepare a master mix solution on ice by combining the following reagents in an autoclaved 0.5 mL thin-walled microtube:

Reagent	Amount (*see* **Note 11**)	Final concentration
RNA	1 µg in up to 9 µL	50 ng/µL
25 mM MgCl$_2$	4 µL	5 mM
Reverse Transcription 10X buffer	2 µL	1X
10 mM dNTPs	2 µL	1 mM
40 U/µL RNAsin ribonuclease inhibitor	0.5 µL	1 U/µL
10 U/µL AMV reverse transcriptase	1.5 µL	15 U/µg RNA
0.5 µg/µL random hexamers	1 µL	0.5 µg/µg RNA
Nuclease-free water	to a final volume of 20 µL	

2. Cap the tubes and vortex gently to mix the solution.
3. Place the tubes in a microcentrifuge and centrifuge them for ~10 s to bring all the liquid to the bottom of the tube.
4. Place in the thermal cycler heating block and incubate for 10 min at 22°C, 45 min at 48°C for the first strand cDNA synthesis, then incubate for 5 min at 99°C to inactivate the AMV reverse transcriptase and prevent it from binding the cDNA. Store the cDNA at +4°C or –20°C until use.

3.4.2. PCR

The cDNA is amplified using specific primers, and detected with the dsDNA binding dye SYBR® Green. Before assaying your samples, it is necessary to optimize the primer concentrations.

3.4.2.1. Optimization of Primer Concentrations

The aim of optimizing the primer concentration is to determine for each primer the minimum concentration that gives the maximum fluorescence and the minimum nonspecific signal.

1. Determine spectrophotometrically the concentration of each primer (1 OD_{260} = 33 µg/mL ssDNA).
2. For each primer, prepare 30 µL of a 10X solution 9 µM, 3 µM and 500 nM in nuclease-free water.
3. In a sterile 1.5 mL microtube, combine 375 µL SYBR® Green master mix, 600 ng cDNA (prepared as described in **Subheading 3.4.1.**, *see* **Note 12**), and nuclease-free water to a final volume of 600 µL. Vortex gently.
4. Add 20 µL of master mix to 27 wells of an optical 96-well plate (*see* **Note 13**).
5. To each well, add 2.5 µL of each 10X primer solution, using the following plate map in triplicates:

Sense Primer Final Concentration (nM)

Antisense primer final concentration (nM)	50	300	900
50	50/50	300/50	900/50
300	50/300	300/300	300/900
900	50/900	300/900	900/900

6. Cap the wells, gently tap the sides of the plate to mix the components and dislodge any air bubbles.
7. Briefly centrifuge the plate (~10 s) to bring all the liquid to the bottom of each well.

3.4.2.2. Amplification

1. Place the 96-well plate in the Applied Biosystems 5700 GeneAmp Sequence Detection System and close the lid.
2. Using the 5700 system software open a new plate document.
3. Click on "Setup," select the "primer/probe" option. Click on "Add" if you are using several different primer pairs in the same plate. Under "acronym" name your primer pairs.
4. In the tray, select all the wells that contain reactions. Click on the pull-down "Type" menu, and define the wells type as "UNKN" (unknowns).
5. Select all the wells corresponding to one primer pair.
6. Click on the "P" icon, assign the corresponding primer pair from the list. Close the window.
7. Select three wells containing identical replicates, enter the sense (sometimes called forward) and antisense (sometimes called reverse) primer concentrations in the "Name" box (*see* **Note 14**).
8. Repeat **steps 5–7** until each well displays a sample type, a primer pair color code and a name.

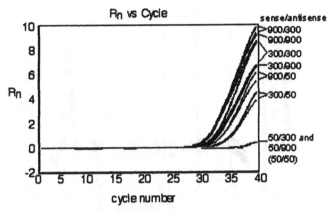

Fig. 2. Example of an experiment to optimize primer concentration. Amplification plots show the relative fluorescence (R_n) of each well as a function of the cycle number. Numbers at the right indicate the concentration of the sense and antisense primers (n*M*).

9. Click on the "Instrument" tab.
10. Change the reaction volume to 25 μL and select the "Dissociation protocol" option.
11. Save the file and click on "Run" to start the amplification reaction.

3.4.2.3. Run Analysis

1. Once the run is finished, select "Results" and then "Amp plot."
2. In the "Analysis" menu, click on "Analyze," select the wells corresponding to one primer pair.
3. Double-click on the *Y* axis, select the linear scale.
4. Determine the cycle number corresponding to the last cycle before fluorescence is detectable above baseline (this defines the baseline).
5. To adjust the baseline correction, click on the "Analysis preferences" button. In the "Baseline" "Stop" box, enter the cycle number determined in **step 4**.
6. Click on "Analyze" in the "Analysis" menu (*see* **Note 15**).
7. By clicking on the wells containing your replicates, visualize the amplification plots of each of the combinations of primer concentrations to determine which concentrations give the highest Rn value and reproducibility (Rn, normalized reporter, is the ratio of the SYBR Green emission intensity to the emission intensity of passive reference 1) (*see* **Fig. 2**). Each time, click on the "Dissociation" tab and check that you have only one peak, indicating that the wells contain only one PCR product (*see* **Fig. 3**) (*see* **Note 16**).
8. Having established the optimal primer concentration, prepare a 25X concentrated solution for each primer in nuclease-free water, and make aliquots of 250 μL in autoclaved microtubes and store at −20°C.

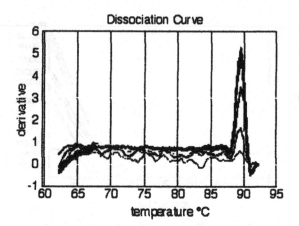

Fig. 3. Dissociation curves of the samples shown in **Fig. 2.** This shows a single peak, which indicates a single product. The different amplitudes reflect the different quantity of product in each sample.

3.4.2.4. Real-Time PCR Measurement of Samples

Each RNA sample is analyzed for ECE-1a, ECE-1b, ECE-1c, ECE-1d and total ECE-1 mRNA content using a SYBR® Green assay. The levels of the 18S ribosomal RNA in each sample is also quantified by using a commercial assay based on the TaqMan® methodology *(30)* . This is used as an internal reference gene for each sample to normalize the results obtained for each ECE-1 isoform or other gene product under investigation.

1. Prepare for each ECE-1 target gene a master mix, by combining in an autoclaved 1.5 mL microtube on ice 500 µL of SYBR® Green PCR master mix, 40 µL of sense primer 25X solution, 40 µL of antisense primer 25X solution, and 220 µL of nuclease-free water (*see* **Note 17**). Vortex gently.
2. Dispense 20 µL of the master mix to 39 wells of a 96-well optical plate (*see* **Notes 13** and **18**).
3. Add 5 µL of sample cDNA (equivalent to 25 ng RNA) to each well. Prepare for triplicate determinations of each sample. Omit the cDNA and instead add 5 µL of nuclease-free water to three wells.
4. Repeat **steps 6** and **7** of **Subheading 3.4.2.1.** and **steps 1–3** of **Subheading 3.4.2.2.,** but without the Dissociation protocol.
5. Select all the wells containing the same primer pairs, click on the "P" icon and assign the corresponding primer pairs from the list. Close the window.
6. Deselect the three wells containing water instead of RNA. Click on the pull-down "Type" menu and define the well type as "UNKN" (unknowns).

7. Select the three wells that contain water instead of RNA, click on the pull-down "Type" menu and define the well type as "NTC" (no template control).
8. Select the wells containing triplicates of one sample, enter the sample name in the "Name" box.
9. Repeat **steps 5–8** above, until each well displays a primer pair color code, a type (NTC or UNKN) and a name.
10. Repeat **steps 9–11** of **Subheading 3.4.2.2.**
11. Prepare for 18S quantification a master mix, by combining, in an autoclaved 1.5 mL microtube on ice 5 μL of 10 μ*M* ribosomal RNA forward primer, 5 μL of 10 μ*M* ribosomal RNA reverse primer, 5 μL ribosomal RNA probe (VIC), 500 μL TaqMan® universal PCR master mix and 285 μL nuclease-free water (*see* **Note 17**). Vortex gently.
12. Repeat **steps 2–10** of **Subheading 3.4.2.4.**, but without the Dissociation protocol.

3.4.2.5. ANALYSIS OF SAMPLE DATA

1. Repeat **steps 1–6** of **Subheading 3.4.2.3.** (*see* **Note 19**).
2. Double-click on the *Y* axis, select the log scale.
3. Determine the *Y* axis value corresponding to the middle of the linear portion of the amplification curves (*see* **Fig. 4**).
4. Select the "Analysis preferences" button and enter the threshold value.
5. Select "Analyze" in the "Analysis" menu (*see* **Note 15**).
6. Select three by three the wells containing replicates of each sample, and check that the threshold is in the linear portion of the amplification plot where the plots are closest. If necessary, modify the threshold value (**steps 4** and **5**, *see* **Note 20**).
7. Click on the "Report" tab. Print the report and export it in a CSV format by clicking on the "Export" button (*see* **Note 21**).

3.4.2.6. ANALYSIS OF THE RESULTS

The analysis of the relative quantity of the target mRNA in each sample is done using the Ct values (cycle number at which an amplification plot reaches the threshold value).

1. Mean the Ct values of the three replicates of each sample for each target mRNA and for the 18S assay.
2. Subtract the 18S mean Ct value from the target mRNA mean Ct value to obtain the ΔCt.
3. Average the ΔCt values of each control sample.
4. Calculate the ΔΔCt value of each sample by subtracting the average ΔCt value of the controls from the mean Ct value of each sample.
5. The relative amount of your target mRNA is expressed as $2^{-\Delta\Delta Ct}$.
6. Express the results as percentage of control, relative to 18S rRNA, following **steps 2–4** of **Subheading 3.3.3.3.**
7. Compare the values obtained for the different treatments using standard statistical methods.

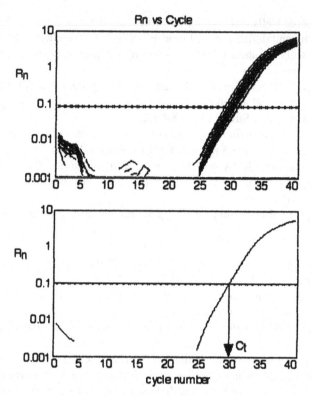

Fig. 4. Amplification plots for ECE-1c mRNA from bovine pulmonary artery smooth muscle cells. The upper panel shows the positioning of the threshold (Ct value) in the linear region of the curves plotted as Log Rn against the number of cycles. The Ct value is defined as the cycle number at which an amplification plot reaches the threshold value (lower panel, Ct = 29.1).

4. Notes

1. Although some of the more obvious safety hazards of the protocols are indicated, all procedures should be risk assessed according to local rules governing the management of laboratory safety. In addition, to avoid contamination of samples, gloves should be worn throughout all laboratory procedures (preferably, these should be powder-free gloves).
2. This protocol was modified from the Stratagene Instruction Manual, Strataprep Total RNA Miniprep Kit, copyright 2001 by Stratagene, Inc.
3. At this stage, the lysates can be stored for 2–3 wk at –80°C for extraction at a later time.
4. Centrifuge at maximum speed in a microcentrifuge indicates a centrifugal force of ~12,000g.

5. The RNA standard solution does not have to originate from the same tissue or cell type as your sample. Extract total RNA from cells grown on a T25 as explained in **Subheading 3.1.** Determine spectrophotometrically the concentration of the RNA solution (1 OD_{260} = 40 µg/mL ssRNA). In an autoclaved tube, dilute the RNA solution with DEPC-treated water to give a final concentration of 2 µg/mL. Prepare aliquots (250 µL) of this RNA standard solution in autoclaved microtubes and store at –80°C. (Or purchase the RiboGreen™ RNA quantification kit from Molecular Probes, R-11490, as this contains the RiboGreen™ dye, some 20X TE buffer and some ribosomal RNA standard solution).

6. The primers are designed so that they hybridize on either site of one (or more) intron(s). Then, if the RNA sample is contaminated with DNA, any amplified product generated from this DNA template will be easily distinguished from the mRNA specific product because of its much larger size. The primers should not hybridize with each other to form dimers, their GC content should be around 40–60% and they should not contain runs of four or more identical nucleotides. There are a number of very helpful computer programs that are commercially available to help design primers (e.g., Primer Designer).

7. In order to obtain semi-quantitative RT-PCR conditions, where the amount of product generated is proportional to the amount of RNA template added to the reaction, the amount of RNA to be included in each reaction should be determined empirically for each cell type or tissue. In an initial experiment, prepare RT-PCR reaction tubes containing no template, 50 ng, 100 ng, 200 ng, and 400 ng RNA template. Perform the RT-PCR, as described in **Subheading 3.3.** Plot the (band density as % volume) for each reaction against the quantity of RNA template (ng). Check that this gives a linear relationship and then use in subsequent experiments a quantity of RNA template in each reaction that is in the middle of the linear part of this plot.

8. To show the specificity of the RT-PCR reaction it is normal practice to include some control samples (at least during the initial evaluation and optimization of a method). The two most common controls are (1) an RNA sample with no reverse transcriptase (particularly important if the primers are not intron spanning), and (2) a sample of nuclease-free water instead of RNA template. The identity of the PCR product obtained with each method that is established should be confirmed by DNA sequencing. Restriction enzyme digestion of PCR products is sometimes performed, but that provides a very limited amount of information compared to DNA sequencing.

9. These instructions apply to the Gel Doc 1000 apparatus operated with Molecular Analyst software. A similar approach is likely with other computer-linked transilluminator workstations.

10. Bright images are required for quantification, but if pixel brightness exceeds the saturation point the relative quantification of the density of each band can not be performed reliably.

11. If you modify the amount of RNA to be reverse transcribed, or the final reaction volume, modify the amount of $MgCl_2$, reverse transcription 10X buffer, dNTPs

and RNasin ribonuclease inhibitor according to the final reaction volume, but keep the ratio of AMV reverse transcriptase units and random hexamers to RNA constant, i.e. always use 0.5 μg primer and 15 U enzyme per μg RNA irrespective of your final reaction volume.

12. For this step, you need to use some cDNA prepared from an RNA sample which you know expresses your target mRNA.

13. Do not make any marks with a marker pen on the optical plate, as the inks may contain some fluorescent compounds that could interfere with the SYBR® Green or TaqMan® quantification.

14. In the Setup file, replicates are defined as wells having the same name.

15. You need to repeat this step each time you make changes in the "Analysis preferences" menu for these changes to become effective.

16. Variations in the amplitude of the peaks in the dissociation plot are acceptable as they correspond to varying amounts of product. Variations in the position of the peaks on the X axis indicate the formation of nonspecific products as each peak represents a different product melting temperature, and/or a change in base composition. This indicates that the primers are not sufficiently specific and new primers should be designed (N.B. real-time PCR works best with short PCR products). Extra peaks may also result from contamination of one of the solutions. This can be checked by running some reactions without the primers, or without the cDNA template, in both cases no product formation should be seen.

17. These volumes are given for 12 samples assayed in triplicates (36 reactions in total), plus 3 controls without template, plus 1 vol to allow for loss of solution when pipeting. Scale up or down these volumes according to your number of samples.

18. To obtain optimal results, run the 18S ribosomal RNA TaqMan® assay and the ECE-1 SYBR® Green assays on different plates, as both assays show considerable differences in the intensity of their fluorescence, which could affect the relative measurements if conducted on the same plate.

19. The default value for the baseline correction is from cycle 6 to cycle 15. The default value of 15 might be too high for 18S amplification plots. To check this, enter a stop value of 9 for baseline correction and determine if the fluorescence increases before the cycle 15. Modify the baseline stop cycle value accordingly.

20. You should aim for a threshold value that gives the highest inter-sample and the lowest intra-sample Ct value differences.

21. You can open the report file saved in a CSV format as a text file in Excel and save it in the Excel format.

References

1. Yanagisawa, M., Kurihara, H., Kimura, S., Tomobe, Y., Kobayashi, M., Mitsui, Y., et al. (1988) A novel potent vasoconstrictor peptide produced by vascular endothelial cells. *Nature* **332,** 411–415.

2. Opgenorth, T. J., Wu-Wong, J. R., and Shiosaki, K. (1992) Endothelin-converting enzymes. *FASEB J.* **6,** 2653–2659.

3. Fukuroda, T., Noguchi, K., Tsuchida, S., Nishikibe, M., Ikemoto, F., Okada, K., and Yano, M. (1990) Inhibition of biological actions of big endothelin-1 by phosphoramidon. *Biochem. Biophys. Res. Commun.* **172,** 390–395.

4. Ikegawa, R., Matsumura, Y., Tsukahara, Y., Takaoka, M., and Morimoto, S. (1990) Phosphoramidon, a metalloproteinase inhibitor, suppresses the secretion of endothelin-1 from cultured endothelial cells by inhibiting a big endothelin-1 converting enzyme. *Biochem. Biophys. Res. Commun.* **171,** 669–675.

5. Matsumura, Y., Hisaki, K., Takaoka, M., and Morimoto, S. (1990) Phosphoramidon, a metalloproteinase inhibitor, suppresses the hypertensive effect of big endothelin-1. *Eur. J. Pharmacol.* **185,** 103–106.

6. Ikegawa, R., Matsumura, Y., Tsukahara, Y., Takaoka, M., and Morimoto, S. (1991) Phosphoramidon inhibits the generation of endothelin-1 from exogenously applied big endothelin-1 in cultured vascular endothelial cells and smooth muscle cells. *FEBS Letts.* **293,** 45–48.

7. Schmidt, M., Kroger, B., Jacob, E., Seulberger, H., Subkowski, T., Otter, R., et al. (1994) Molecular characterization of human and bovine endothelin converting enzyme (ECE-1). *FEBS Letts.* **356,** 238–243.

8. Shimada, K., Takahashi, M., and Tanzawa, K. (1994) Cloning and functional expression of endothelin-converting enzyme from rat endothelial cells. *J. Biol. Chem.* **269,** 18,275–18,278.

9. Xu, D., Emoto, N., Giaid, A., Slaughter, C., Kaw, S., deWit, D., and Yanagisawa, M. (1994) ECE-1: a membrane-bound metalloprotease that catalyzes the proteolytic activation of big endothelin-1. *Cell* **78,** 473–485.

10. Emoto, N. and Yanagisawa, M. (1995) Endothelin-converting enzyme-2 is a membrane-bound, phosphoramidon-sensitive metalloprotease with acidic pH optimum. *J. Biol. Chem.* **270,** 15,262–15,268.

11. Turner, A. J. and Tanzawa, K. (1997) Mammalian membrane metallopeptidases: NEP, ECE, KELL, and PEX. *FASEB J.* **11,** 355–364.

12. Valdenaire, O., Rohrbacher, E., and Mattei, M. G. (1995) Organization of the gene encoding the human endothelin-converting enzyme (ECE-1). *J. Biol. Chem.* **270,** 29,794–29,798.

13. Valdenaire, O., Lepailleur-Enouf, D., Egidy, G., Thouard, A., Barret, A., Vranckx, R., et al. (1999) A fourth isoform of endothelin-converting enzyme (ECE-1) is generated from an additional promoter. Molecular cloning and characterization. *Eur. J. Biochem.* **264,** 341–349.

14. Corder, R. (2001) Identity of endothelin-converting enzyme and other targets for the therapeutic regulation of endothelin biosynthesis. In *Handbook of Experimental Pharmacology, vol. 152* (Warner T. D., ed.), Springer-Verlag, pp. 36–67.

15. Barker, S., Khan, N. Q., Wood, E. G., and Corder, R. (2001) Effect of an antisense oligodeoxynucleotide to endothelin-converting enzyme-1c (ECE-1c) on ECE-1c

mRNA, ECE-1 protein and endothelin-1 synthesis in bovine pulmonary artery smooth muscle cells. *Mol. Pharmacol.* **59**, 163–169.

16. Korth, P., Bohle, R. M., Corvol, P., and Pinet, F. (1999) Cellular distribution of endothelin-converting enzyme-1 in human tissues. *J. Histochem. Cytochem.* **47**, 447–461.

17. Schweizer, A., Valdenaire, O., Nelbock, P., Deuschle, U., Dumas Milne Edwards, J. B., Stumpf, J. G., and Löffler, B. M. (1997) Human endothelin-converting enzyme (ECE-1): three isoforms with distinct subcellular localizations. *Biochem. J.* **328**, 871–877.

18. Corder, R. and Barker, S. (1999) The expression of endothelin-1 and endothelin-converting enzyme-1 (ECE-1) are independently regulated in bovine aortic endothelial cells. *J. Cardiovasc. Pharmacol* **33**, 671–677.

19. Barnes, K., Brown, C., and Turner, A. J. (1998) Endothelin-converting enzyme: ultrastructural localization and its recycling from the cell surface. *Hypertension* **31**, 3–9.

20. Grantham, J. A., Schirger, J. A., Williamson, E. E., Heublein, D. M., Wennberg, P. W., Kirchengast, M., Muenter, K., Subkowski, T., and Burnett, J. C. (1998) Enhanced endothelin-converting enzyme immunoreactivity in early atherosclerosis. *J. Cardiovasc. Pharmacol.* **31 (Suppl 1)**, S22–S26.

21. Minamino, T., Kurihara, H., Takahashi, M., Shimada, K., Maemura, K., Oda, H., et al. (1997) Endothelin-converting enzyme expression in the rat vascular injury model and human coronary atherosclerosis. *Circulation* **95**, 221–230.

22. Wang, X., Douglas, S. A., Louden, C., Vickery-Clark, L. M., Feuerstein, G. Z., and Ohlstein, E. H. (1996) Expression of endothelin-1, endothelin-3, endothelin-converting enzyme-1, and endothelin-A and endothelin-B receptor mRNA after angioplasty-induced neointimal formation in the rat. *Circ. Res.* **78**, 322–328.

23. Harrison, V.J., Barnes, K., Turner, A.J., Wood, E., Corder, R., and Vane, J. R. (1995) Identification of endothelin 1 and big endothelin 1 in secretory vesicles isolated from bovine aortic endothelial cells. *Proc. Natl. Acad. Sci. USA* **92**, 6344–6348.

24. Takahashi, M., Fukuda, K., Shimada, K., Barnes, K., Turner, A. J., et al. (1995) Localization of rat endothelin-converting enzyme to vascular endothelial cells and some secretory cells. *Biochem. J.* **311**, 657–665.

25. Russell, F. D., Skepper, J. N., and Davenport, A. P. (1998) Human endothelial cell storage granules. A novel intracellular site for isoforms of the endothelin-converting enzyme. *Circ. Res.* **83**, 314–321.

26. Brown, C.D., Barnes, K., and Turner, A. J. (1998) Anti-peptide antibodies specific to rat endothelin-converting enzyme-1 isoforms reveal isoform localisation and expression. *FEBS Letts.* **424**, 183–187.

27. Azarani, A., Boileau, G., and Crine, P. (1998) Recombinant human endothelin-converting enzyme ECE-1b is located in an intracellular compartment when expressed in polarized Madin-Darby canine kidney cells. *Biochem. J.* **333**, 439–448.

28. Schweizer, A., Löffler, B. M., and Rohrer, J. (1999) Palmitoylation of the three isoforms of human endothelin-converting enzyme-1. *Biochem. J.* **340,** 649–656.
29. Yanagisawa, H., Yanagisawa, M., Kapur, R. P., Richardson, J. A., Williams, S. C., Clouthier, D. E., et al. (1998) Dual genetic pathways of endothelin-mediated intercellular signaling revealed by targeted disruption of endothelin converting enzyme-1 gene. *Development* **125,** 825–836.
30. Bustin, S. A. (2000) Absolute quantification of mRNA using real-time reverse transcription polymerase chain reaction assays. *J. Mol. Endocrinol.* **25,** 169–193.
31. Lambert, G. L., Barker, S., Lees, D. M., and Corder, R. (2000) Endothelin-2 synthesis is stimulated by the type-1 tumour necrosis factor receptor and cAMP: comparison with endothelin-converting enzyme-1 expression. *J. Mol. Endocrinol* **24,** 273–283.

28. ...
29. ...
30. ...
31. ...

9

Evaluation of Endothelin-Converting Enzyme Inhibitors Using Cultured Cells

Roger Corder

1. Introduction

The concept that endothelin (ET-1) biosynthesis is dependent on specific hydrolysis of the intermediate big endothelin-1 (big ET-1) by an endopeptidase referred to as endothelin-converting enzyme (ECE) originates from the initial description of this peptide by Yanagisawa and colleagues *(1)*. The search for the putative endothelin-converting enzyme soon became the focus of intense research *(2)*. The underlying goal was the drive to identify the target for development of specific ECE inhibitors that could be used therapeutically for treating ET-1 dependent pathologies. These investigations were conducted both on the endogenous production of ET-1 by endothelial cells, and by using cell or tissue homogenates with exogenous big ET-1 as the substrate *(2,3)*. The first clear evidence of a specific physiologically relevant ECE came from studies of the effect of phosphoramidon (N-α-L-rhamnopyranosyloxyhydroxy-phosphinyl-L-Leu-L-Trp) on cultured porcine aortic endothelial cells *(4)*. This was an important breakthrough as it showed that high concentrations of phosphoramidon suppressed ET-1 levels and resulted in increased levels of big ET-1 *(4)*. This inverse relationship between ET-1 and big ET-1 production is an important characteristic of biosynthetic processes as the accumulation of the enzyme's substrate demonstrates the specific inhibition of a key enzymatic step, in this case the physiological ECE. Subsequently other studies have confirmed the effect of phosphoramidon on ET-1 synthesis in a variety of human cell types by using high performance liquid chromatography (HPLC) *(5)* or "double recognition site" sandwich immunoassays *(6)*.

From: *Methods in Molecular Biology, vol. 206: Peptide Research Protocols: Endothelin*
Edited by: J. Maguire and A. Davenport © Humana Press Inc., Totowa, NJ

At the same time as the initial studies of phosphoramidon on cultured endothelial cells, separate investigations showed this compound also inhibited the blood pressure response of systemically administered big ET-1 *(7,8)*, and the conversion of exogenous big ET-1 to ET-1 by cultured endothelial and smooth muscle cells *(9)*. However, phosphoramidon also inhibits a wide variety of metallopeptidases, so it is conceivable that its effects on production of ET-1 from endogenous and exogenous big ET-1 involve actions on several distinct endopeptidases. A further point, which may have some bearing on the identity of the physiological ECE, is that inhibition of endogenous ET-1 synthesis requires phosphoramidon concentrations that are 10–20-fold higher than those needed for preventing the hydrolysis of exogenous big ET-1 *(5,6)*. This indicates that processing of the endogenous peptide occurs intracellularly, which is in agreement with the identification of constitutive secretory vesicles containing ET-1 in cultured endothelial cells *(10)*.

The search for a physiologically relevant ECE progressed rapidly with the purification and cloning of a phosphoramidon-sensitive type II integral membrane peptidase called endothelin-converting enzyme-1 *(ECE-1) (11–13)*. The identification of *ECE-1* in endothelial cells as well as other cells synthesizing endothelins was seen as confirmation that it was the functionally important ECE *(11–13)*. More recently it has been found that ECE-1 gene deletion does not lead to the elimination of ET-1 synthesis even though it produces a phenotype similar to ET-1 knockout *(14)*. Furthermore, treatment of bovine pulmonary artery smooth muscle cells with an antisense oligodeoxynucleotide against ECE-1c (the most abundant *ECE-1* isoform in these cells) caused a marked reduction in *ECE-1* protein levels but had a negligible effect on ET-1 synthesis *(15)*. Consequently, the role of *ECE-1* is now in doubt and the identity of the physiological ECE is uncertain.

In the meantime, ECE inhibitors have been evaluated mainly in biochemical assays using cloned and expressed *ECE-1* with exogenous big ET-1 as the substrate *(16)*. The efficacy of these inhibitors against endogenous synthesis by cultured cells has frequently not been determined. Moreover, measurement of ET-1 production alone by cultured cells may be inadequate because many compounds suppress ET-1 synthesis through effects on gene transcription or translation without inhibiting ECE *(17)*. Hence, conformation of ECE inhibition by measuring the levels of both ET-1 and big ET-1 in the conditioned media is best achieved by specific "double recognition site" sandwich immunoassays *(6,15)*.

The protocols described below provide a fully detailed procedure for the development of sandwich immunoassays for the specific measurement of ET-1 and big ET-1. The principle of both assays is to coat 96-well plates with an affinity-purified rabbit IgG that binds the ET-1 $_{[1-15]}$ sequence. Specific detection of ET-1 or big ET-1 is achieved using anti-ET-1$_{[16-21]}$ IgG and anti-

Endothelin-1 immunoassay

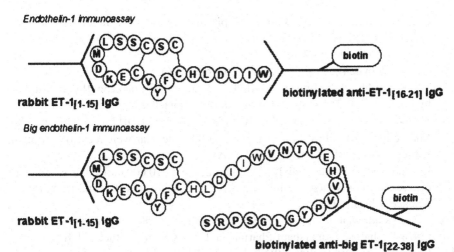

Big endothelin-1 immunoassay

Fig. 1. Schematic representation of "double-recognition site" sandwich immunoassays for ET-1 and big ET-1. Bound peptide is detected with ^{125}I-streptavidin or neutravidin-horseradish peroxidase with a suitable substrate.

human big ET$_{[22-38]}$ IgG respectively (**Fig. 1**). The detection IgG are biotinylated so that the method of quantification can be flexible (e.g., ^{125}I-streptavidin or neutravidin-horseradish peroxidase with chemiluminescent substrate). Because a signal is only detected when the relevant peptide has bound both antibodies, these assays are highly sensitive and specific with negligible crossreactivity (<0.01%) of big ET-1 in the ET-1 assay and vice versa. This is of fundamental importance in the application of these methods to the evaluation of ECE inhibitors on cultured cells. The effect of antigen selective IgG purification on assay specificity is illustrated and the application of these immunoassays in cell experiments is described.

2. Materials

2.1. Reagents and Solutions

1. Custom synthesized peptides: ET-1$_{[1-15]}$ (Formyl-Cys-Ser-Cys-Ser-Ser-Leu-Met-Asp-Nle-Glu-Cys-Val-Tyr-Phe-Cys-Ala-Lys-NH$_2$, disulphide bridges Cys^{1,15} and Cys^{3,11}; Bachem, St Helens, Merseyside, UK) (*see* **Note 1**); ET-1$_{[16-21]}$ (His-Leu-Asp-Ile-Ile-Trp); human big ET-1$_{[22-38]}$ (Val-Asn-Thr-Pro-Glu-His-Val-Val-Pro-Tyr-Gly-Leu-Gly-Ser-Pro-Arg-Ser); human big ET-1 $_{[22-35]}$ (Val-Asn-Thr-Pro-Glu-His-Val-Val-Pro-Tyr-Gly-Leu-Gly-Ser); human big ET-1 $_{[32-38]}$ (Gly-Leu-Gly-Ser-Pro-Arg-Ser).
2. Standard peptides: ET-1, human big ET-1 $_{[1-38]}$, porcine big ET-1 $_{[1-39]}$ (Peptide Institute, Inc., Osaka, Japan).

3. Carrier proteins for immunogen preparation: Keyhole Limpet Hemocyanin (KLH; 20 mg vials–77600ZZ, Pierce, Rockford, IL); bovine thyroglobulin (BTG, T1001; Sigma, Dorset, UK).

4. Glutaraldehyde (25%, G6257, Sigma, Dorset, UK).

5. Water soluble carbodiimide: 1-ethyl-3-[3-dimethylaminopropyl]-carbodiimide hydrochloride (03449 Fluka, Sigma-Aldrich, Dorset, UK).

6. pH Indicator strips 0–6.0 and 5.0–10.0 (31505, 31506; BDH Merck, Dorset, UK).

7. Microcon YM-10 ultrafiltration units (10,000 molecular-weight cut-off; Amicon Bioseparations, Millipore, Bedford, MA).

8. Low nonspecific binding dialysis membranes (e.g., 10,000 molecular-weight cut-off, Spectra/Por Biotech Cellulose Ester, 8-mm width; 131261, Spectrum, Perbio Science, Chester, UK).

9. Freund's adjuvant (complete, F5881; incomplete, F5506; Sigma, Dorset, UK).

10. CNBr Sepharose (Amersham-Pharmacia, Little Chalfont, Bucks., UK).

11. Phosphate-buffered saline (PBS); dissolve 1 PBS tablet (P4417, Sigma, Dorset, UK) in 200 mL water: 0.01 M phosphate buffer, 0.0027 M KCl, 0.137 M NaCl, pH 7.4, at 25°C.

12. Empty chromatography columns (e.g., 7 × 100 mm glass econo-column, 737-0712; column reservoir 731-0003; Bio-Rad, Herts., UK).

13. Biotinylation reagent (e.g., EZ-link NHS-LC-LC-Biotin; Pierce, Rockford, IL).

14. High binding, flat-bottom 96-well plates for immunoassay use (e.g., white opaque plate for immunoassays using ^{125}I-streptavidin and liquid scintillation counting of bound radioactivity, 3922; black for assays using chemiluminescent detection systems, 3601; both plates from Costar, Corning, NY) (*see* **Note 2**).

15. IgG Coating buffer: 50 mM bicarbonate buffer, pH 9.5 (85 mg Na_2CO_3, 143 mg $NaHCO_3$ in 50 mL double-deionized water).

16. Blocking buffer: 150 mg (0.5%) bovine serum albumin (BSA; A7888; Sigma, Dorset, UK) and 15 mg (0.05%) polypep (P-5115; Sigma, Dorset, UK) dissolved in 30 mL coating buffer.

17. Sandwich assay buffer: 1000 mg (0.5%) BSA, 400 mg (0.2%) bovine IgG (G7516; Sigma, Dorset, UK), 400 mg (0.2%) polypep, 100 μL Triton X-100 (X100; Sigma, Dorset, UK), 50 mg NaN_3 dissolved in 200 mL PBS. Filter (0.2 μm) sandwich assay buffer into 50 mL tubes and store frozen at –20°C.

18. ET-1, human big ET-1, and porcine big ET-1 standard solutions (*see* **Note 3**).

19. Assay wash buffer, 0.05% tween-20 (P1379; Sigma, Dorset, UK) in PBS: dissolve one PBS tablet in 200 mL of water and add 100 μL tween-20.

20. ^{125}I-Streptavidin (3.7 MBq, IM236; Amersham-Pharmacia, Bucks., UK). On arrival reconstitute and dilute to 10 mL with sandwich assay buffer. Store 0.5 mL aliquots at –20°C.

21. Neutralization buffer for medium samples: dissolve 363 mg Tris base, 944 mg HEPES free acid, 690 mg BSA, 276 mg bovine IgG, 69μL Triton X-100 in 19.5 mL water (*see* **Note 4**).

22. Ultima Gold MV for liquid scintillation counting and multi-well plate self-adhesive sealing strips (Packard, Berks., UK).

23. Neutravidin-horseradish peroxidase (e.g., Neutravidin-HRP; Pierce, Rockford, IL).
24. Supersignal ELISA pico chemiluminescence substrate (Pierce, Rockford, IL).
25. Dulbecco's Modified Eagles Medium (DMEM; Sigma, Dorset, UK). For use 500 mL DMEM is supplemented with the following stock solutions: 10 mL of antibiotics (penicillin 5000 IU/mL and streptomycin 5000 µg/mL), 5 mL of amphotericin B (250 µg/mL) and 10 mL of L-glutamine (200 mM).
26. DMEM with peptidase inhibitor mix (*see* **Note 5**): To 50 mL of DMEM containing antibiotics and other additives add the following peptidase inhibitors 1 mM bacitracin (71 mg), 10 µM chymostatin (5 µL of 100 mM stock), 10 µM leupeptin (5 µL of 100 mM stock), 1 µM pepstatin A (5 µL of 10 mM stock), and 10 µM thiorphan (5 µL of 100 mM stock).
27. Inhibitor stock solutions (inhibitors obtained from Sigma, Dorset, UK or Peptide Institute, Inc. Japan): chymostatin 100 mM (FW = 600, 25 mg dissolved in 417 µL of DMSO, store at –20°C); pepstatin A 10 mM (FW = 685.9, 5 mg dissolved in 729 µL of DMSO, store at –20°C); leupeptin 100 mM (FW = 426.5, 100 mg dissolved in 2.344 mL of water, store at –20°C); thiorphan 100 mM (FW = 253.3, 5 mg dissolved in 197 µL of DMSO, store at –20°C).
28. Phosphoramidon 100 mM (Peptide Institute, Inc. Japan) (FW = 543.5, 25 mg dissolved in 460 µL sterile PBS, store 100 µL aliquots at –20°C).
29. MTT (Sigma, Dorset, UK) dissolved in DMEM (0.4 mg/mL).

2.2. Equipment

1. HPLC system with gradient elution capability, UV spectrophotometer A_{280}, and fraction collector. A standard reverse phase octadecylsilyl silica column is required (e.g., ODS-120T, 5 µm, 4.6 × 250 mm; Tosohaas, Anachem, Bedfordshire, UK) (*see* **Note 6**).
2. 96-Well plate liquid scintillation counter and luminometer (e.g., Wallac 1450 MicroBeta Trilux).

3. Methods

3.1. Raising Antisera (see Note 7)

3.1.1. Preparation of ET-1$_{[16–21]}$ and Human Big ET-1$_{[22–38]}$ Immunogens

1. Dissolve 2 mg (~2 µmol) ET-1 $_{[16–21]}$ in 2 mL of 0.05 M NaHCO$_3$.
2. Dissolve 5.2 mg (~2 µmol) human big ET-1$_{[22–38]}$ in 2 mL of 0.05 M NaHCO$_3$.
3. Dissolve a 20 mg vial of KLH in 4 mL of 0.05 M NaHCO$_3$ (5 mg/mL). Weigh 10 mg of BTG and dissolve in 2 mL of 0.05 M NaHCO$_3$ (5 mg/mL). Then prepare 2 × 1 mL aliquots (5 mg) of each of these carrier protein solutions.
4. Add 10 µL 25% glutaraldehyde to the solutions of ET-1$_{[16–21]}$ and the solution of human big ET-1$_{[22–38]}$, and leave for 30 min at room temperature in the dark.
5. Add 1 mL glutaraldehyde-activated ET-1$_{[16–21]}$ to 1 mL of KLH (5 mg) and the remaining 1 mL glutaraldehyde-activated ET-1$_{[16–21]}$ to 1 mL of BTG (5 mg). Leave to react at room temperature for 1 h in the dark.
6. Repeat **step 5** with the glutaraldehyde-activated human big ET-1$_{[22–38]}$.

7. To stop the reactions and to block remaining aldehyde groups, after 1 h add 1 mL 0.075 *M* glycine dissolved in 0.3 *M* NaHCO$_3$ to each peptide-glutaraldehyde carrier protein mix prepared in **steps 5** and **6**. Leave to react at room temperature for a further 1 h in the dark.

8. Dilute each immunogen solution with 7 mL of sterile 0.9% saline (=0.1 µmol peptide antigen/mL plus carrier protein or 100 µg/mL ET-1$_{[16-21]}$ and 260 µg/mL big ET-1 $_{[22-38]}$). Freeze each of the immunogens in aliquots of 1 or 2 mL at –80°C for subsequent immunizations.

3.1.2. Preparation of ET-1 Immunogen

1. Dissolve 0.56 mg (0.22 µmol) of ET-1 in 20 µL of DMSO in the vial in which it is supplied. Add 2 mL of water then adjust pH to 4.5–5.0 with 0.1 *M* HCl. Verify by spotting 5 µL onto narrow range pH 0–6.0 indicator strips. If the reaction is to be confirmed by HPLC take a 10 µL reference sample of the ET-1 solution (1 nmol), dilute with HPLC buffer A and inject on to the HPLC system and record peak area of the eluted ET-1 at A_{280} nm (*see* **Note 6**).

2. Dissolve a 20 mg vial of KLH in 4 mL water (5 mg/mL). Adjust pH to 4.5–5.0 with 0.1 *M* HCl as in **step 1** above. Add 1 mL of KLH solution (5 mg) to the 2 mL solution of ET-1.

3. Prepare a solution of 1-ethyl-3-(3-dimethylaminopropyl)-carbodiimide (EDC) hydrochloride in water at a concentration of 4.2 mg/mL (22 µmol/mL).

4. Then add 100 µL of EDC solution to the ET-1/KLH solution and gently vortex. Leave to react for 1 h at room temperature.

5. To confirm successful conjugation of ET-1 to KLH carrier protein, take a 15 µL sample of the reaction mix (equivalent to ≈1 nmol ET-1) and dilute with 200 µL of 10 m*M* NaHCO$_3$ in the filtration unit of a Microcon YM-10 ultrafiltration unit. Centrifuge for 15–30 min in a bench-top microtube centrifuge at ≈12,000*g* until all the ultrafiltrate has passed through the membrane filter. The ET-1/KLH conjugate is retained on the membrane filter.

6. Measure the amount of unreacted ET-1 by HPLC. Dilute the ultrafiltrate with HPLC buffer A and inject onto the HPLC system, record the ET-1 peak area as in **step 1** and quantify.

7. If <70% of the ET-1 has been conjugated to the KLH carrier protein, repeat **steps 4–6**.

8. Dialyze the ET-1/KLH conjugate overnight at 4°C against 500 mL of sterile 0.9% saline. Recover the ET-1 immunogen and dilute to ≈50 µg/mL with sterile 0.9% saline. Freeze aliquots of 1 mL at –80°C for subsequent immunizations.

3.1.3. Rabbit Immunization Protocol (see **Note 8**)

1. Thaw the immunogens and dilute with an equal volume of Complete Freund's adjuvant. Vortex vigorously to create an emulsion. Immunize three rabbits with each antigen: ET-1$_{[16-21]}$, big ET-1$_{[22-38]}$ or ET-1. For ET-1$_{[16-21]}$ and big

ET-1 $_{[22-38]}$ there are two immunogens, therefore the carrier protein is alternated so that rabbits are immunized with the antigen conjugated to KLH, followed 4 wk later by the antigen-BTG conjugate. Inject rabbits subcutaneously at four sites with 0.25 mL of the emulsion (thus, each rabbit receives from 25 to 130 μg of antigen per immunization).

2. Immunize all the rabbits once more 4 wk later. For the second, and subsequent, immunizations Incomplete Freund's adjuvant is used. Prepare the emulsion as above by mixing equal volumes of adjuvant and immunogen.
3. Take a test bleed from each rabbit 2 wk after the second immunization.
4. Continue immunizations every 4 wk for a total of 4–6 mo with test bleeds being taken 2 wk after each immunization. After 6 mo of immunizations (earlier if the titer of test bleeds are studied) collect a terminal bleed of 100–200 mL under deep anaesthesia (*see* **Note 9**).

3.2. Affinity Purification and Biotinylation of Peptide Specific IgG

3.2.1. Conjugation of Peptide Antigens to CNBr Sepharose

1. For each peptide-Sepharose that is to be prepared weigh 1 g CNBr Sepharose and swell with 40 mL 1 mM HCl on a sintered glass filter on top of a vacuum flask. After 2–3 min, apply the vacuum to wash the gel. Repeat this step 5× to wash the gel with a total of 200 mL 1 mM HCl (1 g CNBr Sepharose swells to about 3.5 mL gel) (*see* **Note 10**).
2. Dissolve 14 μmol of each peptide antigen in 7 mL of 0.1 M NaHCO$_3$ containing 0.5 M NaCl in a 15 mL screw-top tube (i.e., the respective amounts to prepare for each peptide-Sepharose are: 7 mg ET-1$_{[16-21]}$; 13.5 mg ET-1$_{[1-15]}$; 10 mg human big ET-1$_{[22-35]}$; 5 mg human big ET-1$_{[32-38]}$).
3. Apply the vacuum to the swollen gel to remove the last 1 mM HCl wash, allow the vacuum to remove all the liquid then transfer the "dry" swollen gel to the peptide solution. Close the tube tightly and mix immediately by repeated inversion of the tube to resuspend the gel in the peptide solution. Mix for 2 h at room temperature using a flat bed roller mixer or end-over-end mixer.
4. After 2 h allow the gel to settle and take a sample of supernatant for assessing reaction efficiency by HPLC (*see* **Note 10**).
5. Add 3.5 mL of 3 M ethanolamine-HCl, pH 8.0, to block remaining active groups. React for a further 1 h at room temperature.
6. Wash the gel on a sintered glass filter (attached to a vacuum flask) with 0.1 M acetic acid (2 × 40 mL) and 0.1% trifluoroacetic/80% acetonitrile (2 × 40 mL) to remove any nonspecifically bound peptide. Turn the vacuum off before the addition of each wash solution, resuspend the gel by gentle stirring with a spatula, and then apply the vacuum to draw each wash solution through the gel.
7. Wash with water (2 × 40 mL) and phosphate-buffered saline (2 × 40 mL). Transfer the vacuum "dry" washed gel to a 15-mL tube. Resuspend the gel with 10 mL of PBS containing 0.02% azide as a preservative. The gel is now ready for affinity purification of IgG. If not to be used immediately the gel should be stored at 4°C.

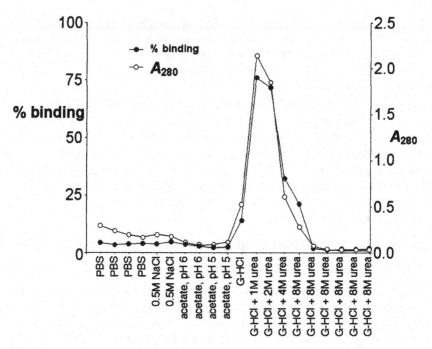

Fig. 2. Affinity purification of rabbit ET-1 IgG on ET-1$_{[1-15]}$-Sepharose. Total rabbit IgG from 100 mL antiserum was passed through a 3 mL column of ET-1$_{[1-15]}$-Sepharose. Elution was performed with the steps indicated (2 mL/fraction); acetate, pH 6.0 = 0.5 M NaCH$_3$COO, pH 6.0; acetate, pH 5.0 = 0.5 M NaCH$_3$COO, pH 5.0; G-HCl = 0.1 M glycine-HCl, pH 2.5. Eluted IgG was monitored spectrophotometrically by measuring A_{280}, 1.4 OD = 1 mg IgG/mL. ^{125}I-ET-1 binding shown to illustrate that the specific binding parallels the IgG concentration (*see* **Note 12**).

3.2.2. Affinity Purification of IgG

1. Thaw antisera of interest and measure 40 mL into a 50-mL screw-top polypropylene tube. Add 7.2 g anhydrous Na$_2$SO$_4$ powder (18% w/v) and mix gently at room temperature until it has all dissolved. When all the Na$_2$SO$_4$ has dissolved the antiserum will be a cloudy suspension. Precipitate the IgG by centrifugation at 2000–3000g, 20°C for 15 min (*see* **Note 11**).
2. Aspirate the supernatant and reconstitute the IgG precipitate by addition of sufficient PBS to obtain the same volume as the original antiserum sample. The IgG solution is now ready for affinity purification.
3. Transfer the peptide-Sepharose gel into an empty column ready for affinity purification. Attach the column reservoir, place 20 mL of PBS in the reservoir, and allow it to drip through the column to waste. Transfer the IgG solution to the reservoir and allow it to drip through the column into a 50-mL tube (the IgG

solution can be reapplied after the column has been eluted to see if further specific IgG is recoverable).

4. Once all the IgG solution has passed through the gel transfer 20–30 mL PBS into the reservoir to wash out unbound IgG. Remove the reservoir once the PBS wash has passed through the gel. The gel is now ready for elution of the specifically bound IgG.

5. Elute the IgG using the following procedure. Place 2 mL of each solution gently on the top of the gel. Allow each solution to run into the gel before adding the next elution step. Collect the eluate from each step into a separate 5 mL tube. Neutralize each acidic fraction with 0.8 M $NaHCO_3$, verify pH by spotting 2–3 µL of each fraction onto pH strips (range 5.0–10.0). Use the following elution steps (repeat as indicated):

   a. 2×2 mL 0.5 M NaCl
   b. 2×2 mL 0.5 M $NaCH_3COO$, pH 6.0
   c. 2×2 mL 0.5 M $NaCH_3COO$, pH 5.0
   d. 1×2 mL 0.1 M glycine HCl, pH 2.5
   e. 1×2 mL 0.1 M glycine HCl, pH 2.5, containing 1 M urea
   f. 1×2 mL 0.1 M glycine HCl, pH 2.5, containing 2 M urea
   g. 1×2 mL 0.1 M glycine HCl, pH 2.5, containing 4 M urea
   h. 5×2 mL 0.1 M glycine HCl, pH 2.5, containing 8 M urea

6. Measure A_{280} of each fraction using a spectrophotometer (1.4 OD = 1 mg/mL of IgG) (*see* example of an elution profile shown in **Fig. 2**) (*see* **Note 12**).

7. Pool peak fractions and dialyze IgG overnight against 1 L of PBS to remove urea.

8. Transfer IgG from dialysis tubing into suitable size tube and centrifuge dialyzed IgG at 2000–3000*g*, 4°C for 15 min, to remove any denatured IgG that has become insoluble.

9. Transfer clarified IgG solution to a fresh tube and measure A_{280} to determine IgG concentration.

10. If the affinity purified IgG is to be used as a plate coating antibody prepare aliquots of 100–200 µg and freeze at –80°C for later use.

3.2.3. Biotinylation of Peptide Specific IgG

1. IgG for biotinylation needs to undergo further dialysis. After centrifugation to clarify the IgG (*see* **Subheading 3.2.2.**, **step 8**), transfer the IgG to fresh dialysis membranes and dialyze 16–18 h against 1 L of 10 mM $NaHCO_3$ containing 0.1 M NaCl. Then change the dialysis buffer to fresh 10 mM $NaHCO_3$ containing 0.1 M NaCl and dialyze for a further 16–18 h (*see* **Note 13**).

2. Recover the IgG from the dialysis membrane and measure A_{280} to determine IgG concentration. Transfer a volume of IgG solution corresponding to 3 mg (20 nmol) of IgG into a separate tube (store the remainder of the IgG at –80°C). Chill the IgG for biotinylation on ice (*see* **Note 14**).

3. Dissolve 5.7 mg EZ-link NHS-LC-LC-Biotin in 250 µL dimethylformamide (handle this solvent in a fume hood wearing gloves) to give a solution of 40 nmol/µL.

4. Transfer 50 µL of biotinylation reagent (2000 nmol, 100-fold excess compared to IgG) to the IgG solution that has been chilled on ice. Vortex gently and leave on ice for 2 h, then transfer to room temperature and leave a further 2 h for the reaction to be completed (*see* **Note 15**).

5. At the end of the reaction transfer the IgG-biotin reaction mixture to dialysis tubing and dialyze for 16–18 h against 1 L of 20 m*M* Tris-HCl, pH 8.0. This eliminates the excess and unbound biotinylation reagent from the biotinylated IgG. If less than 1 mg IgG has been biotinylated add 1 µL Triton X-100 per mL of reaction mix (this will reduce nonspecific losses during dialysis).

6. After dialysis recover the solution of biotinylated IgG from the dialysis membranes, prepare aliquots of 100–200 µL and freeze at –80°C.

3.3. ET-1 and Big ET-1 Sandwich Immunoassays

3.3.1. Sandwich Immunoassays Using ^{125}I-Streptavidin and Liquid Scintillation Counting of Bound Radioactivity

1. Dilute the plate-coating IgG to 3 µg/mL in coating buffer. Take a 96-well high binding white Costar plate and pipet 100 µL of this IgG solution per well leaving two wells without IgG solution. In the remaining two wells, pipet 100 µL of coating buffer so that these wells can provide a nonspecific binding value for the assay. Cover plates and incubate overnight at 4°C.

2. Decant coating buffer and tap the plate gently on paper towel.

3. Pipet 250 µL of blocking buffer into each well. Seal plates in plastic sample bags and incubate for 2 h at 37°C.

4. Decant blocking buffer and tap the plate dry on paper towel.

5. Wash 3× with assay wash buffer (250 µL/well) and tap the plate dry on paper towel between each wash.

6. The plate is now ready to use, but leave the final wash buffer in the plates until ready to continue assay because if the plate should dry out, the coating antibody will become denatured.

7. Dilute standards in sandwich assay buffer to cover the working range of the assay. For example, ET-1 stock standard (10 pmol/mL), 45 µL is diluted in 1.455-mL sandwich assay buffer to give a top standard of 300 fmol/mL. This is serially diluted (1 in 3 dilutions, 0.5 mL + 1 mL) to give the following additional standards: 100, 33.3, 11.1, 3.7, 1.23 fmol/mL.

8. Prepare sufficient biotinylated IgG diluted in sandwich assay buffer for use at 50 µL/well (*see* **Note 16**).

9. You are now ready to continue with the assay. Decant the wash buffer from the final wash and tap plates dry on paper towel. Add immediately 50 µL of diluted biotinylated IgG into all wells of the plate, the plate is now protected from drying out.

10. Pipet 100 µL standard into standard wells, 100 µL buffer into 0 fmol/mL standard and NSB, and 100 µL of samples into the remaining wells (*see* **Note 4**).

11. Cover plates and incubate overnight at 4°C.

12. The following day decant the liquid from the plate and wash 3× with assay wash buffer (250 µL/well). Tap the plate dry on paper towel between each wash.

13. Dilute the stock solution of ^{125}I-streptavidin in sandwich assay buffer to 100,000 cpm/100 μL and pipet 100 μL of this solution per well. Cover plates and incubate for 4 h at room temperature.
14. Aspirate the unbound ^{125}I-streptavidin from each well, and wash 3× with assay wash buffer (250 μL/well). Tap the plate dry on paper towel between each wash.
15. Dispense 100 μL of scintillant per well (Ultima Gold MV). Cover the plate with a self-adhesive sealing strip and measure the bound radioactivity by liquid scintillation counting (Wallac 1450 MicroBeta Trilux counter/luminometer) (**Fig. 3**).

3.3.2. Sandwich Immunoassays with Chemiluminescence Detection

1. Dilute the plate-coating IgG to 3 μg/mL in coating buffer. Pipet 100 μL of this solution per well in a 96-well high binding black Costar plate. (For the measurement of nonspecific binding, two wells should contain coating buffer alone). Cover plates and incubate overnight at 4°C.
2. Perform **steps 2–12** as described in **Subheading 3.3.1.** above.
3. Dilute the neutravidin–HRP to 1 in 40,000 in wash buffer containing 0.5% BSA (*see* **Note 17**), and pipet 100 μL of this solution per well. Incubate plates for 2 h at 4°C.
4. Decant liquid from plates and wash 4× with assay wash buffer (250 μL/well). Tap the plate dry between each wash with clean paper towel to avoid contamination with HRP conjugate.
5. Pipet 100 μL per well of Supersignal ELISA pico-chemiluminescence substrate (50:50 mix of stable peroxide buffer and substrate).
6. Mix gently on a 96-well plate mixer for 5 min.
7. Measure the chemiluminescence 10 min after initial addition of substrate (count 1 s/well) (Wallac 1450 MicroBeta Trilux counter/luminometer).

3.4. Evaluation of ECE Inhibitors on Cultured Cells

3.4.1. Treatment of Cells and Collection of Media

1. Grow the cells under investigation to confluence in 24-well plates in cell growth medium (e.g., DMEM containing 10% fetal calf serum) (*5,15*) (*see* **Note 18**).
2. Warm 50 mL of DMEM containing antibiotics and other additives to 37°C in a water bath.
3. Prepare dilutions of inhibitors to be tested in DMEM containing peptidase inhibitor mix. As a reference ECE inhibitor, dilute the stock solution of phosphoramidon in DMEM containing peptidase inhibitor mix to obtain concentrations of 1 mM, 300 μM, 100 μM, 30 μM, and 10 μM. Warm the diluted inhibitors briefly at 37°C prior to application to the cells.
4. Wash cells with warmed DMEM (0.5 mL/well).
5. Aspirate wash medium and replace with DMEM containing the inhibitors to be studied (300 μL/well).
6. Incubate for 6 h, or 24 h, at 37°C, in a humidified incubator with an atmosphere of 5% CO_2 in air.

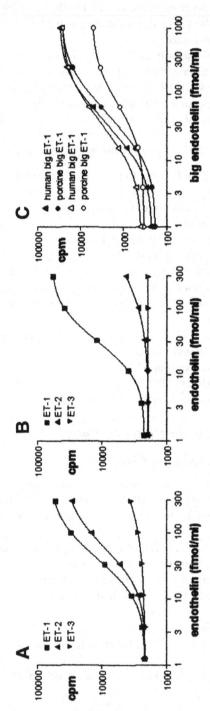

Fig. 3. Examples of different crossreactivities of "double recognition site" sandwich immunoassays for ET-1 peptides. These results demonstrate how affinity purification using different peptide-Sepharoses allows the selection of IgG with a particular antigen specificity, which in turn can be used to develop immunoassays with different specificities. Detection for all assays shown was with ^{125}I-streptavidin. (A) ET-1 immunoassay—plates were coated with ET-1$_{[1–15]}$ IgG and detection of bound peptide was made with biotinylated ET-1$_{[16–21]}$ IgG, crossreactivities of ET-2 and ET-3 were ≈50% and 2% respectively. (B) ET-1 immunoassay—plates were coated with a coating IgG that had been purified from the same antiserum using ET-1$_{[2–13]}$ agarose, detection of bound peptide was made with the same biotinylated ET-1$_{[16–21]}$ IgG as in (A), and crossreactivities of ET-2 and ET-3 were ≈4% and <0.1% respectively. (C) big ET-1 immunoassays—plates were coated with the same ET-1$_{[1–15]}$ IgG as in (A), detection of human and porcine big ET-1 was made with biotinylated anti-human big ET-1$_{[22–38]}$ IgG that had either been purified on human big ET-1$_{[22–35]}$-Sepharose (solid symbols) or on human big ET-1$_{[32–38]}$-Sepharose (open symbols).

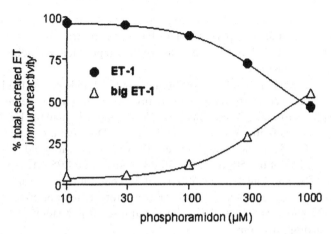

Fig. 4. Representative results from treatment of the human endothelial cell line EA.hy 926 with phosphoramidon for 6 h on the production of ET-1 and big ET-1 measured by specific sandwich immunoassays. A greater degree of inhibition is observed after treatment for 24 h *(5,15)* showing that the effect of phosphoramidon on ET-1 synthesis has a slow onset of action. This is probably because of poor intracellular penetration of phosphoramidon to the relevant site for processing of big ET-1 by the endogenous ECE.

7. Collect the medium (270 µL from each well), heat treat at 80°C for 10 min *(see* **Note 4**). Freeze the medium at $-20°C$ and store for subsequent immunoassay **(Fig 4)**.

3.4.2. Cell Viability Assay

1. Immediately after collection of the medium, aspirate any remaining medium from each well, do not allow the wells to dry out.
2. Add immediately the MTT solution diluted in DMEM (0.4 mg/mL; 250 µL/well) *(see* **Note 19**).
3. Incubate plates for 1h at 37°C in 5% CO_2 incubator.
4. Once the incubation period is completed, aspirate the medium and leave the plates to air-dry at room temperature.
5. Dissolve the insoluble formazan in 300 µL/well DMSO. Transfer 200 µL from each well to a 96-well plate and measure absorbance spectrophotometrically at 550 nm using a 96-well plate reader.

4. Notes

1. This peptide has been developed specifically for affinity purification of anti-ET-1 IgG. The N-terminal is blocked with a formyl group and Lys[9] is replaced by Nle so that there is only one free NH_2 group (Lys[17]-amide) in this peptide. This permits

specific coupling of this peptide to CNBr Sepharose with unrestricted access to the antigen binding site for affinity purification of ET-1$_{[1-15]}$ specific IgG.

2. These plates have been used routinely because of their reproducible binding characteristics and low crosstalk.

3. Standard solutions are required for ET-1, human big ET-1 and porcine big ET-1. These can be prepared reproducibly by using the following scheme with endothelin peptides from the Peptide Institute. For example, human big ET-1: the vial supplied contains 0.56 mg (130 nmol) big ET-1. Dissolve the peptide initially in 20 μL of DMSO, then add sufficient PBS (2.58 mL) to yield a 50 μM stock (50 nmol/mL). Dilute 50 μL of the 50 μM solution in 4.95 mL sandwich assay buffer (=500 pmol/mL), dilute 500 μL of 500 pmol/mL in 24.5 mL sandwich assay buffer to give a stock standard concentration of 10 pmol/mL. Prepare 0.5-mL aliquots and freeze at –20°C. The remaining 50 μM stock peptide is retained for other applications.

4. Medium samples need to be neutralized before assay. The pH of bicarbonate-buffered medium increases progressively during assay incubations to the extent that it may modify the values obtained. To overcome this problem, the following procedure is used. For experiments using 24-well plates, cell incubations are performed with 300 μL of medium per well. At the end of the experiment 270 μL of medium from each well is collected into a 1.5 mL polypropylene microtube, 25 μL of 0.295 mM HCl is added (=25 mM HCl), and the samples are heated at 80°C for 10 min. This heat treatment inactivates peptidases that may interfere in the assay and drives off the CO_2. The HCl facilitates this and partially neutralizes the sample. The amount of HCl required depends on the NaHCO$_3$ concentration in the medium. The method described here is optimized for DMEM containing 44 mM NaHCO$_3$. Once samples have cooled to room temperature to further neutralize each sample add 50 μL of neutralization buffer. This corrects the pH and provides protein and detergent to make the samples compatible with the assay. After immunoassay of the sample, the final ET-1 and big ET-1 values for each sample are corrected for this dilution.

5. Human cells often have high levels of peptidase activity that degrades the secreted ET-1 and big ET-1 immunoreactivity. Therefore, medium containing peptidase inhibitors is used to protect the released peptide. Degradation of ET-1 is not a problem with bovine aortic cells or bovine pulmonary artery smooth muscle cells so studies of these cells can be done without the addition of inhibitors. For other cell types, ET-1 release should be evaluated in the presence and absence of peptidase inhibitors before deciding whether their addition is necessary.

6. The HPLC system is used to purify peptides if required and to verify the success of chemical reactions. It is not essential if all peptides used are >95% purity, but it does provide useful confirmation that reactions have been successful. Depending on the peptide different gradient elution conditions will be required. However, as a general rule elution of 15–75% B over 60 min with buffer A of 0.1% trifluoroacetic acid and buffer B 0.1% trifluoroacetic in 80% acetonitrile/19.9% water will provide adequate resolution.

7. All manipulations to prepare immunogens should be performed using sterile polypropylene tubes, pipet tips and 0.2-μm filtered buffers. These precautions are usually sufficient to reduce the risk of injecting infective agents into the rabbits during the course of raising antisera. Infection can lead to animals becoming sick, with the result that they have to be withdrawn from the immunization schedule.

8. The immunization protocol is described here for rabbits; other species (e.g., sheep or goat) are also suitable. Choice is likely to depend on access to suitable facilities. Normally two or three female New Zealand white rabbits are immunized with each immunogen. The design of the assay does not use second antibody detection systems (**Fig. 1**). This allows both plate-coating IgG and detection IgG to be raised in the same species.

9. Test bleeds are collected into glass tubes and allowed to clot. Serum is separated 1–2 d later. Verification of antibody titer in test bleeds and final bleed can be performed if desired (e.g., by studying ^{125}I-ET-1 binding), but this is not essential as the amount of specific high affinity IgG is quantified spectrophotometrically at the end of the affinity purification step.

10. CNBr Sepharose reacts with free amino groups in peptides (and proteins). For efficient purification of IgG approx 2 μmol of peptide per mL of gel gives the best performance characteristics. The method outlined is a general method that can be applied to each of these peptides. If the efficiency of the reaction is to be confirmed by HPLC, a reference sample of each peptide solution should be taken prior to mixing with the CNBr Sepharose. However, monitoring the reaction is not essential if this method is followed carefully because CNBr Sepharose reacts so efficiently at the reaction ratio of 2 μmol of peptide per mL of gel that it is usual for >95% to react under the conditions described.

11. Sodium sulfate precipitation is a classical method for preparing an IgG precipitate that is relatively free of other serum proteins. Sodium sulfate is only poorly soluble so it needs to be dissolved by gentle mixing at room temperature. The volume of antiserum used can be greater or less than 40 mL—the quantity of sodium sulfate should be adjusted accordingly. Centrifugation of the serum to obtain an IgG precipitate should be carried out at 20°C otherwise the sodium sulfate will come out of solution.

12. Elution of IgG following this procedure may produce more than one peak of IgG. The IgG eluting in the early steps is generally of lower affinity. But late eluting IgG is more likely to be denatured by the procedure and have a consequent loss of affinity. Therefore, peak fractions should be pooled and evaluated separately. If a suitable radioligand is available, it is possible to identify and characterize the different fractions of eluted IgG by performing antibody dilution curves. However, this is unnecessary if the profile of eluted IgG measured spectrophotometrically shows a single peak with abundant levels of IgG (*see* **Fig. 2**).

13. It is important to remove all free NH_2 groups, e.g., residual glycine from the elution procedure as these can interfere with the biotinylation procedure. The reaction needs to be conducted at pH 8.0.

14. The quantity of IgG that is biotinylated can be as little as 100 μg. The quantity of the reactants need to be adjusted accordingly.

15. *N*-hydroxysuccinimide (NHS) esters, such as the biotinylation reagent being used here, are active esters that react with free NH_2 groups such as the ε-NH_2 group of Lys residues. They are unstable in aqueous solution, therefore, to favor the desired reaction and slow hydrolysis of the ester, these reactions are usually started at 4°C.

16. The ideal choice of dilution for a biotinylated IgG needs to be determined empirically by setting up a number of standard curves and testing a range of biotinylated antibody dilutions. Typically 50 µL per well in the range of 0.2–1 µg/mL of biotinylated IgG provides a suitable dilution.

17. Incubations with horseradish peroxidase (HRP) conjugates need to be performed in the absence of azide. Therefore the sandwich assay buffer is not suitable. Avidin-HRP and streptavidin-HRP are available from many suppliers. The working dilution for each HRP-conjugate should be determined by setting up a series of standard curves (including nonspecific binding) for evaluation of different conjugate dilutions. Selection of the optimal HRP-conjugate dilution is then based on the signal to noise ratio for each standard curve.

18. The methods described are applicable for any type of cell in culture that produces sufficient ET-1 for measurement by immunoassay. The EA.hy 926 cell line (results shown in **Fig. 4**) are grown to confluence in DMEM containing 10% fetal calf serum. Release studies over 6 h are conducted in serum free medium. For longer periods 1% fetal calf serum is added. Subcultures are prepared by treating confluent cultures in a T-75 flask with trypsin (0.05%) to detach cells. The cells are seeded onto 24-well plates for use when confluent. The method can be adapted for other cell types. For instance, human umbilical vein endothelial cells can be isolated from human umbilical cords and cultured using the following procedure. The umbilical vein is cannulated, flushed with Hanks balanced salt solution, and then filled with Dispase II (2.4 U/mL, Boehringer Mannheim). After incubation at 37°C for 30 min, detached cells are washed out and precipitated by centrifugation (5 min, 250*g*). The cell pellet is resuspended in endothelial cell growth medium (EGM-2; Clonetics, BioWhittaker, Walkersville, MD), and seeded onto plates precoated with gelatin (0.5%, overnight at 37°C). Inhibitor studies are performed in endothelial cell basal medium (EBM-2; Clonetics). Subcultures can be prepared by trypsinization of confluent cultures.

19. At the end of the incubation period, it is important to determine which test agents have had cytotoxic effects. This is done by using the MTT test to measure mitochondrial dehydrogenase activity by conversion of MTT to insoluble formazan, which is quantified spectrophotometrically. Reduced formazan production indicates a loss of viable cells and hence a cytotoxic effect of the agent under investigation.

Acknowledgments

I am indebted to Ms. N. Khan for her excellent technical assistance with these methods.

References

1. Yanagisawa, M., Kurihara, H., Kimura, S., Tomobe, Y., Kobayashi, M., Mitsui, Y., et al. (1988) A novel potent vasoconstrictor peptide produced by vascular endothelial cells. *Nature* **332,** 411–415.
2. Opgenorth, T. J., Wu-Wong, J. R., and Shiosaki, K. (1992) Endothelin-converting enzymes. *FASEB J.* **6,** 2653–2659.
3. Ohlstein, E. H., Arleth, A., Ezekiel, M., Horohonich, S., Ator, M. A., Caltabiano, M. M., and Sung, C. P. (1990) Biosynthesis and modulation of endothelin from bovine pulmonary arterial endothelial cells. *Life Sci.* **46,** 181–188.
4. Ikegawa, R., Matsumura, Y., Tsukahara, Y., Takaoka, M., and Morimoto, S. (1990) Phosphoramidon, a metalloproteinase inhibitor, suppresses the secretion of endothelin-1 from cultured endothelial cells by inhibiting a big endothelin-1 converting enzyme. *Biochem. Biophys. Res. Commun.* **171,** 669–675.
5. Corder, R., Khan, N., and Harrison, V. J. (1995) A simple method for isolating human endothelin converting enzyme (ECE-1) free from contamination by neutral endopeptidase 24.11. *Biochem. Biophys. Res. Commun.* **207,** 355–362.
6. Woods, M., Mitchell, J. A., Wood, E. G., Barker, S., Walcot, N. R., Rees, G. M., and Warner, T. D. (1999) Endothelin-1 is induced by cytokines in human vascular smooth muscle cells: Evidence for intracellular endothelin-converting enzyme. *Mol. Pharmacol.* **55,** 902–909.
7. Fukuroda, T., Noguchi, K., Tsuchida, S., Nishikibe, M., Ikemoto, F., Okada, K., and Yano, M. (1990) Inhibition of biological actions of big endothelin-1 by phosphoramidon. *Biochem. Biophys. Res. Commun.* **172,** 390–395.
8. Matsumura, Y., Hisaki, K., Takaoka, M., and Morimoto, S. (1990) Phosphoramidon, a metalloproteinase inhibitor, suppresses the hypertensive effect of big endothelin-1. *Eur. J. Pharmacol.* **185,** 103–106.
9. Ikegawa, R., Matsumura, Y., Tsukahara, Y., Takaoka, M., and Morimoto, S. (1991) Phosphoramidon inhibits the generation of endothelin-1 from exogenously applied big endothelin-1 in cultured vascular endothelial cells and smooth muscle cells. *FEBS Letts.* **293,** 45–48.
10. Harrison, V. J., Barnes, K., Turner, A. J., Wood, E. Corder. R., and Vane, J. R. (1995) Identification of endothelin 1 and big endothelin 1 in secretory vesicles isolated from bovine aortic endothelial cells. *Proc. Natl. Acad. Sci. USA* **92,** 6344–6348.
11. Schmidt, M., Kroger, B., Jacob, E., Seulberger, H., Subkowski, T., Otter, R., et al. (1994) Molecular characterization of human and bovine endothelin converting enzyme (ECE-1). *FEBS Letts.* **356,** 238–243.
12. Shimada, K., Takahashi, M., and Tanzawa, K. (1994) Cloning and functional expression of endothelin-converting enzyme from rat endothelial cells. *J. Biol. Chem.* **269,** 18,275–18,278.
13. Xu, D., Emoto, N., Giaid, A., Slaughter, C., Kaw, S., deWit, D., and Yanagisawa, M. (1994) ECE-1: a membrane-bound metalloprotease that catalyzes the proteolytic activation of big endothelin-1. *Cell* **78,** 473–485.

14. Yanagisawa, H., Yanagisawa, M., Kapur, R. P., Richardson, J. A., Williams, S. C., Clouthier, D. E., et al. (1998) Dual genetic pathways of endothelin-mediated intercellular signaling revealed by targeted disruption of endothelin converting enzyme-1 gene. *Development* **25,** 825–836.

15. Barker, S., Khan, N. Q., Wood, E. G., and Corder, R. (2001) Effect of an antisense oligodeoxynucleotide to endothelin-converting enzyme-1c (ECE-1c) on ECE-1c mRNA, ECE-1 protein and endothelin-1 synthesis in bovine pulmonary artery smooth muscle cells. *Mol. Pharmacol.* **59,** 163–169.

16. Jeng, A. Y., De Lombaert, S., Beil, M. E., Bruseo, C. W., Savage, P., Chou, M., and Trapani, A. J. (2001) Design and synthesis of a potent and selective endothelin-converting enzyme inhibitor, CGS 35066. *J. Cardiovasc. Pharmacol.* **36 (Suppl. 1),** S36–S39.

17. Corder, R. (2001) Identity of endothelin-converting enzyme and other targets for the therapeutic regulation of endothelin biosynthesis, in *Handbook of Experimental Pharmacology, vol. 152* (Warner, T. D., ed.) Springer-Verlag, pp. 35–67.

10

Endothelin-Converting Enzyme Activity in Vascular Smooth Muscle Preparations In Vitro

Janet J. Maguire

1. Introduction

The synthesis of ET-1, by the specific cleavage of its larger precursor big ET-1, by one or more endothelin-converting enzymes (ECE) has been discussed in Chapter 7. In the human vasculature ET-1, big ET-1 and ECE-1 are localized to secretory and storage granules *(1)* within endothelial cells *(2)*. ET-1 is released via the constitutive and stimulated pathways, together with big ET-1 *(3)*, and it is possible that additional conversion of this released big ET-1 occurs on the surface of the underlying smooth muscle cells. This is predicted by the observation that big ET-1, infused into the human forearm, significantly increases plasma levels of immunoreactive ET and decreases forearm blood flow in a phosphoramidon-sensitive manner. The hemodynamic response to big ET-1 occurred too quickly for appreciable amounts of phosphoramidon to have penetrated cell membranes, suggesting that the ECE responsible for conversion of infused big ET-1 is probably an ectoenzyme. As endothelial ECE has a predominantly intracellular localization *(1)*, expression of ECE on the surface of human smooth muscle cells may account for the rapid response to exogenous big ET-1. This is consistent with reports that, in isolated vascular preparations, removal of the endothelium does not alter responses to big ET-1 *(5–8)* implying the presence of a nonendothelial, presumably smooth muscle enzyme. Indeed, ECE activity has been reported in cultured vascular smooth muscle cells *(9,10)* and one isoform of ECE-1, ECE-1b, has been localized to the smooth muscle cell plasma membrane *(11)*.

Earlier reports indicated an apparent lack of immunoreactive ECE observed in smooth muscle cells *(12)* although we detect low levels of staining in adult

From: *Methods in Molecular Biology, vol. 206: Peptide Research Protocols: Endothelin*
Edited by: J. Maguire and A. Davenport © Humana Press Inc., Totowa, NJ

smooth muscle cells with more prominent localization of immunoreactive ECE in the fetal smooth muscle cells of the human umbilical vein *(1)*. A physiological role for this putative smooth muscle ECE remains to be determined. However, in human umbilical vein this enzyme will convert big ET-1, big ET-$2_{(1-37)}$, big ET-$2_{(1-38)}$ and big ET-3 to their respective mature, biologically active forms *(13)*. ET-2 and ET-3 are not synthesized by the endothelium *(14)*, but their precursors are present in human plasma *(15)*. We have therefore postulated that circulating big ET-2 and big ET-3, together with big ET-1 that is released from the endothelium, may be converted at their target organs, e.g., by smooth muscle cells in the vasculature.

In patients with coronary artery disease, plasma levels of ET-1 are raised *(16)*, and there are reports of increased ET-1 production in human atherosclerotic lesions *(17,18)*. ECE isoforms have been localized to coronary artery atherectomy specimens *(19)* and ECE-1c, ECE-1b and ECE-2 are associated with macrophages infiltrating atherosclerotic plaques within diseased arteries *(20)*. Increased expression or activity of ECE on smooth muscle cells, or other cell types present in atherosclerotic tissue, may therefore contribute to the increased plasma and tissue levels of the peptide seen in coronary artery disease. Using the protocol described in this chapter we demonstrated, for the first time, functional upregulation of ECE activity in atherosclerotic human coronary artery in vitro, compared to nondiseased vessels *(21)*. The enhanced vasoconstrictor response to big ET-1 that we measured in the diseased artery was associated with an increase in mature ET levels detected in the bathing medium. Control experiments indicated that the responses to ET-1 were not different in healthy and diseased vessels. Therefore, the increased response to big ET-1 in the atherosclerotic tissue must be due to increased cleavage to ET-1 and not to any increased response to ET-1 itself. Animal models of atherosclerosis also show an increase in ECE mRNA or protein levels in addition to an increase in enzyme activity *(19,22)*. We have subsequently used the selective ECE inhibitor PD159790 *(23)* to confirm a role for smooth muscle ECE in the conversion of big ET-1 to ET-1 in human coronary artery in vitro *(24)*.

Recent publications have indicated that smooth muscle conversion of big ET-1 to ET-1 may be attributable to enzymes other than the known ECEs *(25)*. The availability of selective ECE inhibitors will allow us to use vascular in vitro experiments, such as that described in this chapter, to identify novel enzymatic activity that may also contribute to smooth muscle ET-1 generation *(26)*, as has been controversially suggested for angiotensin II synthesis *(27–29)*. This may have implications for the development of mixed enzyme inhibitors as effective drugs for reducing the overproduction of ET-1 in cardiovascular disease.

This chapter describes the use of endothelium-denuded vascular preparations to construct concentration-response curves to the ET-1 precursor, big ET-1, in the presence and absence of known enzyme inhibitors or test compounds to determine the extent of nonendothelial ECE activity and its functional characteristics. In the absence of selective inhibitors, ECE activity was originally characterized using the selective neutral endopeptidase (NEP) inhibitor thiorphan and the mixed NEP/ECE inhibitor phosphoramidon *(30)*. Thus, ECE activity was described as the thiorphan-insensitive, but phosphoramidon-sensitive, conversion of big ET-1 to ET-1. In the in vitro vascular experiments, the observed vasoconstrictor response is presumably elicited by the ET-1 generated by smooth muscle cell conversion of the exogenously added big ET-1. Therefore, it is important when demonstrating the effect or lack of effect of enzyme inhibitors (novel or known) on big ET-1 vasoconstriction that a control experiment is carried out to show a lack of effect of the inhibitor on ET-1. Only if this is carried out can any effect on big ET-1 be attributable to an attenuation of ECE activity and not to any subsequent effect on the ET-1 peptide that is generated by the tissue. **Figure 1** shows concentration-response curves to big ET-1 and ET-1 in the absence and presence of thiorphan and phosphoramidon illustrating the experimental protocol outlined below. After the functional experiments are terminated, the bathing medium from each bath is collected for subsequent analysis by radioimmunoassay, using the protocol described in Chapter 2. The presence of ET-1 in the bathing medium confirms that conversion of big ET-1 to ET-1 has occurred. This protocol may be followed for human or animal vascular preparations (arteries and veins) or indeed nonvascular preparations including human bronchus *(31)*, rat uterus *(32)* and guinea pig lung parenchyma *(33)*.

2. Materials

1. Vascular tissue.
2. In vitro pharmacology equipment comprising heated organ baths (*see* **Note 1**), isometric force transducers (*see* **Note 2**) with vernier control (to adjust preload), amplifiers, chart recorder and/or computerized data acquisition system, circulating water bath (**Fig. 2**).
3. Krebs' solution: 20 L of solution A is prepared from concentrated stocks of individual salts that are made up in double distilled water and kept at 4°C.
   To 16755 mL double distilled water add 1 L of NaCl (104.2 g/L), 1 L of NaHCO$_3$ (48.8 g/L), 400 mL of KCl (18.6 g/L), 400 mL of MgSO$_4$·7H$_2$O (6 g/L) and 400 mL of Na$_2$HPO$_4$·2H$_2$O (8.9 g/L). Bubble continuously (for at least 15 min) with 95% O$_2$/5% CO$_2$ to reduce pH and slowly add 45 mL 1 M CaCl$_2$ solution. Solution A is then stored at 4°C.
   Solution B is prepared as follows. To 1 L double distilled water (in a 2-L beaker as this mixture effervesces) add 63 g NaHCO$_3$, then slowly add 29 g fumaric acid. Stir, add 36.75 g glutamic acid and when this has dissolved add 90.5 g glucose and 27.5 g sodium pyruvate. Solution B is stored in 20 mL aliquots at −20°C until required.

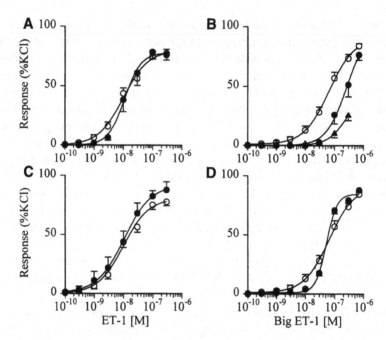

Fig. 1. Concentration-response curves in endothelium-denuded human umbilical vein to **(A)** ET-1 in the absence (○) and presence (●) of 10 μ*M* phosphoramidon; **(B)** big ET-1 in absence (○) and presence of 10 μ*M* (●) and 100 μ*M* (▲) phosphoramidon; **(C)** ET-1 in the absence (○) and presence (●) of 10 μ*M* thiorphan; **(D)** big ET-1 in the absence (○) and presence (●) of 10 μ*M* thiorphan. The data show the lack of effect of both inhibitors on the response to ET-1 (A,C), the lack of effect of thiorphan on big ET-1 (D), but the concentration-dependent inhibition of big ET-1 by phosphoramidon (B) (*see* **ref. *13*).

To make up Krebs' solution, defrost solution B and add 20 mL to each liter of solution A. The final composition of this Krebs' solution is: 90 m*M* NaCl, 5 m*M* KCl, 0.5 m*M* MgSO$_4$, 1 m*M* NaHPO$_4$, 45 m*M* NaHCO$_3$, 10 m*M* glucose, 5 m*M* Na pyruvate, 5 m*M* glutamic acid; 5 m*M* fumaric acid; 2.25 m*M* CaCl$_2$.

4. 1 *M* KCL Solution stored at 4°C.

5. Endothelin peptides (ET-1, big ET-1) are from Peptide Institute (Osaka, Japan) (*see* **Note 3**) and are prepared according to their instructions in 0.01% acetic acid as 10^{-4} *M* stock solutions. These are dispensed as 50–100 μL aliquots and kept at –20°C. Dilutions (1 in 10 from 10^{-4} *M* to 10^{-8} *M*) are prepared in deionized water and kept on ice during the experiment.

6. Phosphoramidon (Peptide Institute, Osaka, Japan) is prepared as a 10^{-2} *M* stock solution in deionized water and stored as aliquots at –20°C. Thiorphan (Sigma Aldrich, Poole, Dorset, UK) is prepared as a 10^{-2} *M* solution in dimethyl sulfoxide. Test inhibitors/novel compounds are made up as appropriate.

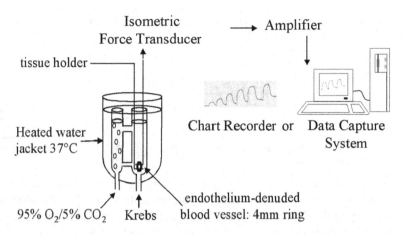

Fig. 2. Schematic representation of equipment used for in vitro pharmacology experiments.

7. Glass barrelled fixed needle syringes (e.g., Hamilton Microliter™ Syringe 705N) to dispense microliter volumes of peptides into organ bath, or similar.
8. Ice bucket and ice.
9. Dissecting scissors, forceps, seeker, small Petri dishes and single edge blades.
10. Polypropylene tubes and caps to store samples of bath contents at –20°C.
11. Curve-fitting program, e.g., Fig P (Biosoft, Cambridge, UK) or similar, or semi-log graph paper.

3. Methods

1. Turn on the organ bath equipment, warm up and oxygenate the Krebs' solution (37°C, 95% O_2/5%CO_2), warm up and calibrate the transducers (*see* **Note 4**), set up the chart recorder and/or data capture system. Allow the 1 M KCl solution to come to room temperature.
2. Dissect out the blood vessel from surrounding connective tissue. Take care not to damage the smooth muscle layer. Cut into 4-mm lengths using a single-edged blade. Place the rings in oxygenated, Krebs' solution in a Petri dish. Use a blunt metal seeker to gently rub the luminal side of each ring to disrupt the endothelium. Transfer the rings to the organ baths and place on tissue holders without tension. Leave to equilibrate for 30–60 min (*see* **Note 5**).
3. Carry out a normalization (resting tension-active tension) procedure to determine the appropriate resting tension for each ring (*see* **Note 6**). Use the vernier control to place 1–5 gf (~10–50 mN) (the amount will depend on blood vessel type, size and wall thickness; less than 1 gf should be used on very small, thin walled vessels) on each ring and add 1 M KCl to give a final bath concentration of 100 mM (account for the 5 mM KCl in the Krebs' solution, i.e., add 480 μL of 1 M KCl to a 5 mL bath). Allow the KCl response to plateau and then wash out and replace

Grams force developed   2.9gf   5.2gf   8.4gf   10.1gf   11.3gf   11.1gf

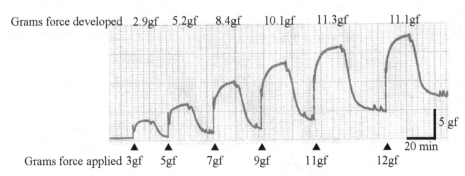

Grams force applied 3gf   5gf   7gf   9gf   11gf   12gf

Fig. 3. An example of the normalization procedure for the determination of optimal resting tension in endothelium-denuded human saphenous vein. Responses are obtained to 100 mM KCl at incrementally increasing level of basal tension (grams force applied) until no further increase in KCl response (grams force developed) is obtained.

with fresh Krebs. Once the baseline has stabilized, increase the basal tension by a further 1–5 gf increment and repeat the KCl response. Continue in this manner until successive responses to KCl are comparable (within approx 10%) (**Fig. 3**). Wash preparations and allow them to equilibrate for a further 30–60 min before starting the experiment (*see* **Note 7**).

4. Lack of functional endothelium can be determined by addition of a submaximal concentration of an appropriate vasoconstrictor such as noradrenaline (~3 × 10^{-7} M) or phenylephrine (~10^{-5} M). Once the constrictor response has reached a plateau add an endothelium-dependant vasodilator such as acetylcholine or bradykinin (both at ~10^{-6} M). No response to the vasodilator confirms the absence of a functional endothelium (*see* **Note 8**). Wash the preparations and leave to reequilibrate in fresh Krebs' solution for 10–20 min.

5. If ECE inhibitors/test compounds are being investigated, add these to the bathing medium at the appropriate concentration and leave for 30 min or a time determined in other assays (*see* **Note 9**). Ideally, the inhibitors will be tested at more than one concentration.

6. Set up appropriate control baths for the radioimmunoassay. These should include (a) tissue set up for which no ET-1/big ET-1 curve is constructed, this is used to determine any basal release of ET from the tissue into the Krebs' solution during the time course of the experiment; (b) a bath in which no tissue is set up, but big ET-1 is added to determine if big ET-1 spontaneously breaks down to ET-1 in the Krebs' medium and (c) a bath in which no tissue is set up and no peptides are added (blank).

7. Construct cumulative concentration-response curves to ET-1 and big ET-1 in the absence (controls) and presence of the inhibitors. Add peptides to the bathing medium at concentrations increasing by half a log unit. Allow each response to reach a maximum before the next is added. When addition of the next concentration of agonist elicits no further increase in response, the experiment is termi-

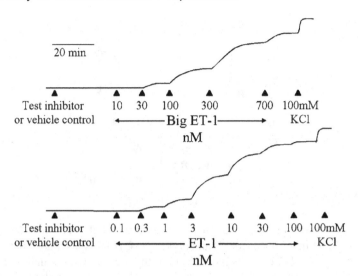

Fig. 4. Schematic representation of an experiment to determine the effect of a test ECE inhibitor on big ET-1 vascular smooth muscle vasoconstriction in vitro. Cumulative concentration response curves are constructed to ET-1 and big ET-1 in the absence (vehicle control) and presence of the inhibitor in rings of endothelium-denuded blood vessel, from the same animal or patient, set up in adjacent tissue baths.

nated by addition of 1 M KCl to give a bath concentration of 100 mM; this determines the maximum possible contractile response of each vascular ring (**Fig. 4**) (*see* **Note 10**).

8. Transfer the Krebs' solution from each bath to polypropylene tubes, cap, label and store at –20°C. for subsequent analysis of ET-1 content by radioimmunoassay (*see* Chapter 2).

9. For data analysis, the agonist responses are derived manually from the pen-recorder chart or from the data capture system used, e.g., the Biopac MP100 system (Biopac, Santa Barbara, CA). From the raw data construct concentration-response graphs with the agonist response expressed either (a) in gf (or mN) or (b) as a percentage of the maximal KCl response obtained prior to the concentration-response curve or (c) as a percentage of the terminal KCl response (**Fig. 1**) (*see* **Note 11**).

10. Analyze data curves for ET-1 and big ET-1 in the absence and presence of inhibitors using a nonlinear, iterative curve-fitting program, such as Fig P (Biosoft, Cambridge, UK), to give values of pD_2 (or EC_{50}) and E_{max}. Express values of pD_2 and E_{max} from a number of experiments as arithmetic mean ± s.e. mean. This allows control values to be compared to those obtained in the presence of an inhibitor using appropriate statistical tests. Where the effect of an inhibitor is such that it is not possible to complete a concentration-response curve to ET-1 or big ET-1 in the presence of that inhibitor (because of constraints on the amount

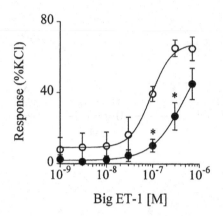

Fig. 5. Concentration-response curves in human endothelium-denuded coronary artery to big ET-1 in the absence (○) and presence (●) of 100 μ*M* phosphoramidon. In this tissue, the big ET-1 curve is incomplete in the presence of the inhibitor over the concentration range of big ET-1 that can be achieved. The effect of phosphoramidon is therefore expressed as a significant reduction in response to 100 n*M* and 300 n*M* big ET-1 (*) compared to control, determined using Student's *t*-test.

of peptide available), then it is reasonable to compare the response of a single concentration of ET-1 or big ET-1 to that obtained in the presence of the inhibitor and show a significant attenuation of response (**Fig. 5**).

11. Confirmation of the conversion of big ET-1 to ET-1 in vascular smooth muscle preparations may be obtained by the detection of mature ET in the bathing medium by radioimmunoassay as described in Chapter 2 (*see* **Note 12**). We detected significantly higher levels of mature ET in the bathing medium from human atherosclerotic coronary arteries compared to nondiseased vessels *(21)*. However, it should be remembered that these levels reflect amounts of ET present in the bathing medium and not receptor bound or nonspecifically bound ET. Therefore, the differences observed are relative rather than absolute.

4. Notes

1. Small volume organ baths of approx 5 mL are most appropriate for experiments using peptides, as these are prohibitively expensive if used in conjunction with baths of 10–50 mL volume. If possible, baths can be coated with Sigmacote (Sigma-Aldrich, Poole, Dorset, UK) to reduce adherence of peptide to the glass, although this does not appear to be a problem with the endothelin peptides. We use a 5-mL bath (Linton Instrumentation, Diss, UK) that incorporates a side chamber housing the O_2/CO_2 inlet. Separating tissue chamber from gas inlet chamber reduces bubble artefacts (*see* **Fig. 2**). Commercial sources of organ bath equipment include Linton Instrumentation (Diss, UK) and Hugo Sachs Elektronik (March-Hugstetten, Germany).

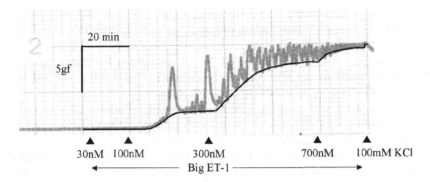

Fig. 6. Original trace illustrating the development of spontaneous activity in a 4-mm ring of endothelium-denuded human umbilical vein during the construction of a big ET-1 concentration-response curve. The solid black line indicates the tonic response that is measured to increasing concentrations of the peptide, upon which the spontaneous phasic contractions are superimposed. At the higher concentrations of big ET-1, the amplitude of the phasic response is reduced, but the frequency of oscillation is increased as previously reported for other vasoconstrictors in, e.g., human coronary artery *(34)*.

2. The force transducer used should have sufficient range to measure the tension developed by different vascular preparations to agonists/KCl. For most vascular preparations, a range of 30gf is sufficient, e.g., the F30 (Hugo Sachs Elektronik, March-Hugstetten, Germany).
3. Peptides are available from several different commercial sources. We recommend the Peptide Institute (Osaka, Japan) as the peptides are supplied as net peptide content and instructions are provided for making the peptides up as solutions of a given concentration. Always check if a peptide is provided as net peptide content, if not account for this, and peptide purity, when making up stock solutions. The concentration of a peptide solution may be confirmed by spectrophotometry.
4. The transducers are calibrated either in gf or mN.
5. Vascular ring preparations sometimes develop phasic spontaneous activity that makes measurement of drug responses more difficult. These may commence at any time during the experiment, e.g., immediately tension is applied to the tissue, during the normalization procedure, during the equilibration period post-KCl normalization or following addition of inhibitors/agonists (at the beginning or mid-way through the concentration-response curve). As they are not directly related to the action of the test compounds (usually commencing before addition of these), but are most likely elicited by the physical manipulation of the tissue, we measure the agonist responses as changes in basal tension upon which the phasic, spontaneous activity may be superimposed. Sufficient time must therefore be allowed between agonist additions for the phasic spontaneous contractions to return to their basal level to determine if the effect of the agonist on basal tone is completed (**Fig. 6**). Stork and Cocks have written a very useful and rel-

evant paper that discusses the occurrence and possible ionic basis of spontaneous activity in human coronary artery *(34)* that has wider applicability.

6. If possible a resting tension-passive tension normalization procedure can be carried out that sets the resting tension to 90% of the tension the vascular tissue would be under in vivo. For convenience, this usually requires an automated vernier control system attached to the tissue holder.

7. For particular vascular preparations once the normalization procedure has been carried out on two or three separate occasions, the amount of tension a ring of a particular blood vessel is capable of developing and the approximate value of the optimal basal tension should become apparent. The appropriate initial tension to be applied and the incremental tension increases with subsequent KCl additions can then be determined to reduce this part of the experiment to three or four applications of KCl.

8. We have generally confirmed destruction of the endothelial cell layer by histological examination of frozen sections of the prepared vascular tissue to show a lack of staining with the endothelial cell marker von-Willebrand factor *(13)*.

9. Inhibitors or test compounds should be added to the baths in volumes of less than 1% of total bath volume. If dissolved in anything other than water or Krebs' solution then the solvent should be tested, at the appropriate volume, for nonspecific effects on responses to ET-1 and big ET-1.

10. For each different smooth muscle preparation, control concentration-response curves should be constructed to KCl in tissue from several animals/patients to determine the concentration that elicits the maximum contractile response. For the human large diameter blood vessels that we study this is typically 100 mM.

11. In our experience, in control experiments (i.e., ET-1 or big ET-1 concentration-response curves in absence of inhibitors) the magnitude of the terminal KCl response (post-KCl) is not significantly different from that obtained at the beginning of the experiment following normalization (pre-KCl). In studies investigating the effects of enzyme inhibitors, this post-KCl/pre-KCl ratio can be extremely useful in identifying nonspecific effects of the test compounds on vascular function.

12. Measurement of the levels of mature ET in the bathing medium reflects only the free concentration of peptide present and does not account for receptor-bound or nonspecifically bound peptide.

Acknowledgments

We thank the British Heart Foundation for support.

References

1. Russell, F. D., Skepper, J. N., and Davenport, A. P. (1998) Human endothelial cell storage granules: a novel intracellular site for isoforms of the endothelin-converting enzyme. *Circ. Res.* **80,** 314–321.

2. Davenport, A. P., Kuc, R. E., Plumpton, C., Mockridge, J. W., Barker, P. J., and Huskinsson, N. S. (1998) Endothelin-converting enzyme in human tissue. *Histochem. J.* **30,** 1–16.

3. Plumpton, C., Kalinka, S., Martin, R. C., Horton, J. K., and Davenport, A. P. (1994) Effects of phosphoramidon and pepstatin A on the secretion of endothelin-1 and big

endothelin-1 by human umbilical vein endothelial cells: measurement by two-site enzyme-linked immunosorbent assays. *Clin. Sci.* **87**, 245–251.

4. Plumpton, C., Haynes, W. G., Webb, D. J., and Davenport, A. P. (1995) Phosphoramidon inhibition of the in vivo conversion of big endothelin-1 to endothelin-1 in the human forearm. *Br. J. Pharmacol.* **116**, 1821–1828.

5. Fukuroda, T., Noguchi, K., Tsuchida, S., Nishikibe, M., Ikemoto, F., Okada, K., and Yano, M. (1990) Inhibition of biological actions of big endothelin-1 by phosphoramidon. *Biochem. Biophys. Res. Commun.* **172**, 390–395.

6. Yano, M., Okada, K., Takada, J., Hioki, Y., Matsuyama, K., Fukuroda, T., et al. (1991) Endothelin-converting enzyme and its in vitro and in vivo inhibition. *J. Cardiovasc. Pharmacol.* **17(Suppl. 7)**, S26–S28.

7. Hisaki, K., Matsumura, Y., Nishiguchi, S., Fujita, K., Takaoka, M., and Morimoto, S. (1993) Endothelium-independent pressor effect of Big endothelin-1 and its inhibition by phosphoramidon in rat mesenteric artery. *Eur. J. Pharmacol.* **241**, 75–81.

8. Mombouli, J.-V., Le, S.Q., Wasserstrum, N., and Vanhoutte, P. (1993) Endothelins 1 and 3 and big endothelin-1 contract isolated human placental veins. *J. Cardiovasc. Pharmacol.* **22(Suppl.8)**, S278–S281.

9. Kent, A. and Keenan, A. K. (1995) Evidence for signalling by big endothelin-1 via conversion to endothelin-1 in pulmonary-artery smooth-muscle cells. *Life Sci.* **57**, 1191–1196.

10. Yu, J. C. M. and Davenport, A. P. (1995) Secretion of endothelin-1 and endothelin-3 by human cultured vascular smooth-muscle cells. *Br. J. Pharmacol.* **114**, 551–557.

11. Emoto, N., Nurhantari, Y., Alimsardjono, H., Xie, J., Yamada, T., Yanagisawa, M., and Matsuo, M. (1999) Constitutive lysosomal targeting and degradation of bovine endothelin-converting enzyme-1a mediated by novel signals in its alternatively spliced cytoplasmic tail. *J. Biol. Chem.* **274**, 1509–1518.

12. Takahashi, M., Fukuda, K., Shimada, K., Barnes, K., Turner, A.J., Ikeda, M., et al. (1995) Localization of rat endothelin-converting enzyme to vascular endothelial cells and some secretory cells. *Biochem. J.* **311**, 657–665.

13. Maguire, J. J., Johnson, C. M., Mockridge, J. W., and Davenport, A. P. (1997) Endothelin converting enzyme (ECE) activity in human vascular smooth muscle. *Br. J. Pharmacol.* **122**, 1647–1654.

14. Plumpton, C., Ashby, M. J., Kuc, R. E., O'Reilly, G., and Davenport, A. P. (1996) Expression of endothelin peptides and mRNA in the human heart. *Clin. Sci.* **90**, 37–46.

15. Matsumoto, H., Suzuki, N., Kitada, C., and Fujino, M. (1994) Endothelin family peptides in human plasma and urine: their molecular form and concentration. *Peptides* **15**, 505–510.

16. Lerman, A., Edwards, B. S., Hallett, J. W., Heublein. D. M., Sandberg, S. M., and Burnett, J. C. (1991) Circulating and tissue endothelin immunoreactivity in advanced atherosclerosis. *N. Engl. J. Med.* **325**, 997–1001.

17. Zeiher, A. M., Goebel, H., Schächinger, V., and Ihling, C. (1995) Tissue endothelin-1 immunoreactivity in the active coronary atherosclerotic plaque. A clue to the mechanism of increased vasoreactivity of the culprit lesion in unstable angina. *Circulation* **91**, 941–947.

18. Bacon, C. R., Cary, N. R. B., and Davenport, A. P. (1996) Endothelin peptide and receptors in human atherosclerotic coronary artery and aorta. *Circ. Res.* **79,** 794–801.

19. Minamino, T., Kurihara, H., Takahashi, M., Shimada, K., Maemura, K., Oda, H., et al. (1997) Endothelin-converting enzyme expression in the rat vascular injury model and human coronary atherosclerosis. *Circulation* **95,** 221–230.

20. Davenport, A. P. and Kuc, R. E. (2000) Cellular expression of isoforms of endothelin-converting enzyme-1 (ECE-1c, ECE-1b and ECE-1a) and endothelin-converting enzyme-2. *J. Cardiovasc. Pharmacol.* **36(Suppl. 1),** S12–S14.

21. Maguire, J. J. and Davenport, A. P. (1998) Increased response to big endothelin-1 in atherosclerotic human coronary artery: functional evidence for up-regulation of endothelin-converting enzyme activity in disease. *Br. J. Pharmacol.* **125,** 238–240.

22. Grantham, J. A., Schirger, J. A., Williamson, E. E., Heublein, D., Wennberg, P. W., Kirchengast, M., et al. (1998) Enhanced endothelin-converting enzyme immunoreactivity in early atherosclerosis. *J. Cardiovasc. Pharmacol.* **31(Suppl.1),** S22–S26.

23. Ahn, K., Sisneros, A. M., Herman, S. B., Pan, S. M., Hupe, D., Lee, C., et al. (1998) Novel selective quinazoline inhibitors of endothelin converting enzyme-1. *Biochem. Biophys. Res. Commum.* **243,** 184–190.

24. Maguire, J. J., Ahn, K., and Davenport, A. P. (1999) Inhibition of big endothelin-1 (big ET-1) responses in endothelium-denuded human coronary artery by the selective endothelin-converting enzyme-1 (ECE-1) inhibitor PD159790. *Br. J. Pharmacol.* **126,** U102.

25. Barker, S., Khan, N. G., Wood, E. G., and Corder, R. (2001) Effect of an antisense oligodeoxynucleotide to endothelin-converting enzyme-1c (ECE-1c) on ECE-1c mRNA, ECE-1 protein and endothelin-1 synthesis in bovine pulmonary artery smooth muscle cells. *Mol. Pharmacol.* **59,** 163–169.

26. Maguire, J. J., Kuc, R. E., and Davenport, A. P. (2001) Vasoconstrictor activity of novel endothelin peptide, ET-1$_{(1-31)}$, in human mammary and coronary arteries in vitro. *Br. J. Pharmacol.* **134,** 1360–1366.

27. Urata, H., Kinoshita, A., Misono, K. S., Bumpus, F. M., and Husain, A. (1990) Identification of a highly specific chymase as the major angiotensin II-forming enzyme in the human heart. *J. Biol. Chem.* **265,** 22,348–22,357.

28. Zisman, L. S., Abraham, W. T., Meixell, G. E., Vamvakias, B. N., Quaife, R. A., Lowes, B. D., et al. (1995) Angiotensin II formation in the intact human heart: predominance of the angiotensin-converting enzyme pathway. *J. Clin. Invest.* **95,** 1490–1498.

29. Kokkonen, J. O., Saarinen, J., and Kovanen, P. T. (1998) Angiotensin II formation in the human heart: an ACE or nonACE-mediated pathway? *Ann. Med.* **30(Suppl. 1),** 9–13.

30. Turner, A. J. and Murphy, L. J. (1996) Molecular pharmacology of endothelin converting enzymes. *Biochem. Pharmacol.* **51,** 91–102.

31. Yap, E. Y. S., Battistini, B., and McKay, K. O. (2000) Contraction to big endothelin-1, big endothelin-2 and big endothelin-3, and endothelin-converting enzyme inhibition in human isolated bronchi. *Br. J. Pharmacol.* **129,** 170–176.

32. Rae, G. A., Calixto, J. B., and D'Orléans-Juste, P. D. (1993) Conversion of big endothelin-1 in rat uterus causes contraction mediated by ET_A receptors. *J. Cardiovasc. Pharmacol.* **22(Suppl. 8),** S192–S195.
33. Battistini, B., Brown, M., and Vane, J. R. (1995) Selective proteolitic activation and degradation of ETs and Big ETs in parenchymal strips of guinea-pig lung. *Biochem. Biophys. Res. Commum.* **207,** 675–681.
34. Stork, A. P. and Cocks, T. M. (1994) Pharmacological reactivity of human epicardial coronary arteries: phasic and tonic responses to vasoconstrictor agents differentiated by nifedipine. *Br. J. Pharmacol.* **113,** 1093–1098.

IV

IN VITRO FUNCTIONAL ASSAYS

11

Characterization of a New Endothelin Receptor Ligand by In Vitro Assays

J. Ruth Wu-Wong

1. Introduction

Following the discovery of endothelin *(1)*, functional characterization of the three endothelin (ET) isoforms (ET-1, ET-2 and ET-3) predicted that two mammalian receptor subtypes are present: the ET_A receptor that is selective for ET-1, and the ET_B receptor that has equal affinity for the three isoforms *(2)*. The existence of the two distinct high-affinity ET receptor subtypes has been confirmed by cloning. Unique cDNAs that code for ET_A and ET_B belonging to the G-protein linked heptahelical receptor superfamily are identified in human, bovine and rat tissues *(3–6)*. While pharmacological studies suggest that there may be more ET receptor subtypes *(7)*, no additional homologous mammalian cDNAs have been identified.

In tissues and cells, ET binding initiates a complex signal transduction cascade *(8)*. ET-1 binding activates phospholipases C and D, causing increases in inositol 1,4,5-trisphosphate and neutral 1,2-diacylglycerol which are associated with a biphasic increase in the intracellular Ca^{2+} concentration and activation of various kinase-mediated pathways involved in mitogenic responses *(9,10)*. Recent evidence suggests that ETs may play a role in modulating apoptosis of endothelial and smooth muscle cells *(11,12)*. ET-1 may play a pivotal role in the pathogenesis of cardiovascular diseases and cell growth disorders such as cancer *(13)*.

A major advance was made in the ET field with the development of ET receptor antagonists. In particular, BQ-123 *(14)* and FR139317 *(15)* have been important tools in studying ET-mediated pathophysiology. Both are ET_A receptor-selective, but are peptidic compounds and have poor pharmacokinetics with limited utility as therapeutic agents. Following the peptidic compounds,

From: *Methods in Molecular Biology, vol. 206: Peptide Research Protocols: Endothelin*
Edited by: J. Maguire and A. Davenport © Humana Press Inc., Totowa, NJ

many pharmaceutical companies reported the discovery of a number of nonpeptide antagonists with greatly improved pharmacokinetics, such as Ro 47-0203, SB 209670, PD 151242, ABT-627, and so on (*see* Fig. 1 and Table 1 in Chapter 5). Some of these antagonists are being investigated in human clinical trials.

Previously we have reported the characterization of new ET receptor antagonists developed by Abbott Laboratories *(16,17)*. The purpose of this chapter is to compile information on some of the well-established in vitro assays in order to provide guidelines to researchers who need to characterize a new ET receptor ligand.

The following factors shall be considered when characterizing a new ET receptor ligand: (1) procedures for handling ET receptor ligands, (2) using receptor binding studies to characterize the new ligand, (3) using functional assays to characterize the new ligand, and (4) other characteristics of the new ligand.

1.1. Procedures for Handling ET Receptor Ligands

As mentioned in Chapter 5, ET receptor agonists and antagonists are by nature very sticky. These agents stick to the walls of test tubes or containers easily. Therefore, in order to obtain accurate information when conducting ET studies, precautions should be taken when making and handling stock solutions or dilutions of ET receptor ligands. The procedures followed in our own laboratory for handling these ligands are described in details under Subheading 3.1. in Chapter 5.

1.2. Using Receptor Binding Studies to Characterize the New Ligand

The questions to ask when first characterizing a new ligand are: How potent is this compound in antagonizing ET-1 binding to ET_A and ET_B receptors? How selective is this ligand to ET_A vs ET_B receptor? To answer these questions, an effective approach is to conduct receptor binding studies using membranes prepared from tissues or cells. Two types of membranes should be used: one that contains ET_A exclusively, and the other that contains ET_B exclusively. If the membranes contain both ET_A and ET_B receptors, it will make data interpretation more difficult. So, using membranes that only contain either ET_A or ET_B is highly recommended. A good practice is to use membranes prepared from mammalian cells transfected with only ET_A or ET_B receptor. In our own laboratories, we have cloned human ET receptors and expressed them in CHO cells for this very purpose. The methods for generating CHO cells with ET_A or ET_B receptor have been described previously *(18)*. If CHO cells transfected with ET_A or ET_B receptor are not available, it is quite acceptable to use a tissue or a cell line that expresses either ET_A or ET_B receptor. When a natural source of

Table 1
Cells or Tissues that Express ET_A or ET_B Receptor

Cell/tissue type	Receptor subtype	Reference
Astrocytoma U138MG (human)	ET_A	*19*
Astrocytoma U373MG (human)	ET_B	*20*
Cerebellum (porcine)	ET_B	*21*
Fibroblast IMR90 cells (human)	ET_A	*22*
Fibroblast 3T3-L1 (mouse)	ET_A	*23*
Fibroblast Swiss 3T3 (mouse)	ET_A	*24*
MMQ from pituitary tumor (rat)	ET_A	*25*
Prostatic carcinoma (human)	ET_A	*26*
Umbilical vein endothelial cells (human)	ET_B	*27*

ET_A or ET_B receptor is used, make sure that the receptor density is adequate for obtaining good counts. Detailed characterization of the receptor is important. The method for characterizing an ET receptor in a tissue or cell line is described in Chapter 5. **Table 1** shows a short list of cells and tissues that express either ET_A or ET_B receptor.

Once a source with the right subtype of ET receptor is identified, the next step is to prepare membranes. Methods for membrane preparation from cells and tissues are described in Chapter 5 (*see* Subheading 3.3.1.). After membranes are prepared, it may be necessary to determine the amount of membrane proteins required to achieve good counts. Even from the same tissue or cell source, every time a batch of membranes is prepared, it is often necessary to conduct a study to determine the amount of membrane proteins needed in a binding study. Because of this, membranes should be prepared in as large a quantity as possible in order to reduce efforts in having to go through the characterization process frequently. The method for testing the binding capacity of a membrane preparation is described below (*see* **Subheading 3.1.2.**).

When the membranes and other ingredients are ready, then a competition binding study can be conducted to determine the IC_{50} value of the ligand in antagonizing the binding of [^{125}I]ET-1 or [^{125}I]ET-3. We use [^{125}I]ET-1 for membranes expressing ET_A and [^{125}I]ET-3 for ET_B. It is acceptable to use [^{125}I]ET-1 for ET_B since [^{125}I]ET-1 can bind to both ET_A and ET_B receptors. Once the IC_{50} value is obtained, it can be compared with IC_{50} values of other known antagonists (*see* **Note 1**). Better yet, the new ligand can be compared with a known antagonist in the same competition binding study to determine the potency. The known antagonist also serves as the positive control to ensure the binding study is done correctly.

From the IC_{50}, the K_i of the ligand can be calculated by using the following equation if the K_d of ET-1 or ET-3 binding to that tissue/cell is known.

$$IC_{50} = K_i (1 + [L]/K_d)$$

L, concentration of $[^{125}I]$ET-1 used; K_d, equilibrium dissociation constant of ET-1.

As an example, the IC_{50} value of A-216546 (ABT-546), an ET_A-selective antagonist, is 0.49 nM when determined using CHO cells transfected with human ET_A receptor. Assuming the K_d of ET-1 binding to human ET_A is 0.1 nM (calculated by Scatchard analysis. *See* Chapter 5 for discussion on the pros and cons of using Scatchard analysis to determine K_d), then the K_i of ABT-546 is determined to be 0.25 nM when 0.1 nM $[^{125}I]$ET-1 is used in the competition binding study.

To determine the true K_i value of a ligand, a more accurate approach is to conduct $[^{125}I]$ET-1 or $[^{125}I]$ET-3 saturation binding studies in the presence of several different concentrations of the test ligand. Using this approach, the K_i value is no longer dependent on the concentration of $[^{125}I]$ET-1 used. In addition, from the data, the mode of inhibition for the compound can be determined. For example, if a compound decreases the binding affinity (K_d) of ET-1 without affecting the receptor density (B_{max}), likely it is a competitive inhibitor of ET-1 binding. The method for determining K_i is described under **Subheading 3.1.4.** Using this approach, the K_i value of A-216546 is determined to be 0.46 nM.

From the IC_{50}, the selectivity of the ligand can also be determined. The ratio between the IC_{50} values of ET_A compared to ET_B indicates how selective this ligand is for one receptor over the other. For example, if the IC_{50} values of the ligand for ET_A and ET_B are 1 nM and 1000 nM respectively, then it is an ET_A selective ligand with a 1000-fold selectivity for ET_A. If the IC_{50} ratio between ET_A and ET_B is less than 100-fold, the ligand is nonselective. The differentiation becomes more ambiguous if the ratio is less than 500-fold but more than 100-fold. Depending on information from functional studies, such a ligand is sometimes classified as nonselective.

1.3. Using Functional Assays to Characterize the New Ligand

Once the potency and selectivity are determined by binding studies, the next step is to determine whether the ligand of interest is an antagonist or an agonist. In general, if the ligand can induce a biological response by itself and the effect can be blocked by a known ET receptor antagonist, it is an ET receptor agonist. On the other hand, if the ligand antagonizes biological responses induced by ET-1 or ET-3, it is not necessarily an antagonist. A partial agonist can sometimes antagonize ET-1-induced biological responses. Also, a toxic agent may inhibit

Table 2
ET-Induced DNA Synthesis in Cultured Cells

Cell type	Receptor subtype	Reference
Astrocytoma U138MG (human)	ET_A	*19*
Endothelial cells (bovine and human)	ET_B	*28*
Fibroblast IMR90 cells (human)	ET_A	*22*
Melanoma (human)	ET_B	*29*
Ovarian carcinoma (human)	ET_A	*30*
Prostatic carcinoma (human)	ET_A	*26*
Smooth muscle cells (human)*	ET_A	*31*

*Most smooth muscle cells express both ET_A and ET_B receptors. However, ET-1-induced DNA synthesis seems to be mediated predominantly by ET_A.

ET-1-induced biological responses. A true ET receptor antagonist is one that does not evoke any biological response by itself, and at the same time can specifically and effectively block ET-1 or ET-3 induced biological responses.

To determine whether a ligand is an antagonist or agonist, it is necessary to set up assays that measure biological responses induced by ETs. There are many assays available for this purpose. For example, it can be an ex vivo assay that measures ET-1-induced vasoconstriction in isolated rat aortic rings (mediated mainly by ET_A receptors) or rabbit pulmonary artery rings (mediated mainly by ET_B receptors). It can also be an in vivo assay that measures ET-1-induced changes in mean arterial pressure in the rat. Detailed discussion for the ex vivo and in vivo assays are beyond the scope of this chapter, and information on these assays has been provided previously *(16,17)*.

Another approach is to use a cell-based system to measure ET-1-induced biological responses. A cell-based assay offers many advantages over ex vivo or in vivo assays. It is easier to set up and the cost is usually lower. More importantly, it is possible to select cells in which the ET-1-induced effect is mediated exclusively by either ET_A or ET_B receptors. In ex vivo assays using tissues or in vivo assays using whole animals, an ET-1-induced response is more likely to be mediated by both ET_A and ET_B, which tends to complicate data interpretation.

In general, the following factors shall be considered when choosing a cell-based base for the purpose of characterizing a new ligand: (1) the assay shall be as cheap and simple as possible regarding the requirement of equipment and setups, (2) the assay shall allow a large number of samples to be processed at the same time, (3) the assay shall give good sensitivity for the detection of an effect, (4) the assay shall be specific so that noise from interfering materials is minimal, (5) the effect is mediated by only one type of ET receptor. We have looked at several cell-based assays such as MAP kinase activation, phosphatidylinositol (PI) hydrolysis, arachidonic acid release, elevation of intracellular cAMP, calcium mobilization, and DNA synthesis. Some of these assays are too tedious, costly, and/or labor-intensive to be suitable for high-throughput testing purposes. From our experience, assays measuring DNA synthesis, PI hydrolysis, and arachidonic acid release are useful for testing a new ligand, although each has its pros and cons as discussed below.

1.3.1. DNA Synthesis

It is well documented that ETs stimulate DNA synthesis in a variety of cells and tissues. **Table 2** shows a list of cells in which ETs stimulate DNA synthesis mediated by either ET_A or ET_B receptor. DNA synthesis can be determined by measuring incorporation of radiolabeled thymidine into DNA (*see* **Subheading 3.1.5.**). The method is well established, easy, and straightforward. The downside of using this assay is that the effect of ET-1 on stimulating DNA synthesis in many cells may be at most 2–3-fold of control. Thus, sensitivity can be an issue.

1.3.2. PI Hydrolysis

This assay measures the phosphoinositide turnover in cells. ET receptors are known to be coupled to phospholipase C via G proteins in many different types of cells. ET binding will activate phospholipase C, which in turn breaks down phosphatidylinositol 4,5-bisphosphate to form inositol 1,4,5-triphosphate and 1,2-diacylglycerol. Inositol 1,4,5-triphosphate can be further phosphorylated or dephosphorylated to form other inositol lipid metabolites. Two enzymes that are involved in the dephosphorylation of inositol phosphates, the inositol polyphosphate 1-phosphatase and inositol monophosphatase, are inhibited by treating cells with lithium ions in the mM range. As a result, the accumulation of inositol phosphates, especially inositol monophosphates, can be measured using the assay described in **Subheading 3.1.6. Table 3** shows a list of cells in which ET-1 stimulates PI hydrolysis. In some cells, e.g., 3T3-L1 cells, the increase in PI hydrolysis induced by ET-1 can be fivefold of control, making the assay suitable for detecting the effect of an antagonist. The downside of this assay is that the process is rather tedious and labor intensive when compared to the DNA synthesis and arachidonic acid release assays.

1.3.3. Arachidonic Acid Release

Table 4 shows a list of cells in which ET-1 stimulates arachidonic acid release mediated by either ET_A or ET_B receptor. ETs are known to be coupled to phospholipase A_2 via G proteins in a variety of cells. Phospholipase A_2, upon activation, hydrolyzes phospholipids to release a fatty acid such as arachidonic acid and a lysophospholipid. The assay is very simple and suitable for

Table 3
ET-Induced PI Hydrolysis in Cultured Cells

Cell type	Receptor subtype	Reference
Aortic A7r5 smooth muscle cells (rat)	ET$_A$	*32*
Ciliary muscle cells (human)	ET$_A$	*35*
Fibroblast 3T3-L1 (mouse)	ET$_A$	*23*
MMQ cells (rat)	ET$_A$	*25*
Osteoblast-like MC3T3-E1 cells	ET$_A$	*37*
Pericardial smooth muscle cells (human)	ET$_A$	*38*

testing a large number of samples at the same time. The downside of this assay is that many different factors may contribute to the release of arachidonic acid and thus compromise the specificity of the assay in response to ETs. In addition, this assay is more suitable for cells that form monolayers in culture.

1.4. Other Characteristics of the New Ligand

Other information about the compound of interest, e.g., protein binding characteristic, the pharmacokinetic profile, the toxicity profile, the in vivo efficacy, and the biological duration, is important and should be obtained. However, they are beyond the scope of this chapter. Some of these methods have been described previously *(16,17)*.

To determine whether the compound of interest is specific for ET receptors, the compound should be assessed in assays testing a few different proteins such as angiotensin AT1 receptor, insulin receptor, or adenosine A$_1$ receptor. If the compound of interest shows promising characteristics and there is interest for developing it further, it may be necessary to test the specificity of the compound in a wide variety of assays to rule out the possibility that the compound interferes with other systems. There are companies that specialize in this very matter. We usually send out our compounds to be assessed in a large number of different types of assays *(see* **Note 2***)*.

2. Materials
2.1. ET Receptor Ligands

For information on the availability and handling of ET receptor ligands, please refer to Chapter 5.

2.2. Functional Studies

1. Radiolabeled materials: Myo-[^{3}H]inositol, [^{3}H]thymidine, and [^{3}H]arachidonic acid are commercially available.
2. Lithium chloride (LiCl).

Table 4
ET-Induced Arachidonic Acid Release in Cultured Cells

Cell type	Receptor Subtype	Reference
Aortic endothelial cells (rat)	ET_B	*32*
Aortic A7r5 smooth muscle cells (rat)	ET_A	*33*
Brain capillary endothelial cells (rat)	ET_B	*34*
Ciliary muscle cells (human)	ET_A	*35*
Iris sphincter smooth muscle cells (cat)	ET_A	*36*
Osteoblast-like MC3T3-E1 cells	ET_A	*37*
Pericardial smooth muscle cells (human)	ET_A	*38*

3. Protease inhibitors: Phosphoramidon, EDTA, phenylmethylsulfonyl fluoride, Pepstatin A.
4. Anion-exchange resin AG1-X8.

2.3. Binding Studies

For information on equipment and buffers used in binding studies, please refer to Chapter 5.

2.4. Cell-Based Functional Studies

1. Earle's solution: 140 mM NaCl, 5 mM KCl, 1.8 mM CaCl$_2$, 0.8 mM MgSO$_4$, 5 mM glucose, buffered with 25 mM HEPES, pH 7.4.
2. Scintillation counter.
3. Cell culture set-up.
4. Buffer/reagent used in DNA synthesis: PBS; 10% TCA; 0.1 N NaOH.
5. Buffer/reagent/equipment used in PI hydrolysis: (1) Batch chromatograph set-up: the Disposaflex Column Rack System (Kontes, cat. no. 420200-0000). The system includes columns, racks and a waste collection tank. (2) Reagent for washing and storing anion-exchange resin AG1-X8: 1 N formic acid. (3) Reagent for regenerating anion-exchange resin AG1-X8: 1 N NaOH; 1 N formic acid. (4) Buffer/reagent for eluting samples from the column: (a) 5 mM inositol, (b) 60 mM sodium formate and 5 mM sodium tetraborate, (c) 1 M ammonium formate plus 0.1 N formic acid. (5) Chloroform/methanol (1:2, v/v).

3. Methods

3.1. Radioligand Binding to Membranes

3.1.1. Preparation of Membranes

For information on how to make membrane preparations, please refer to Chapter 5.

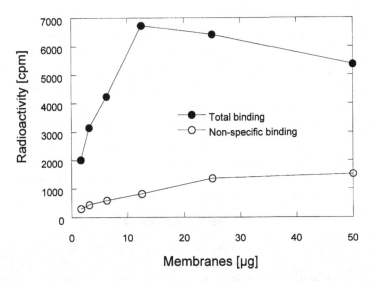

Fig. 1. Testing the membrane preparation. Membranes prepared from CHO cells stably transfected with the human ET_A receptor (2–50 μg) are incubated with 0.1 nM [^{125}I]ET-1 in the presence or absence of 1 μM ET-1 at room temperature for 3 h.

3.1.2. Determining the Binding Capacity of a Membrane Preparation

1. Incubate different amounts of membranes (2–500 μg depending on the tissue and cell type) with 0.1 nM [^{125}I]ET-1 for 4 h at 25°C in 96-well microtiter plates precoated with 0.1% bovine serum albumin. The binding study is conducted as described in Chapter 5.
2. Plot radioactivity against the amount of membranes. An example is shown in **Fig. 1**. In this particular study, an amount of 10 μg was deemed adequate (*see* **Note 3**).

3.1.3. Competition Radioligand Binding Studies for the Determination of IC_{50}

1. Competition radioligand binding studies are carried out as described in Chapter 5.
2. **Figure 2** shows the result from a typical competition binding study. The test compound inhibited [^{125}I]ET-1 binding to the human ET_A receptor with an IC_{50} value of 0.57 nM.
3. To analyze data, nonspecific binding, as determined in the presence of 1 μM of ET-1, is subtracted from total binding to give specific binding. The specific [^{125}I]ET-1 binding in the absence of the test agent (Control) is shown as 100%, and the specific [^{125}I]ET-1 binding in the presence of the test agent is normalized as % of Control.

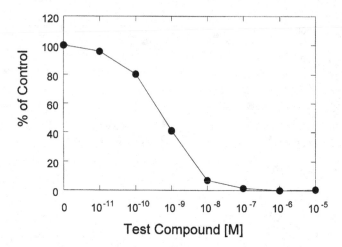

Fig. 2. Competition binding studies. Membranes (10 µg) prepared from CHO cells stably transfected with the human ET_A receptor are incubated with 0.1 nM [^{125}I]ET-1 in the absence (Control) or presence of increasing concentrations of an antagonist at room temperature for 3 h. Nonspecific binding, 680 cpm as determined in the presence of 1 µM of ET-1, is subtracted from total binding to give specific binding. Results are expressed as % of control (specific binding in the absence of unlabeled ligand).

3.1.4. Saturation Radioligand Binding Studies for the Determination of K_i

1. Saturation binding studies are carried out as described in Chapter 5.
2. To determine the K_i value, the compound of interest should be tested at a minimum of three different concentrations. An example for the layout of wells and plates in a saturation binding study testing ABT-627 at 0.1, 0.2 and 0.4 nM with each condition tested in duplicates is shown in **Fig. 3**.
3. After the data are collected, binding results can be analyzed using the radioligand binding analysis program "EBDA & LIGAND" (Biosoft, MO) to calculate K_d' values of ET-1 binding at each antagonist concentration (*see* **Subheading 3.1.4.** in Chapter 4). Alternatively, K_d values for ET-1 binding at each antagonist concentration can be determined by Scatchard analysis (*see* **Subheading 3.3.2.** in Chapter 5).
4. To calculate the K_i value, K_d' is plotted against the antagonist concentrations, [I], to determine the slopes.

$$K_{d'} = K_d \text{ when } [I] = 0. \text{ Since } K_{d'} = (1 + \frac{[I]}{K_i})K_d, K_i = \frac{K_d}{\text{slope}}$$

See **Fig. 4** for an example.

3.1.5. ET-1-Induced DNA Synthesis

The assay described below is suitable for cells that form a monolayer in culture.

Plate #1

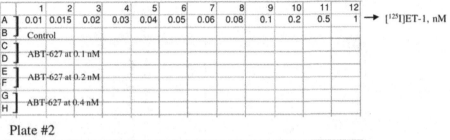

	1	2	3	4	5	6	7	8	9	10	11	12	
A	0.01	0.015	0.02	0.03	0.04	0.05	0.06	0.08	0.1	0.2	0.5	1	→ [^{125}I]ET-1, nM
B	Control												
C													
D	ABT-627 at 0.1 nM												
E													
F	ABT-627 at 0.2 nM												
G													
H	ABT-627 at 0.4 nM												

Plate #2

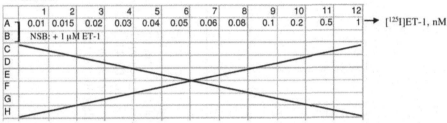

	1	2	3	4	5	6	7	8	9	10	11	12	
A	0.01	0.015	0.02	0.03	0.04	0.05	0.06	0.08	0.1	0.2	0.5	1	→ [^{125}I]ET-1, nM
B	NSB: + 1 µM ET-1												
C													
D													
E													
F													
G													
H													

Fig. 3. An example of the plate and well layout for determining the K_i of ABT-627.

1. Grow human coronary artery smooth muscle cells (*see* **Note 4**) in SmGM media containing 5% fetal bovine serum (FBS) (*see* **Note 5**).
2. Incubate cells at approx 60% confluency in 48-well plates (*see* **Note 6**) in serum-free medium for 24 h (*see* **Note 7**), treated with 1 nM ET-1 (*see* **Note 8**) in the presence or absence of different concentrations of the test agent for 20 h, followed by incubation with [^{3}H]thymidine (1 µCi/well) for another 4 h at 37°C (*see* **Note 9**).
3. After the incubation, wash each well with 1 mL of PBS, and then wash with 0.5 mL of ice-cold 10% trichloroacetic acid (TCA) for 30 min at 4°C (*see* **Note 10**). Wash each well again with 0.5 mL of 10% TCA.
4. Dissolve materials not soluble in TCA in 0.1 *N* NaOH for scintillation counting.
5. To calculate data (*see* **Note 11**), first subtract the background (radioactivity in wells receiving no treatment). The net increase in DNA synthesis stimulated by ET-1 in the absence of the test agent is 100% (Control). Normalize the increase in DNA synthesis in the presence of ET-1 and the test agent as % of Control. Ideally, if the test agent is an antagonist that has no toxic effect on cells, the wells treated with the test agent alone will give the same result as the background.

3.1.6. ET-1-Induced Phosphatidylinositol Hydrolysis

1. Label MMQ cells (0.4 × 10^6 cells/mL) with 10 µCi/mL of myo-[^{3}H]inositol in RPMI for 16–24 h (*see* **Note 12**).
2. Wash cells with PBS and resuspend into Earle's solution (*see* **Note 13**) containing protease inhibitors (3 m*M* EDTA, 0.1 m*M* phenylmethylsulfonyl fluoride, and 5 µg/mL pepstatin A) and 10 m*M* LiCl and then incubate for 60 min at 37°C.

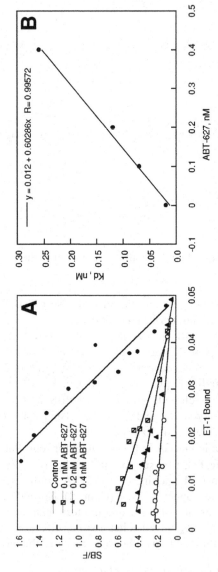

Fig. 4. Determining the K_i of the ABT-627 by $[^{125}I]ET$-1 saturation binding studies. Membranes (15 μg) from CHO cells stably transfected with the human ET_A receptors are incubated with increasing concentrations of $[^{125}I]ET$-1 in the presence of ABT-627 (concentrations as indicated) for 4 h at 25°C. Nonspecific binding is determined by adding 1 μM unlabeled ET-1 and is subtracted from total binding to give specific binding. (**A**) Scatchard plots. (**B**) Determination of K_i value (0.033 nM) as described in the text.

3. Challenge the cells (0.5 mL per tube) with 1 nM ET-1 in the presence or absence of the test agent for 30 min at 37°C.
4. Terminate the ET-1 challenge by the addition of 1.5 mL of chloroform/methanol (1:2, v/v) (*see* **Note 14**).
5. Extract total water-soluble inositol phosphates by addition of 0.5 mL chloroform and 0.4 mL water (*see* **Note 15**).
6. Transfer the upper aqueous phase (1 mL) to a clean tube and count a small portion (100 μL) (*see* **Note 16**).
7. Transfer the rest of the aqueous sample onto an anion-exchange resin AG1-X8 column (*see* **Note 17**). Rinse the sample tube with 2 mL water and add the rinse onto the same column. Wash the column with 20 mL of 5 mM inositol, followed by 6 mL of 60 mM sodium formate and 5 mM sodium tetraborate. Elute the column with 6 mL of 1 M ammonium formate plus 0.1 N formic acid. Collect the eluent for scintillation counting.
8. To calculate the data, subtract the basal signal obtained from untreated wells, and normalize the increase in signal stimulated by ET-1 in the presence of the test agent as a % of Control (the increase stimulated by ET-1 in the absence of the test agent).

3.1.7. ET-1-Induced Arachidonic Acid Release

1. Label human pericardial smooth muscle cells in 48-well culture plates at 80% confluency (*see* **Note 18**) with 0.4 μCi/well of [^{3}H]arachidonic acid in DMEM with 10% fetal bovine serum for 16–24 h.
2. Incubate cells with DMEM plus 0.2% bovine serum albumin (0.5 mL/well) for 30 min.
3. After the incubation, remove the medium and add 0.3 mL DMEM with 0.2% bovine serum albumin plus 10 nM BQ-788, an ET$_B$ receptor-selective antagonist *(39)*, to each well (*see* **Note 19**).
4. Add the test agent at different concentrations and finally add 1 nM ET-1.
5. Incubate cells at 37°C for another 30 min and collect the incubation medium to determine radioactivity (*see* **Note 20**). Calculate data as described in **Sub-heading 3.1.6.**

4. Notes

1. When comparing IC$_{50}$ values obtained from different labs, check to make sure that the experimental conditions used to generate the values are similar. *See* Sub-heading 1.3. in Chapter 5 for discussion on this subject.
2. We sent ABT-546 (A-216546) to Cerep (Celle L'Evescault, France) to be tested in 73 different assays.
3. We usually pick a membrane concentration that gives counts in the range of 5000–7000 cpm. With this level of radioactivity, the nonspecific binding (as determined by addition of 1 μM ET-1) is ~10% of total binding.
4. We have tested human coronary artery smooth muscle cells purchased from Clonetics (San Diego, CA). We have also prepared cells from normal human

coronary artery and human coronary artery neointima tissue sections by explant culturing. In human coronary artery smooth muscle cells, the effect of ET-1 on stimulating DNA synthesis is at most twofold. If human tissues are unavailable, cells can be prepared from pig or rat coronary arteries. From our experience, smooth muscle cells prepared from the rat grow better, express a higher density of ET receptors, and respond more profoundly to ET-1 stimulation. However, for our purposes we routinely use human cells if there is a choice.

5. The cell culture conditions are dependent on the cell type. The condition described here is for culturing human coronary artery smooth muscle cells. When using different cell types, make sure the right medium and conditions are used.

6. Dependent on the response to ET-1, different sizes of plates and/or different cell density may be used.

7. For some cells, it is necessary to serum-starve for 48 h in order to make the cells go into the quiescent state.

8. It is necessary to first conduct a ET-1 dose-dependent study to learn how cells respond to ET-1. The EC_{50} of ET-1 to stimulate a biological response such as DNA synthesis is likely in the range of $0.1-1$ nM depending on the experimental conditions. As described in Chapter 5, if bovine serum albumin is used in the assay buffer, the concentration of serum albumin will affect the EC_{50}. The higher the serum albumin concentration is, the higher the EC_{50} will be. After the response of cells to ET-1 is determined, a fixed concentration of ET-1 can be chosen in functional studies to evaluate the test compound. We like to use an ET-1 concentration that is at or below 1 nM, and elicits >90% of the maximal response. As discussed in Chapter 5, since ET-1 binding is much less reversible than antagonist binding, if the ET-1 concentration used to evoke a response is too high, a weak antagonist may fail to block the effect of ET-1 no matter how high the antagonist concentration is.

9. In some studies, we add [^{3}H]thymidine together with ET-1 and the test agent, and let the cells incubate for 24 h at 37°C. The goal is to obtain enough counts in order to see an effect, but at the same time keep the background (the basal level of radioactivity) as low as possible.

10. If the background radioactivity (radioactivity in wells that are not treated with ET-1 and the test agent) is high, wash cells with 1 mL PBS for a few times. However, some cells are very sensitive to rinsing and may peel off if washed too much.

11. To test whether the compound alone affects DNA synthesis, proper controls should be included in the same assay. We always include wells that receive no treatment (no ET-1, no test agent), ET-1 alone, ET-1 and the test compound, and the test compound alone. If necessary, we treat some cells with 5% FBS as the positive control. Some agents may inhibit DNA synthesis via other mechanisms that are completely independent of ET-1. By including different control conditions, it is possible to see from the data whether the test agent specifically blocks ET-1-induced DNA synthesis.

12. The MMQ cells are cultured in suspension. For cells that form a monolayer, such as fibroblast 3T3-L1, culture cells in 48-well-plates and label each well with

1 μCi/well of myo-[^{3}H]inositol. Although it is often suggested that special medium should be used during the myo-[^{3}H]inositol incubation period, we find that normal culture medium works just fine, at least for MMQ cells and fibroblast 3T3-L1.

13. Adjust the volume of Earle's solution used to resuspend cells to get a higher or lower cell density according to the requirements of the study.

14. A time course study should be conducted to determine how long cells need to be challenged with ET-1 to achieve a good response. In MMQ cells, a 30-min incubation time with ET-1 is determined as adequate. Because of the use of chloroform, process the samples in glass tubes. For cells in suspension, we usually make aliquots of cells into glass tubes after cells are resuspended into the Earle's solution. The sample volume in each tube is 0.5 mL. If cells in monolayers are used, incubate cells in 0.5 mL/well of Earle's solution plus LiCl, and replace EDTA with phosphoramidon (0.1 mM). After challenging cells with ET-1, add 50 μL/well of 1 N NaOH to terminate the ET-1 effect and to dissolve cells. Then add a volume of 50 μL/well 1 N HCl to neutralize the mixture before transferring the sample from the well to a glass tube for chloroform treatment.

15. Dependent on the starting sample volume, different amounts of the chloroform/methanol mixture, chloroform and water may be added. The goal is to achieve final proportions of chloroform/methanol/water of 1:1:0.9 (v/v/v).

16. The radioactivity determined from this small portion (100 μL) of the sample serves as a control for checking whether there is sample-to-sample variation in cell labeling.

17. AG1-X8 is purchased from Bio-Rad (Hercules, CA). Wash the AG1-X8 resin thoroughly with 1 N formic acid and store at 4°C. Pack the resin into 1 mL-disposable columns with about 0.7 mL solid resin per column. Each column can be used for 5–7×. After each use, wash the resin sequentially with 20 mL 1 N NaOH, 20 mL water, 20 mL 1 N formic acid and 20 mL water before reuse. We prepare a big batch of columns in order to process a large number of samples at the same time. The batch chromatography can be achieved using the Disposaflex Column Rack System (Kontes, cat. no. 420200-0000).

18. Cell density has a significant effect on the amount of radioactivity released into media in response to ET-1. For example, in human pericardial smooth muscle cells, when cells at 80% confluency are used, basal radioactivity released in control (no drug treatment) after 30 min of incubation is typically in the range of 1000–5000 counts/min (cpm) and is 0.5–1.0% of total radioactivity. ET at 10 nM can increase the amount of released radioactivity to 200–400% of control. When cells from the same preparations are used at 100% confluency, basal radioactivity remains in the range of 1000–5000 cpm. However, the stimulation by ET could increase to 600–1400% of control.

19. Human pericardial smooth muscle cells express both ET_A and ET_B receptors. Addition of BQ-788 is to block the ET_B receptor so that the effect of a compound on antagonizing the ET_A-mediated response can be assessed without the complication of the ET_B factor. As discussed above, ideally a cell line that expresses only one type of ET receptor should be used. Human pericardial smooth muscle cells are used as an example here to demonstrate that it is possible to use cell

lines that express both ET_A and ET_B receptors to achieve desired results, if steps are taken to block the effect from the unwanted receptor subtype.

20. This assay described here measures the change in radioactivity released into the incubation medium. The assay is useful for measuring the effect of a test agent on an ET-1-induced biological response. It is not meant as an assay to measure the activation of phospholipase A_2 and the generation of arachidonate. Analytical methods such as HPLC are required to confirm the identity of the radioactive material released into the medium.

References

1. Yanagisawa, M., Kurihara, H., Kimura, S., Tomobe, Y., Kobayashi, M., Mitsui, Y., et al. (1988) A novel potent vasoconstrictor peptide produced by vascular endothelial cells. *Nature* **332,** 411–414.

2. Opgenorth, T. J. (1995) Endothelin receptor antagonism. *Adv. Pharmacol.* **33,** 1–65.

3. Arai, H., Hori, S., Aramori, I., Ohkubo, H., and Nakanishi, S. (1990) Cloning and expression of a cDNA encoding an ET receptor. *Nature* **348,** 730–732.

4. Sakurai, T., Yanagisawa, M., Takuwa, Y., Miyazaki, H., Kimura, S., Goto, K., and Masaki, T. (1990) Cloning of a cDNA encoding a nonisopeptide-selective subtype of the endothelin receptor. *Nature* **348,** 732–735.

5. Arai, H., Nakao, K., Takaya, K., Hosoda, K., Ogawa, Y., Nakanishi, S., and Imura, H. (1993) The human endothelin-B receptor gene. *J. Biol. Chem.* **268,** 3463–3470.

6. Elshourbagy, N. A., Korman, D. R., Wu, H.-L., Sylvester, D. R., Lee, J. A., Nuthalaganti, P., et al. (1993) Molecular characterization and regulation of the human endothelin receptors. *J. Biol. Chem.* **268,** 3873–3879.

7. Bax, W. and Saxena, P. (1994) The current endothelin receptor classification: time for reconsideration? *Trends Pharmacol. Sci.* **15,** 379–386.

8. Simonson, M. S. (1993) Endothelins: Multifunctional renal peptides. *Physiol. Rev.* **73,** 375–411.

9. Wu-Wong, J. R. and Opgenorth, T. J. (2002) The roles of endothelins in proliferation, apoptosis, and angiogenesis. *Handbook of Experimental Pharmacology,* in press.

10. Wu-Wong, J. R. and Opgenorth, T. J. (1998) Endothelin and isoproterenol counter-regulate cAMP and mitogen-activated protein kinases. *J. Cardiovasc. Pharmacol.* **31,** S185–S191.

11. Wu-Wong, J. R., Chiou, W., Dickinson, R. and Opgenorth, T. J. (1997) Endothelin attenuates apoptosis in human smooth muscle cells. *Biochem. J.* **28,** 733–737.

12. Shichiri, M., Kato, H., Marumo, F., and Hirata, Y. (1998) Endothelin-B receptor-mediated suppression of endothelial apoptosis. *J. Cardiovasc. Pharmacol.* **31,** S138–S141.

13. Webb, D. J., Monge, J. C., Rabelink, T. J., and Yanagisawa, M. (1998) Endothelin: new discoveries and rapid progress in the clinic. *Trends Pharmacol. Sci.* **19,** 5–8.

14. Ihara, M., Noguchi, K., Saeki, T., Fukuroda, T., Tsuchida, S., Kimura, S., et al. (1991) Biological profile of highly potent novel endothelin antagonists selective for the ET_A receptor. *Life Sci.* **50,** 247–255.

15. Sogabe, K., Nirei, H., Shoubo, M., Nomoto, A., Ao, S., Notsu, T., and Ono, T. (1993) Pharmacological profile of FR139317, a novel, potent, endothelin ET_A receptor antagonist. *J. Pharmacol. Exp. Ther.* **264,** 1040–1046.

16. Opgenorth, T. J., Adler, A. L., Calzadilla, S., Chiou, W. J., Dayton, B. D., Dixon, D. B., et al. (1996) Pharmacological Characterization of A-127722: An orally active and highly potent ET_A-selective receptor antagonist. *J. Pharmacol. Exp. Ther.* **276,** 473–481.

17. Wu-Wong, J. R., Dixon, D. B., Chiou, W. J., Dayton, B. D., Novosad, E. I., Adler, A. L., et al. (1999) Pharmacology of A-216546: A Highly Selective Antagonist for The Type-A Endothelin Receptor. *Eur. J. Pharmacol.* **366,** 189–201.

18. Chiou, W., Magnuson, S. R., Dixon, D. B., Sundy, S., Opgenorth, T. J., and Wu-Wong, J. R. (1997) Dissociation characteristics of endothelin receptor agonists and antagonists in cloned human type-B endothelin receptor. *Endothelium: J. Endothelial Cell Res.* **5,** 179–189.

19. Wu-Wong, J. R., Chiu, W., Magnuson, J. R., Bianchi, B. R., and Lin, C. W. (1996) Human astrocytoma U138MG cells express predominantly type-A endothelin receptors. *Biochem. Biophys. Acta* **1311,** 155–163.

20. Wu-Wong, J. R., Chiou, W., Magnuson, S. R., and Opgenorth, T. J. (1995) Endothelin Receptor in Human Astrocytoma U373MG Cells: Binding, Dissociation, Receptor Internalization. *J. Pharmacol. Exp. Ther.* **274,** 499–507.

21. Wu-Wong, J. R., Chiou, W., Magnuson, S. R., and Opgenorth, T. J. (1994) Endothelin receptor agonists and antagonists exhibit different dissociation characteristics. *Biochem. Biophys. Acta* **1224,** 288–294.

22. Chiou, W. J., Wang, J., Berg, C. E., and Wu-Wong, J. R. (1999) SV40 virus transformation down-regulates endothelin receptor. *Biochem. Biophys. Acta* **1450,** 35–44.

23. Wu-Wong, J. R., Berg, C. E., Wang, J., Chiou, W. J., and Fissel, B. (1999) Endothelin Stimulates Glucose Uptake and GLUT4 Translocation Via Activation of Endothelin ET_A Receptor in 3T3-L1 Adipocytes. *J. Biol. Chem.* **274,** 8103–8110.

24. Wu-Wong, J. R., Chiou, W., and Opgenorth, T. J. (1993) Phosphoramidon modulates the number of endothelin receptors in cultured Swiss 3T3 fibroblasts. *Mol. Pharmacol.* **44,** 422–429.

25. Wu-Wong, J. R., Chiou, W., Magnuson, S. R., Witte, D. G., and Lin, C. W. (1993) Identification and characterization of type A endothelin receptor in MMQ cells. *Mol. Pharmacol.* **44,** 285–291.

26. Nelson, J. B., Hedican, S. P., George, D. J., Reddi, A. H., Piantadosi, S., Eisenberger, M. A., and Simons, J. W. (1995) Identification of endothelin-1 in the pathophysiology of metastatic adenocarcinoma of the prostate. *Nature Med.* **1,** 944–949.

27. Tsukahara, H., Ende, H., Magazine, H. I., Bahou, W. F., and Goligorsky, M. S. (1994) Molecular and functional characterization of the nonisopeptide-selective ET_B receptor in endothelial cells. Receptor coupling to nitric oxide synthase. *J. Biol. Chem.* **269,** 21,778–21,785.

28. Morbidelli, L., Orlando, C., Maggi, C. A., Ledda, F., and Ziche, M. (1995) Proliferation and migration of endothelial cells is promoted by endothelins via activation of ET$_B$ receptors. *Am. J. Physiol.* **269,** H686–H695.
29. Lahav, R., Heffner, G., and Patterson, P. H. (1999) An endothelin receptor B antagonist inhibits growth and induces cell death in human melanoma cells in vitro and in vivo. *Proc. Natl. Acad. Sci.* **96,** 11496–11500.
30. Bagnato, A., Tecce, R., Di Castro, V., and Catt, K. J. (1997) Activation of mitogenic signaling by endothelin 1 in ovarian carcinoma cells. *Cancer Res.* **57,** 1306–1311.
31. Wu-Wong, J. R., Chiou, W., Huang, Z.-J., Vidal, M. J., and Opgenorth, T. J. (1994) Endothelin receptor in human pericardium smooth muscle cells: antagonist potency differs on agonist-evoked responses. *Amer. J. Physiol.* **267,** C1185–C1195.
32. Oriji, G. K. (1999) Endothelin-induced prostacyclin production in rat aortic endothelial cells is mediated by protein kinase C. *Prostaglandins Leukot. Essent. Fatty Acids* **60,** 263–268.
33. Cioffi, C. L. and Garay, M. (1993) Short-term regulation of endothelin receptor-mediated phosphoinositide hydrolysis and arachidonic acid release in A7r5 smooth-muscle cells. *J. Cardiovasc. Pharmacol.* **22,** S168–S170.
34. Vigne, P. and Frelin, C. (1994) Endothelins activate phospholipase A$_2$ in brain capillary endothelial cells. *Brain Res.* **651,** 342–344.
35. Yousufzai, S. Y. and Abdel-latif, A. A. (1997) Endothelin-1 stimulates the release of arachidonic acid and prostaglandins in cultured human ciliary muscle cells: activation of phospholipase A$_2$. *Exp. Eye Res.* **65,** 73–81.
36. Abdel-Latif, A. A., Husain, S., and Yousufzai, S. Y. (2000) Role of protein kinase C alpha and mitogen-activated protein kinases in endothelin-1-stimulation of cytosolic phospholipase A$_2$ in iris sphincter smooth muscle. *J. Cardiovasc. Pharmacol.* **36,** S117–S119.
37. Suzuki, A., Shinoda, J., Watanabe-Tomita, Y., Ozaki, N., Oiso, Y., and Kozawa, O. (1997) ET$_A$ receptor mediates the signaling of endothelin-1 in osteoblast-like cells. *Bone* **21,** 143–146.
38. Wu-Wong, J. R., Dayton, B. D., and Opgenorth, T. J. (1996) Endothelin-1-evoked arachidonic acid release: a Ca$^{(2+)}$-dependent pathway. *Am. J. Physiol.* **271,** C869–C877.
39. Ishikawa, K., Ihara, M., Noguchi, K., Mase, T., Mino, N., Saeki, T., et al. (1994) Biochemical and pharmacological profile of a potent and selective endothelin B-receptor antagonist, BQ-788. *Proc. Natl. Acad. Sci.* **91,** 4892–4896.

12

Use of In Vitro Organ Cultures of Human Saphenous Vein as a Model for Intimal Proliferation

Karen E. Porter

1. Introduction

The autologous internal mammary artery and the long saphenous vein are the most frequently used conduits as bypass grafts in the management of occlusive arterial disease in both the coronary and lower limb circulations. However, significant stenosis occurs in over a third of lower limb reconstructions in the first postoperative year *(1)*, and the patency rate for coronary bypass grafts is only 50% after 5 yr *(2)*. The underlying pathological lesion of such stenoses is intimal hyperplasia (IH). IH is characterized by excessive smooth muscle cell migration and proliferation in the intima of the vessel wall, together with an accumulation of extracellular matrix. This in turn results in a significant loss in lumenal area with a subsequent reduced blood flow to the tissues.

The widespread use of animal models of IH has provided a valuable experimental tool, and although such studies have undoubtedly increased our understanding of the etiology of this condition, the results, particularly in small animals, have not been reproducible in human studies. Likewise, isolated cell culture techniques have provided a wealth of information in the study of the function of endothelial and smooth muscle cells under normal and pathophysiological conditions, but the interactions of the different cell types are probably better studied in an organ culture system. Organ culture implies a three-dimensional culture of intact tissue retaining some or all of its in vivo histological features *(3)*. In organ culture, whole organs or representative parts, are maintained as small fragments in culture, thus retaining the spatial distribution of the participating cells, without which it may be difficult to reproduce the characteristic cell behavior of the tissue.

From: *Methods in Molecular Biology, vol. 206: Peptide Research Protocols: Endothelin*
Edited by: J. Maguire and A. Davenport © Humana Press Inc., Totowa, NJ

The technique of organ culture is by no means new; it was first described in the Strangeways laboratories in 1926 *(4)*. At that time the method was chiefly used for the culture of embryonic organs which could be cultured whole and were able to survive the anoxic conditions which prevailed in such cultures. It was almost 30 yr later that Trowell studied the behavior of a variety of segments of mature organs *(5)* and concluded that explants that were naturally thin or flat survived better than those which were spherical or cuboid, because superior diffusion of oxygen and nutrients could be achieved in thin tissues. With respect to vascular tissue, he reported that the histological appearance of rat arteries following a 9-d culture period was perfectly preserved, with healthy endothelium, media, and adventitia being observed.

Later studies further developed the technique of organ culture in rabbit *(6)* and porcine arteries *(7,8)* and were able to demonstrate a stimulation of smooth muscle cell proliferation by the endothelium resulting in the development of a cellular neointima. In 1979, Barrett first described intimal proliferation of smooth muscle cells in cultured human aorta *(9)*, representing an important advance in the study of atherosclerosis. The first description of human saphenous vein organ culture came from Soyombo and colleagues in 1990 *(10)*, who showed that the cultured vein remained viable over a 14-d culture period. They further reported the appearance of an intimally-directed smooth muscle cell proliferation, resulting in the formation of a cellular sub-endothelial layer or "neointima." Vein culture is therefore a potentially useful model for the study of bypass graft intimal hyperplasia, and the use of human tissue in such studies avoids the problems of interpreting results from animal models *(11)*. Furthermore, the studies that will be described here utilize the exact tissue associated with the clinical problem; namely, the human long saphenous vein. As with all in vitro studies, caution is required in interpreting the results, the most obvious being that this model is one of static culture without flow conditions. Nevertheless, the advantage that organ culture offers is that it maintains the integrity and architecture of the vein wall in order that interactions between the endothelium and smooth muscle cells may be studied.

2. Materials

2.1. Source of Saphenous Vein and Collection Procedure

1. Segments of saphenous vein are obtained from patients undergoing surgery for carotid endarterectomy, lower limb bypass grafting, or coronary artery bypass grafting. Local ethical committee approval and patient consent is required for this. The length of vein available is dictated by clinical requirements, but 2–3 cm is usual. The surgeon exposes the vein using a no-touch technique, avoiding distension and keeping handling to a minimum.
2. After harvesting, place the vein for culture directly into a sterile transport medium, for example, calcium-free Krebs physiological saline: 118 mM NaCl,

4.7 mM KCl, 1.2 mM MgSO$_4$, 1.2 mM KH$_2$PO$_4$, 25 mM NaHCO$_3$, 11.1 mM glucose (*see* **Note 1**) and transfer immediately to the laboratory.

2.2. Preculture Assessment

1. All veins designated for culture should be macroscopically normal; calcified and varicose veins are unsuitable.
2. For assessing endothelial integrity a 0.2% solution of Trypan blue is required (Sigma).

2.3. Equipment for Setting up Cultures

Note that unless otherwise stated, all equipment must be sterile and procedures are performed aseptically in a class II laminar flow hood. The following equipment should be prepared for setting up the organ cultures:

1. Organ culture dishes (for details regarding preparation, *see* **Note 2**).
2. A1 Minuten pins (Watkins & Doncaster, Cranbrook, Kent, UK) (*see* **Note 3**).
3. 500 μm Polyester mesh-cut into pieces of approx 1–2 cm^2 (*see* **Note 4**).
4. 90-mm Plastic Petri dishes.
5. Micro-dissecting scissors (Richardsons, Leicester, UK) (*see* **Note 5**), fine curved forceps, scalpel blades (size 23).
6. Dissecting microscope.
7. Complete vein culture medium: RPMI 1640, 30% v/v fetal calf serum, penicillin 50 U/mL, streptomycin 50 μg/mL, L-glutamine 2 mM (All Gibco-BRL, Paisley, UK). Store all prepared media in a refrigerator at 4°C.
8. 5-mL Pipets and pipet filler.
9. Humidified tissue culture incubator supplied with 5% CO$_2$ in air.
10. 10% Formalin solution for fixation.

2.4. Pharmacological Agents for Inhibitor Studies

1. Any potential agent under evaluation as an inhibitor of neointima formation must be prepared in an appropriate vehicle (usually recommended by the manufacturer) (*see* **Note 6**).
2. Prepare drugs at 50X the concentration required in the final culture medium, and filter-sterilize by passing through a 0.22-μm filter. By preparing a 50X concentrated stock, a volume of 100 μL of drug can be added to a total volume of 5 mL of culture medium on the vein segment.
3. It is advisable to store the drugs (usually this will be at –20°C) in sterile vials in small aliquots. In this way, repeated freeze-thaw cycles are avoided. In the studies to be described here the drugs chosen were:
   a. Bosentan, a specific, but nonselective ET receptor antagonist *(12)* (Actelion Pharmaceuticals Ltd., Allschwil, Switzerland). Soluble in water.
   b. BQ123, a selective ET$_A$ receptor antagonist *(13)* (CN Biosciences, Nottingham, UK). Soluble in water.
   c. BQ788, a selective ET$_B$ receptor antagonist *(14)* (CN Biosciences, Nottingham, UK). Soluble in dimethylsulfoxide (DMSO).

2.5. Histopathology Facilities and Monoclonal Antibodies

Processing equipment for paraffin-embedding (normally an automated process) and section cutting of fixed vein segments (microtome) is required. Such facilities should be routinely available in any pathology department (*see* **Note 7**). Also required are monoclonal antibodies:

1. Anti α-smooth muscle actin (clone 1A4, DAKO).
2. Anti Endothelin-1 (clone MA3-005, Cambridge Bioscience).
3. Millers elastin stain (BDH).
4. Measurement of endothelin-1 in culture medium is performed using an ELISA (enzyme-linked-immunosorbant assay) kit (Biochemica, Austria [UK supplier Cozart, cat. no. BI 20052]). Measurement of endothelin peptides by ELISA is covered in detail in Chapter 2.

3. Methods
3.1. Saphenous Vein Organ Culture
3.1.1. Determination of Endothelial Integrity

1. Cultures should be established as soon as possible after harvesting the saphenous veins and always within 1–2 h (*see* **Note 8**).
2. Transfer the harvested vein, together with the transport medium, into a 90-mm sterile Petri dish in the class II cabinet. Using the fine dissecting scissors and forceps, carefully clean off any excess fat and adventitial tissue (**Fig. 1A**). Excise the potentially damaged ends with a scalpel blade and discard. Visually check that there is no other physical injury (e.g., clamp injury) to the vein. Divide the remaining length of vein into segments of approx 5 mm with a scalpel blade, and then open each up longitudinally with the dissecting scissors (**Fig. 1B**).
3. Set one segment aside into a clean Petri dish to rapidly assess endothelial coverage as follows. With the lumenal surface facing up, pipet sufficient trypan blue solution over the surface of the vein to completely cover it. After 1–2 min, aspirate off the trypan blue and gently wash the surface of the vein using physiological saline. Observe under a dissecting microscope; areas of endothelial loss or damage will stain blue (**Fig. 1C**), whereas intact endothelium will exclude the stain (**Fig. 1D**). Any vein which is estimated to have greater than about 40% endothelial loss or damage is not suitable for organ culture.

3.1.2. Establishment of Vein Cultures

Providing endothelial integrity is satisfactory, the remaining vein segments can be set up for culture.

1. Using one dish for each segment, pin out the segment to approx the *in situ* length, luminal surface uppermost, on a 500-μm mesh mat resting on the layer of Sylgard resin. This pinning stage should be completed rapidly to avoid any drying out of the endothelial layer using one pin at each corner of the segment.

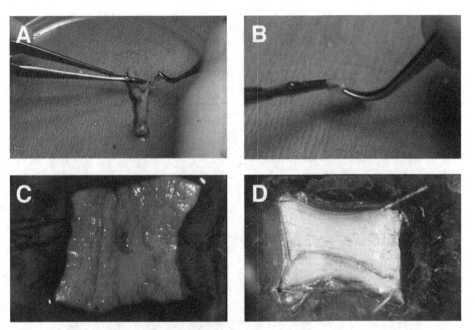

Fig. 1. (**A**) Under sterile conditions the vein is cleared of any fat and adventitial tissue. (**B**) After dividing into lengths of approx 5 mm, the segments are carefully opened longitudinally using microdissecting scissors. (**C**) Endothelium-denuded or damaged vein will take up trypan blue stain and is therefore unsuitable for culture. (**D**) Vein with well-preserved endothelium will exclude trypan blue and is ideal for organ culture. Generally, most veins will have some degree of endothelial loss/damage but if this is estimated at 40% or less, such segments are also suitable for culture.

2. Use one segment of pinned-out vein as an uncultured "control" by fixing immediately in a solution of 10% formalin for 18 h at room temperature.
3. Immediately cover the veins to be cultured with 5 mL of complete culture medium (**Fig. 2**) and replace the lid. Maintain cultures at 37°C in a humidified atmosphere of 5% CO_2 in air for 14 d.
4. Every 2–3 d, aspirate the medium off each culture, discard (or snap-freeze as required for further analysis), and replace with 5 mL of fresh medium.

3.1.3. Processing and Immunohistochemistry

1. At the end of the culture period (d 14), remove all of the medium from the segments and immediately cover the pinned segment with 10% formalin in the culture dish, for 18–24 h at room temperature (*see* **Note 9**).
2. Sections are then automatically dehydrated through 70–100% alcohol, cleared in chloroform, and then impregnated with paraffin wax.

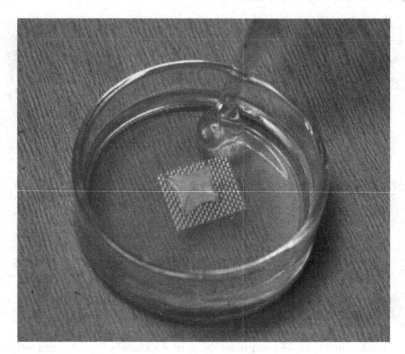

Fig. 2. The vein segment is stretched to approx its *in situ* length and pinned at each corner onto the mesh mat with the endothelial surface uppermost. Culture medium (5 mL) is then added to completely immerse the segment.

3. From the paraffin blocks, transverse sections of 4 μm thickness are cut and mounted onto 3-aminopropyltriethoxysilane (silane) -coated microscope slides (*see* **Note 10**). Unless such facilities are readily available in your own laboratory, it is advisable to seek the help of a histopathology laboratory.
4. Slide-mounted sections are immunostained using a combination of anti-smooth muscle α-actin and Millers elastin stain. This particular staining protocol was developed in our own laboratory *(15)* such that clear delineation of the layers of the vessel wall could be observed. The staining procedure uses an indirect immunoperoxidase method to localize smooth muscle actin, which is achieved by incubation with monoclonal anti-α smooth muscle actin at 1:400 dilution (DAKO, High Wycombe, UK). Color development is effected using diaminobenzidine (DAKO) and counterstaining with acid hematoxylin. This is followed by the application of a Millers elastin stain to localize the internal elastic lamina *(16)*. For a detailed protocol of this technique, *see* **Note 11**.

3.1.4. Measurement of Neointimal Thickness

1. Microscopic examination of cultured vein segments will reveal the development of a cellular smooth muscle actin-positive layer, or "neointima." This new layer

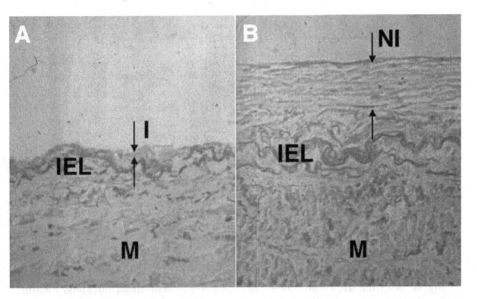

Fig. 3. (**A**) Transverse segment of freshly isolated vein stained with smooth muscle actin/Millers elastin. The layers of the vein wall are clearly delineated (I, intima; M, media; IEL, internal elastic lamina). (**B**) After 14 d in culture a neointima (NI) has developed, comprising of several layers of smooth muscle actin-positive cells that are readily distinguishable from the original intima.

    (**Fig. 3B**, arrowed) is clearly distinguishable from the original intima and is not present on the freshly isolated, uncultured segments (**Fig. 3A**).

2. Perform neointimal thickness measurements using a computer-assisted image analysis system. We use a "RasterOps" video-imaging program (Improvision, Coventry, UK). Taking two consecutive sections, measure the thickness of the neointima at uniform intervals across transverse sections of the vein. Four individual measurements across each high power (×160 magnification) field are ideal (**Fig. 4**). Repeat this procedure across the full width of the sections, such that at least 30 individual measurements have been made.

3. Input the measurements into a computer spreadsheet package to facilitate computation of the results. Using an appropriate formula, calculate the median and range of neointimal thickness for each vein.

3.2. Evaluation of Endothelin-1 as a Mediator of Intimal Hyperplasia in the Saphenous Vein Organ Culture Model

    The neotima that develops in vitro over 14 d shares many of the features of the stenotic lesion which occurs in vivo in graft stenoses, which we have described in detail elsewhere (*17*). Common features of graft stenosis and the cultured vein neointima include smooth muscle cell proliferation, phenotypic

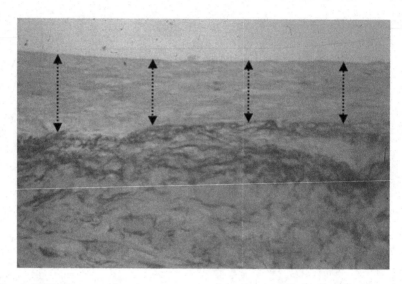

Fig. 4. With the use of an image-analysis system, neointimal thickness measurements are made at evenly spaced intervals across the full width of each transverse section. For example, four measurements for each high power (×160) field are ideal (designated by the arrows).

modulation and extracellular matrix deposition. The organ-cultured saphenous vein therefore offers potential in the investigation of proposed mediators of IH, e.g., endothelin-1 (ET-1), and in evaluating possible therapeutic agents for the prevention of stenosis. The remainder of this section will focus exclusively on the potential of endothelin-1 as a mediator of IH, and investigate whether ET receptor antagonists could be potentially useful therapeutic agents.

3.2.1. Measurement of Secreted ET-1 from Cultured Saphenous Vein

1. Prepare veins and culture in standard culture medium (described in **Subheading 3.1.2.**) for a 14-d period.
2. At each medium change (every 48 h), snap-freeze a sample of "conditioned" medium, taken from the cultured segment, in liquid N_2 and store at $-80°C$ for measurement of ET-1 levels. Take an additional aliquot of fresh medium to act as a control.
3. Measure ET-1 levels in the culture media using ELISA according to the manufacturer's instructions (*see* **Subheading 2.5.**). We found that ET-1 is virtually undetectable in fresh culture medium (0.24 pg/mL), but elevated levels (2.77 pg/mL) are observed in the conditioned medium of cultured vein segments measured over an 18-h period between d 5 and 6 in culture (**Fig. 5**). In our laboratory, we have shown that ET-1 secretion reaches a maximum level between d 6 and 8 in culture, an effect that precedes maximum proliferation, which occurs between d 10 and 14 *(17)*.

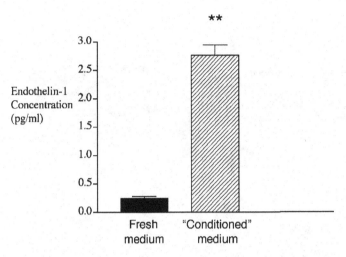

Fig. 5. Bar graph showing elevated levels of endothelin-1 (ET-1) in the medium of organ-cultured vein segments (2.77 +/– 0.17 pg/mL). Samples were taken following an 18-h "conditioning" period between d 5 and 6 in culture. By comparison, ET-1 levels in fresh culture medium are negligible (0.24 +/– 0.035 pg/mL). $^{**}p = 0.004$ (paired t-test).

3.2.2. Cellular Localization of ET-1 in Cultured Saphenous Vein

1. Using 4 µm sections of cultured vein segments, immunohistochemistry is performed using a mouse monoclonal antibody to human ET-1 (Cambridge Bioscience, Cambridge, UK).
2. The protocol for immunostaining is similar to that described for smooth muscle actin (*see* **Note 11**), although "antigen retrieval" is a necessary step for visualization of ET-1 (*see* **Note 12**). We found that a 1:250 dilution of the primary antibody gives optimum positive ET-1 staining, with a minimum of "background" staining. Strong, positive staining is observed in both the endothelium and the smooth muscle cells of the neointima, but not the smooth muscle cells of the intima or media (**Fig. 6**).

3.2.3. Evaluation of Endothelin Antagonists as Inhibitors of Intimal Hyperplasia

The neointima of cultured vein in vitro closely resembles the stenotic lesion in vivo *(17)*. Furthermore ET-1 is produced and secreted by cultured vein. Numerous studies have shown that ET-1 is a mitogen for vascular smooth muscle cells *(18–20)*. The organ culture model therefore lends itself to the evaluation of potential therapeutic agents that antagonize the effects of ET-1 and may therefore inhibit neointimal formation by reducing smooth muscle cell proliferation.

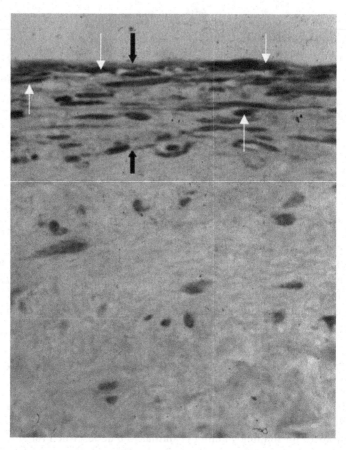

Fig. 6. Immunostaining for ET-1 in 14-d cultured vein segments. Black arrows mark out the neointima. Strong positive staining can be observed in the endothelium and neointimal smooth muscle cells (white arrows).

Two receptor subtypes have been identified for ET-1, designated ET_A and ET_B *(21,22)*. Many drug companies have for several years been actively engaged in the design and synthesis of receptor antagonists. Specific agents are available that are antagonists at both the ET_A and ET_B receptor (nonselective antagonists) or act only at the ET_A or the ET_B receptor (selective antagonists). This section will describe how to evaluate the effectiveness of the endothelin receptor antagonists bosentan, BQ123 and BQ 788 (introduced in **Subheading 2.4.**), in their ability to inhibit neointima formation in cultured vein segments. Solubilization and preparation of pharmacological agents are described in **Subheading 2.4.** In the studies described here, the concentrations of drugs chosen were 10 μ*M* for bosentan, and 3 μ*M* for both BQ788 and

BQ123. The bosentan concentration has been shown to be in the mid-range of therapeutic serum levels after oral administration *(23)* and the selected concentrations of the BQ compounds have been associated with significant and selective ET receptor antagonism *(24)*.

1. Collect vein specimens and prepare for culture as described in **Subheading 3.1.2.** For each drug under study, vein from at least ten patients should be obtained. The number of segments required from each vein will depend upon how many concentrations of drug are to be evaluated, plus a control (no drug) segment (*see* **Note 13**). For example, two drug concentrations plus a control will require three separate cultures from one piece of vein. Remember that the segments should be at least 5-mm square.

2. Add 5 mL of culture medium to each segment and then add the drug (or vehicle for control) in a volume of 100 µL into the 5 mL of culture medium.

3. Incubate the vessels exactly as described in **Subheading 3.1.2.**, and perform a complete medium change and replenishment of the drug or vehicle every 48 h.

4. At the end of the 14-d culture interval, fix, process and prepare sections for neointimal thickness measurements exactly as described in **Subheadings 3.1.3.** and **3.1.4.**

5. After making a series of at least 30 neointima measurements for each segment, calculate the median neointimal thickness of each. Input the data into a suitable computer graphics/statistics package, for example GraphPad Prism (GraphPad Software Inc.). Generate a "scatter plot" and calculate the median neointimal thickness for each cultured segment. Differences between medians of the control and treatment groups are compared using a Wilcoxon paired rank test, with significance assumed at the 95% confidence level ($p < 0.05$).

In our hands, the nonselective antagonist bosentan significantly reduced neointima formation (data not shown). A significant reduction in neointimal thickness was also achieved using the ET_B-selective antagonist BQ 788, although in contrast, the ET_A-selective antagonist BQ123 had no effect on neointima formation. We were therefore able to conclude that it is the ET_B receptor playing a central role in the development of intimal hyperplasia in this model. Representative scatter plots of data generated from these studies are shown in **Fig. 7**.

3.3. Organ Culture—A Valuable Experimental Model?

Culture of segments of the long saphenous vein for 14 d in serum-supplemented medium results in the development of a sub-endothelial "neointima" comprising several layers of smooth muscle actin-positive cells. Furthermore, this neointimal thickening shares many of the characteristics of the stenotic lesion that develops in saphenous vein bypass grafts. For further reading, *see* **ref. *17***. Although this is an in vitro model, a major advantage is that it uses the

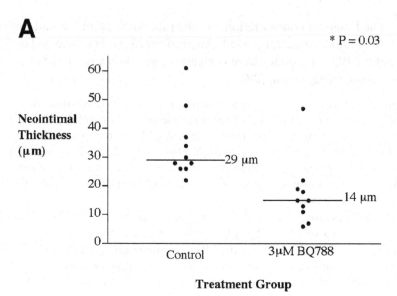

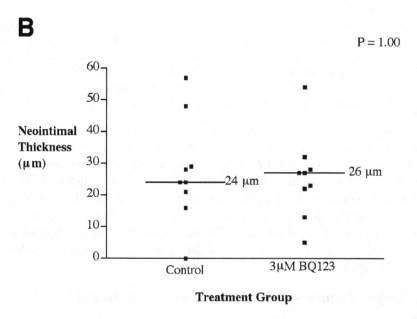

Fig. 7. Representative scatter plots comparing the effect of selective endothelin receptor antagonists on the development of neointimal thickening. (A) BQ788, a selective ET_B receptor antagonist significantly reduced neointima formation ($^*p = 0.03$, Wilcoxon paired rank test) compared with control. (B) BQ123, a selective ET_A receptor antagonist had no significant effect on the development of neointima compared with control ($p = 1.00$, Wilcoxon paired rank test).

exact tissue in which the human clinical problem occurs, namely the long saphenous vein.

The studies described here relate specifically to endothelin-1 as a mediator of IH and the effect of endothelin receptor antagonists upon its development. It is an equally useful and versatile model for the investigation of other potential candidate molecules involved in the development of IH and the evaluation of possible preventative strategies in the amelioration of vein bypass graft stenosis.

4. Notes

1. Prepare transport medium in bulk (e.g., 1 L), sterilize by filtration using a 0.22 μm filter and aliquot approx 10–15 mL into 20 mL sterile universal tubes. Cap tightly and store at 4°C for up to 1 mo. Use one aliquot for each vein sample to be collected.

2. Culture dishes for organ culture are prepared using 60 × 20 mm Duran glass Petri dishes. Prepare Sylgard 184 elastomer (BDH, Poole, UK) as per the manufacturer's instructions and cast a layer into each dish to a depth of approx 5 mm. Stand dishes on a completely level surface and allow resin to "cure." This is best achieved by incubating the dishes at 40°C for approx 24 h in a clean, dust-free atmosphere. Wash the dishes in 10% acetic acid for 1 h, rinse in distilled water, and dry in the oven. This acid washing step is necessary to prevent unpleasant vapors being emitted when the dishes are autoclaved for the first time. Replace lids onto dishes, double-wrap each dish individually in autoclave bags, and sterilize by autoclaving at 120°C for 20 min. The culture dishes are now ready for use and can be repeatedly washed, sterilized, and reused many times. With repeated washing the Sylgard will discolor, but this in no way affects its performance.

3. A1 minuten pins are very difficult to handle. The best way to prepare them for use is to make a "pincushion" by almost filling an autoclavable specimen pot with Sylgard resin (prepared as above). Using curved, fine forceps press a hundred or more pins into the resin individually, replace the lid onto the pot and sterilize by autoclaving. Open the pot only inside a Class II cabinet and use only sterile forceps to remove pins as required. Store unused pins with the lid tightly closed.

4. A mesh size of 500 μm is not crucial. Any polyester mesh will serve the purpose, which is merely to allow a small space between the vein and the silicone resin so that nutrients are accessible to the adventitial surface of the vein.

5. Ophthalmic scissors are used for opening up vein segments. "Noyes" straight vanna 3-inch scissors (Richardsons, Leicester, UK, cat. no. D2044) are ideal for this purpose.

6. Antagonists should be solubilized according to the manufacturer's recommendations in a suitable vehicle. Ensure that the vehicle itself is not toxic to the vein culture. We have found that a final concentration of up to 2%, DMSO has no detrimental effect on the cultures.

7. Paraffin-embedding, unless carried out routinely in your own laboratory, is best performed by an experienced histopathology department. After fixation and dehydration, the vein segment should be divided in half with a sharp blade and embed-

ded in the paraffin block *longitudinally* with the cut edges of the vein facing towards you. When the trimmed paraffin block is then placed on the microtome, two consecutive transverse sections are transferred onto the microscope slide.

8. If, for any reason, there is likely to be a delay in setting up the organ cultures, we have found that collection of the vein directly into complete culture medium (i.e., 30% serum) and storage at 4°C will preserve good viability for several (up to six) hours.

9. Fixing the vein segments while still pinned-out in the dish minimizes any shrinkage artefact and therefore facilitates more accurate measurements of neointimal thickness.

10. To prepare silane-coated slides place the required number of microscope slides into racks. In a fume-cupboard prepare four glass staining dishes and into the first place 350 mL acetone and 3 mL 3-aminopropyltriethoxy silane (Sigma, Poole, UK). Fill the second dish with acetone, and the remaining two with ultra-pure water. Immerse slide racks into each dish in order for approx 5 s with gentle agitation. Drain onto tissue and dry at 42°C overnight. Slides can then be stored in a clean, dry atmosphere (back in the original boxes) and used as required.

11. We have found that the use of a combined stain for smooth muscle and elastin greatly facilitates delineation of the layers of the vein wall and hence allows precise and reproducible measurements of neointimal thickness, which is of central importance in inhibitor studies.

   The method employed for detection of smooth muscle and elastic fibres is fundamentally an "ABC complex/HRP" technique, which is a standard procedure in any histopathology laboratory. Our method is as follows. Unless specifically stated, all incubations are performed at room temperature.

   a. Dewax and rehydrate slide-mounted sections by placing sequentially into 99% xylene, 95% xylene, 99% ethanol, 95% ethanol (5 min in each).

   b. Wash in water for 2 min.

   c. Place into 6% hydrogen peroxide for 10 min (to block endogenous peroxidase activity).

   d. Wash in water (2 min), followed by Tris-buffered saline (TBS, 2 min).

   e. Dry around the sections with a tissue and lay slides in a humidified chamber (moist tissues in the bottom). Cover each section with a few drops of normal goat serum (diluted 1:20 with TBS) for 10 min. This blocks any nonspecific binding of the primary antibody. During this period, prepare the primary SMA antibody in TBS at a 1:400 dilution.

   f. Drain off the goat serum (*do not wipe!*) and add 100 µL of primary antibody to each section. Incubate in the humidified chamber at 4°C overnight.

   g. Place slides into a rack and wash in phosphate-buffered saline (PBS) for 20 min.

   h. Shake off excess moisture, wipe around the sections with tissue and cover each section with the secondary antibody (goat anti-mouse immunoglobulins) for 30 min. We use a Streptavidin ABComplex/HRP Duet (mouse/rabbit) complete kit for the secondary and tertiary antibodies (DAKO). In this case, the secondary antibody is labeled "C" and should be prepared according to the instructions.

   i. Wash slides in PBS for 20 min. During this period prepare the tertiary antibody (ABC complex, labeled "A" and "B" in the kit).

    j. Wipe around the sections with tissue and place 100 μL of the complex onto each section. Incubate for 30 min.

    k. Wash the slides in PBS (2 × 15 min). During these washes prepare the diaminobenzidine (DAB) according to the manufacturer's instructions in PBS.

    l. After the wash periods, place the slides onto a rack over a sink. Immediately add 70 μL of 3% hydrogen peroxide to the DAB/PBS, mix and filter onto the slides. Leave for 5 min, then wash in water.

    m. Immerse the slides into Millers (elastin) stain for 30 min.

    n. Wash slides with 95% ethanol, then finally dehydrate by performing sequential 5-min washes in 95% ethanol, 99% ethanol, 95% xylene, and 99% xylene.

    o. Mount and coverslip the sections.

    p. When viewed under the microscope, smooth muscle is stained brown and elastic fibers dark blue/black.

12. "Antigen retrieval" requires pretreatment of slide-mounted sections with 1% (w/v) trypsin solution. This is prepared by dissolving 0.3 g of trypsin and 0.36 g of granular calcium chloride in 300 mL of water at 37°C. Adjust to pH 7.8 using a weak sodium hydroxide (NaOH) solution. Following **step 2** in the ABC protocol, immerse slides in the trypsin solution for 10 min at 37°C. Wash in water for 2 min, and then proceed with **steps 11c–p** as for the ABC protocol.

13. The inhibitor studies described here were all performed separately, with their own individual controls. This was principally a result of limitations on the length of vein available. In theory, if the amount of vein available is sufficient to divide into many segments, then each antagonist could be evaluated within one study against a single control segment.

References

1. Mattos, M. K., van Bemmelen, P. S., Hodgson, K. J., Ramsey, D. E., Barkmeier, L. D., and Sumner, D. S. (1993) Does correction of stenoses identified with colour duplex scanning improve infrainguinal graft patency? *J. Vasc. Surg.* **17,** 54–66.

2. Angelini, G. D. and Newby, A. C. (1989) The future of saphenous vein as a coronary artery bypass conduit. *Eur. Heart J.* **10,** 273–280.

3. Freshney, R. I. (1987) *Culture of Animal Cells*, 2nd ed., Alan R. Liss Inc., New York, pp. 298–305.

4. Strangeways, T. S. P. and Fell, H. B. (1926) Experimental studies on the differentiation of embryonic tissues growing in vivo and in vitro *Proc. Royal Soc. London* **99,** 340–366.

5. Trowell, O. A. (1959) The culture of mature organs in a synthetic medium. *Exp. Cell Res.* **16,** 118–147.

6. Pederson, D. C. and Bowyer, D. E. (1985) Endothelial injury and healing in vitro. Studies using an organ culture system. *Am. J. Pathol.* **119,** 264–272.

7. Koo, E. W. Y. and Gotlieb, A. I. (1989) Endothelial stimulation of intimal cell proliferation in a porcine aortic organ culture. *Am. J. Pathol.* **134,** 497–503.

8. Koo, E. W. Y. and Gotlieb, A. I. (1991) Neointimal formation in the porcine aortic organ culture. *Lab. Invest.* **64,** 743–753.

9. Barrett, L. A., Mergner, W. J., and Trump, B. F. (1979). Long term culture of human aortas. *In Vitro* **15**, 957–966.

10. Soyombo, A. A., Angelini, G. D., Bryan, A. J., Jasani, B., and Newby, A. C. (1990) Intimal proliferation in an organ culture of human saphenous vein. *Am. J. Pathol.* **137**, 1401–1410.

11. Ferrell, M., Fuster, V., Gold, H. K., and Chesebro, J. H. (1992) A dilemma for the 1990's. Choosing appropriate experimental models for the prevention of restenosis. *Circulation* **85**, 1630–1631.

12. Clozel, M., Breu, V., Gray, G. A., Kalina, B., Loffler, B. M., Burri, K., et al. (1994) Pharmacological characterisation of bosentan, a new potent orally active nonpeptide endothelin receptor antagonist. *J. Pharmacol. Exp. Ther.* **270**, 228–235.

13. Ihara, M., Ishikawa, K., Fukuroda, T., Saeki, T., Funabashi, K., Fukami, T., et al. (1992) In vitro biological profile of a highly potent novel endothelin (ET) antagonist BQ-123 selective for the ET_A receptor. *J. Cardiovasc. Pharmacol.* **20**, 511–514.

14. Ishikawa, K., Ihara, M., Noguchi, K., Mase, T., Mino, N., Saeki, T., et al. (1994) Biochemical and pharmacological profile of a potent and selective endothelin B-receptor antagonist, BQ-788. *Proc. Natl. Acad. Sci. USA* **91**, 4892–4896.

15. Sayers, R. D., Jones, L., Varty, K., Allen, K., Morgan, J. D. T., Bell, P. R. F., and London, N.J.M. (1993) The histopathology of infrainguinal vein graft stenoses. *Eur. J. Vasc. Surg.* **7**, 16–20.

16. Miller, R. J. (1971) An elastin stain. *Med. Lab. Tech.* **28**, 148–154.

17. Porter, K. E., Varty, K., Jones, L., Bell, P. R. F., and London, N. J. M. (1996) Human saphenous vein organ culture: A useful model of intimal hyperplasia? *Eur. J. Vasc. Endovasc. Surg.* **11**, 48–58.

18. Bobik, A., Grooms, A., Millar, J. A., and Grinpukel, S. (1990) Growth factor activity of endothelin on vascular smooth muscle. *Am. J. Physiol.* **258**, C408–C415.

19. Hirata, Y., Takagi, Y., Fukuda, Y., and Marumo, F. (1989) Endothelin is a potent mitogen for rat vascular smooth muscle cells. *Atherosclerosis* **78**, 225–228.

20. Masood, I., Porter, K. E., and London, N. J. M. (1997) Endothelin-1 is a mediator of intimal hyperplasia in an organ culture of human saphenous vein. *Br. J. Surg.* **84**, 499–503.

21. Arai, H., Hori, S., Aramori, I., Ohkubo, H., and Nakanishi, S. (1990) Cloning and expression of a cDNA encoding an endothelin receptor. *Nature* **348**, 730–732.

22. Sakurai, T., Yanagisawa, M., Takuwa, Y., Miyazaki, H., Kimura, S., Goto, K., and Masaki, T. (1990) Cloning of a cDNA encoding a nonisopeptide-selective subtype of the endothelin receptor. *Nature* **348**, 732–735.

23. Weber, C., Schmitt, R., Birnboeck, H., Hopfgartner, G., Vanmarle, S. P., Peeters, P. A. M., et al. (1996) Pharmacokinetics and pharmacodynamics of the endothelin receptor antagonist bosentan in healthy human subjects. *Clin. Pharmacol. Ther.* **60**, 124–137.

24. Douglas, S. A., Vickery-Clark, L. M., Louden, C., Elliot, J. D., and Ohlstein, E. H. (1995) Endothelin receptor subtypes in the pathogenesis of angioplasty-induced neointima formation in the rat - A comparison of selective ET(A) receptor antagonism and dual ET(A)/ET(B) receptor antagonism using BQ123 and SB204670. *J. Cardiovasc. Pharmacol.* **26**, S186–S189.

V

In Vivo Functional Assays

13

Investigation of the Endothelin System in Experimental Heart Failure

Gillian A. Gray and Lorcan Sherry

1. Introduction

The first evidence that endothelin-1 (ET-1) was implicated in the pathophysiology of chronic heart failure (CHF) came from studies demonstrating elevated plasma concentrations of the mature peptide in patients with CHF *(1)* Subsequent studies showed that plasma levels of ET-1 and particularly of its precursor big ET-1 correlated with the severity of CHF *(2)* and were able to predict the necessity for heart transplant *(3)*. The ET system has since been studied in CHF patients using acute administration of inhibitors of ET formation, ET receptor agonists and ET receptor antagonists either locally into the forearm or hand vein *(4,5, see* Chapter 14) or systemically *(6,7)*. These hemodynamic studies provided an indication that blockade of the ET system might be of therapeutic benefit in CHF. However, these types of studies are unable to answer questions relating to tissue expression of the ET-1 synthesizing pathway or ET receptors and how these might be altered during disease progression. These questions can be best addressed initially using experimental models, which also permit detailed histological and molecular analysis of the pathways modified by ET system blockade and can be followed through to a mortality endpoint. Studies in experimental animals provided the first evidence that ET receptor antagonists might improve survival in heart failure *(8)* and these observations are now being followed through into clinical trials in CHF patients *(9)*.

There are many experimental models of heart failure, all of which have their particular advantages and disadvantages, these have been reviewed recently *(10,11)*. The ET system has been studied using several of these models, some examples are given in **Table 1** *(8,12–24)*. Complete coverage of the findings of

From: *Methods in Molecular Biology, vol. 206: Peptide Research Protocols: Endothelin*
Edited by: J. Maguire and A. Davenport © Humana Press Inc., Totowa, NJ

Table 1
Examples of Experimental Heart Failure Models and Their Use in the Investigation of the Endothelin System in Heart Failure

Experimental model	Species	Ref. no.
Coronary artery ligation	Rat	*8,12–16*
Coronary artery ligation	Rabbit	*17*
Rapid pacing	Dog	*18*
Pressure overload	Rat	*19*
Salt-induced hypertension	Rat	*20*
Cardiomyopathy	Hamster	*21*
Chronic catecholamine infusion	Rabbit	*22*
Volume overload	Rabbit	*23*
Viral myocarditis	Mouse	*24*

these studies is beyond the scope of this chapter, and interested readers are referred to recent reviews of ET system activation in CHF for further information *(25)*.

This chapter describes the rat coronary artery ligation (CAL) model of heart failure, a model of CHF resulting from ischaemic heart disease, originally described by Selye in 1960 *(26)* and subsequently modified by Pfeffer *(27)*. This is among the most widely studied models of CHF, perhaps because responses to treatment in this model have been shown to translate to benefit in patients, particularly in the case of angiotensin-converting enzyme (ACE) inhibitors *(28)*, suggesting that it is a reasonable model for the human condition.

While each of the research groups using this model to study the ET system follows the same general protocol, i.e., ligation of the left main coronary artery, the outcomes are often quite different. For example, in the model used by the Sakai and colleagues *(8,12)* mortality immediately post-CAL is very high (>60%), the animals have very large infarcts (>50% left ventricular free wall) and many of the animals die within a study period of 8 wk. The authors have reported increased expression of pre-pro-ET-1, ET_A and ET_B receptor mRNA in this model *(12)*, as well as inhibition of hypertrophy and mortality by ET_A receptor antagonist *(8)*. In contrast, the model that we ourselves use is more moderate with mortality of <20% immediately post-CAL, smaller infarcts (close to 40% left ventricular free wall) and no mortality up to 12 wk post-CAL *(13)*. While our model does develop CHF (as indicated by elevated left ventricular end-diastolic pressure), the model is clearly less severe than that of Sakai and colleagues and this is reflected in more selective activation of the ET system. We have found, e.g., that ET_B receptor mRNA is selectively upregulated in the non-infarcted left-ventricle at 12 wk post-CAL and in small blood vessels from the same animals *(13)*. Others using similar models have also reported selective ET_B receptor upregulation in the ventricle *(14)*. ET receptor antagonist studies in the moderate model provide further evidence for differential activation of the ET system *(15,16)*. Taken together these studies suggest a relationship between infarct size, disease severity and activation of the ET system in heart failure, consistent with clinical studies. The variation between the models is largely owing to the position of placement of the ligature on the coronary artery, with more severe models and faster disease progression resulting from a ligation placed near to the root of the coronary artery. We, and others, have found that placement of the ligature approx 1/3 down the length of the artery produces CHF but with low initial mortality and more gradual development of CHF *(13–16)*.

Our own studies using this model have been directed at investigation of expression of pre-pro-ET-1 and its receptors in the blood vessels and the heart using *in situ* hybridization *(29)* and immunocytochemistry, as well as vascular function *(13)*. These methods are not described here as they are dealt with in some detail in other chapters of this book. We have, however, chosen to describe the surgical technique for coronary artery ligation and also the methods for hemodynamic and histological assessment of the model. We are indebted to Professor Jos Smits and his staff in University Hospital, Maastricht, the Netherlands for their generous assistance with training and establishment of this model, and more recently the mouse CAL model of heart failure, in our laboratory.

2. Materials

2.1. Surgery and Hemodynamic Analysis

1. A room licensed for animal procedures containing a heated table, good room lighting, and adequate space for a small animal ventilator and heated recovery boxes.
2. Surgical instruments for ligation surgery: needle holders, round-ended curved scissors (10-cm length), De Bakey tissue forceps, curved forceps (8-cm length), micro-dissecting retractor.
3. Surgical instruments for hemodynamic analysis: 2 pairs curved forceps, round-ended curved scissors, small artery clamp, watchmakers forceps for arterial cannulation, curved sharp-ended Vannas microscissors, 2 pairs hemostatic forceps.
4. Small animal ventilator (Harvard Apparatus).
5. A cold light source with fibre optic flexible light, e.g., Schott KL1500 electronic light source.
6. A system for delivery of O_2 by a gas regulator including small animal masks.
7. 1 mL Syringes, assorted needles for intraperitoneal and subcutaneous injection, sterile gauze, sterile 0.9% saline, gloves, mask and surgical gown, 70% alcohol.
8. Assorted Portex plastic cannulas red (FG 5, 1.65 mm) for intubation during surgery, blue (FG3, 0.75 mm) for chest drainage post-surgery and for vessel can-

nulation and white (F4, 1.3 mm) or pink (F3, 1 mm) for exsanguination via the dorsal aorta.

9. Sodium pentobarbital (60 mg/mL Sagatal, Rhone Merieux Ltd., Essex, UK) for anesthesia and buprenorphine hydrochloride (Vetergesic®, 0.3 mg/mL; Reckitt & Colman) for analgesia.
10. A small coat clipper.
11. Surgical needles with sutures attached from Ethicon: 10-mm round bodied (5/0 Mersilk W595) for coronary ligation, 16-mm round bodied (3/0 Mersilk W546) for closure of the chest muscle and 25-mm round bodied (3/0 Mersilene W6591) for skin closure.
12. An autoclave for sterilization of instruments.
13. Pressure transducer-tipped catheter (2F, Model SPR-407, Millar Instruments, Texas) for ventricular pressure measurement post-surgery, attached to a suitable recording system.

2.2. Tissue and Blood Collection

1. 10% Phosphate-buffered formalin if collecting tissue for histology or immuno-cytochemistry (plus access to tissue processing and embedding facilities).
2. Liquid nitrogen (if collecting tissue for molecular analysis).
3. Chilled tubes containing 0.5% EDTA for blood collection and centrifugation.
4. Chilled bench top centrifuge for separation of plasma.
5. −70°C Freezer for storage of blood and tissue samples.

2.3. Post-Surgical Assays

2.3.1. Radioimmunoassay of Plasma ET-1 and Big ET-1 Concentration

Method described in Chapter 2.

2.3.2. Immunocytochemical Localization of ET-1

Method described in Chapter 1.

2.3.3. Investigation of ET Receptor Function in Isolated Blood Vessels

Methods similar to those described elsewhere in this book (*see* Chapter 10).

2.3.4. Measurement of Plasma Lactate Dehydrogenase

The plasma concentration of lactate dehydrogenase was assayed to confirm successful infarction using a commercial kit from Boehringer-Mannheim (MPR 2, 1442597).

2.3.5. Histological Staining

For histological staining to measure infarct size the following items are required:

1. Microtome for tissue sectioning.
2. Floating out bath.
3. TESPA (3-aminopropyltriethoxy-saline) coated glass slides.
4. Glass Coplin jars containing xylene, 100, 90, and 70% alcohol, Celestine blue nuclear stain, or van Giesons stain (50 mL saturated aqueous picric acid solution, 9 mL 1% aqueous acid fuschin solution, 50 mL distilled H_2O).
5. Slide holders and glass boxes for slide rinsing.
6. Light microscope and image analysis system.

3. Methods

3.1. Coronary Artery Ligation Surgery in the Rat

Male Wistar rats (ideally 250–280 g) are subjected to ligation of the proximal portion of the left coronary artery and infarction of the left ventricular free wall according to the method first described by Selye et al. *(26)* and subsequently modified by Pfeffer et al. *(27)*. Rats are allowed access to normal rat chow and water ad libitum prior to surgery.

1. On the day of surgery, weigh the rats and anesthetise using sodium pentobarbital (60 mg kg^{-1} i.p.), which will maintain anesthesia for 3–4 h.
2. Shave the front right area of the rat's chest and clean with 70% alcohol. Place the rat on a thermostatically controlled heating pad (*see* **Note 1**) and then intubate (1.5-mm diameter plastic cannula, Portex Ltd., UK) via the mouth (*see* **Note 2**). Begin mechanical ventilation immediately (using room air mixed with 100% O_2 at a rate of 60 cycles/min and a tidal volume of 1 mL/100 g body weight).
3. Use sterile instruments to cut a 2-cm long area of the skin parallel to the direction of the ribs at a level between the fourth and fifth ribs. Gently separate the underlying muscle layers using blunt scissors and hold in position by smooth stainless steel clips, revealing the rib cage. Perform a left thoracotomy between the fourth and fifth ribs exposing the inner chest cavity. To avoid damage to the lungs during surgery, collapse the left lung by folding a small square of sterilized gauze and use it to cover the lung, which is then gently pushed downward and away from the heart. Cut the pericardium and gently and rapidly exteriorize the heart by gentle application of pressure to the thorax. Place a 10-mm round-bodied needle under the proximal left coronary artery at the level of the base of the left atrium and pull through leaving suture in position untied. Return the heart to its position in the thorax, and leave for 10 min to permit recovery of the blood pressure, which drops during externalization of the heart. Tie the ligature, checking that there is no bleeding from the ventricular wall that would indicate damage to the artery.
4. Subject sham-operated rats to the same protocol, except the ligature is not tied, but pulled through under the coronary artery.
5. Before closing the ribcage (*see* **Note 3**), place a 0.75-mm diameter plastic cannula in the chest cavity, and remove the small square of sterilized gauze retaining the

lung. Gently squeeze the chest cavity to remove air before inserting 2 sutures (16-mm round-bodied needle) to bring the ribs together and close the rib cage. Release the chest muscle back over the rib cage and close the skin with 4 sutures (25-mm round-bodied needle). Connect the plastic cannula in the chest cavity to a 1-mL syringe and use to extract any remaining air from the chest after closure, then remove gently.

6. Take the rat off the ventilator and, when spontaneous ventilation is reestablished, place on a heated pad in a recovery box. During recovery, place a mask delivering 100% O_2 close to the animals head so that it is breathing oxygen-enriched air. Remove the tracheal cannula upon initial signs of recovery from anesthesia and leave the animals to fully recover (usually 3–4 h after initial anesthesia) before returning to their cages. Administer buprenorphine hydrochloride (Vetergesic) subcutaneously upon recovery from anesthetic and again the following day for analgesia.

7. When it is necessary to ensure that infarction has been successful, e.g., for assignment of animals to drug treatment groups, a small piece of tail (2–3 mm) can be removed during the final stages of recovery from anesthetic and after analgesic administration. This permits collection of 0.5 mL blood for assay of lactate dehydrogenase (LDH, using the kit listed above).

3.2. Hemodynamics, Echocardiography, and Tissue Sampling

1. After the allocated period of ligation or sham-operation, weigh the rats and then anesthetize using Na pentobarbital (60 mg kg^{-1} i.p.).

2. If the equipment is available, echocardiography should be used to measure cardiac dimensions in CHF compared to sham animals (*see* **refs. *12–17***). Lightly anesthetize the rat and place in the left lateral position. Shave a small area of the anterior chest wall and obtain images in the short-axis with a 7.5 MHz probe using a standard ultrasound machine (e.g., Acuson XP10). Measure left ventricular dimensions and fractional shortening from M-mode images. Store images on videotape and use two independent observers, blinded to which group the animal belonged, to analyze them.

3. For subsequent hemodynamic analysis, locate the left carotid artery, dissect free of extraneous tissue and cannulate with a Millar pressure transducer-tipped catheter (Model SPR-407, Millar Instruments, Texas), attached to a recording system (e.g., the Powerlab online data acquisition system, AD Instruments). Measure arterial blood pressure when the catheter is in position in the carotid artery. Advance the cannula into the left ventricle for measurement of left ventricular pressures (*see* **Fig. 1**), heart failure is usually recognized by the elevation of the LV end-diastolic from approx 5 mm Hg to more than 15 mm Hg.

4. If blood is to be collected for assay of endothelin-1 and big endothelin-1 then the rat is exsanguinated via a needle (1-mm diameter, Microlance®, Becton Dickinson, Ireland) or a cannula of similar dimensions placed in the dorsal aorta. Collect the blood into a 10 mL syringe prerinsed with heparin (100 U/mL final concentration, Multiparin®, CP Pharmaceuticals, Wrexham, UK) then aliquot into

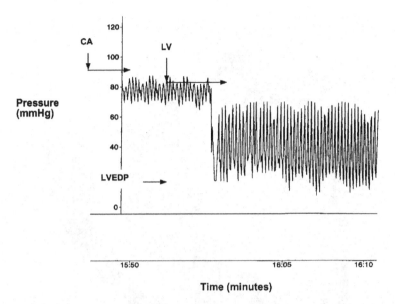

Fig. 1. A sample trace from pressure recording using a pressure-transducer tipped catheter, showing mean arterial blood pressure recorded when the catheter tip is placed into the carotid artery (CA), and the left ventricular end-diastolic pressure (LVEDP) when it is advanced into the left ventricle (LV). From each animal LVEDP value is calculated by averaging the pressure reading from the troughs of 20 pressure spikes along the trace.

prechilled test tubes containing 50 μL of 10 mmol/L final concentration EDTA and centrifuge immediately (2000g, 4°C, 20 min). For future plasma ET-1 and big ET-1 analysis by radioimmunoasay plasma is be stored at −70°C (*see* Chapter 2).

5. Dissect out required tissues (heart, blood vessels, etc.), rinse in ice-cooled physiological saline and weigh. Fresh tissue may then be used immediately for functional studies (e.g., *see* Chapter 10) or for the measurement of endothelin peptides by ELISA or radioimmunoassay (*see* Chapter 2). Alternatively, tissues may be placed into fixative (10% neutral-buffered formalin or similar) for histological analysis (*see* **Subheading 3.3.** below) or into liquid nitrogen for analysis of endothelin peptides, receptors or converting enzymes at the protein (*see* Chapters 1 and 4) or molecular (*see* Chapters 6 and 8) level (*see* **Note 4**).

3.3. Histological Staining and Measurement of Infarct Size

1. Cut hearts in two from apex to base through the infarcted region, fix for 24 h in 10% neutral-buffered formalin then process and wax embed using standard procedures.

2. For measurement of infarct size, section wax-embedded hearts at 3 μm and float out on a water bath set at 48°C. Place sections on TESPA (3-Amino-

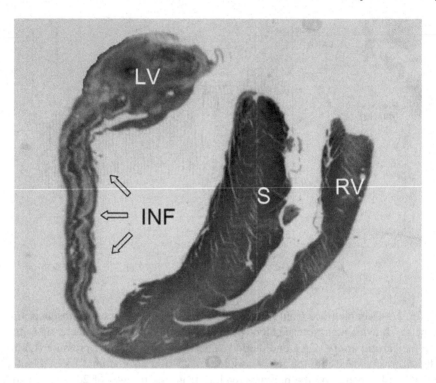

Fig. 2. Image of a typical longitudinal section of a heart from an animal that has undergone coronary artery ligation. Infarct parameters are measured using image analysis software as described in the text. LV, left ventricle; RV, right ventricle, S, septum; INF, area of infarction.

propyltriethoxy-saline; Sigma, UK)-coated slides and allow to adhere overnight in an oven at 37°C.

3. For collagen staining, initially dewax sections through xylene and rehydrate through 100%, 90%, and 70% alcohol solutions before placing in water for 15 min. Dip sections in celestine blue nuclear stain for 2 min, immerse in van Gieson's stain for 3 min, then dehydrate through 70%, 90%, and 100% alcohol solutions and xylene and mount in DePeX mounting medium (BDH Laboratory Supplies, UK). Using this staining method, the infarction containing large amounts of collagen can be differentiated from healthy tissue. The collagen fibrils stain pink with van Geison stain while healthy myocardium is stained yellow.

4. For measurement of infarct size place sections under a CCD video camera module attached to a microscope with a ×20 lens, and bring an image of the heart (*see* **Fig. 2**) up on the image analysis system computer. Determine the endocardial and epicardial circumferences of the infarcted tissue and of the remaining left ventricle with the image analysis software (e.g., Zeiss Kontron 300 image analysis package, Image Associates, Thame, UK). Infarct size is calculated as:

$$\frac{\text{[endocardial + epicardial circumference of the infarcted free left ventricle (mm)]}}{\text{[endocardial + epicardial circumference of the whole free left ventricle (mm)]}}$$

and is expressed as a percentage. To measure infarct thickness, randomly select 4 points along the length of the infarct and calculate an average value in mm. The myocardial/collagen content of the infarct is measured in the infarct wall by identifying areas of collagen and myocardium in the infarct zone using the light microscope. Measure the area of each (in mm^2) and calculate the ratio of myocardium to collagen. All sections from different groups within the same study must be examined blind, with heart numbers and corresponding group reserved from the investigator until the analysis is complete.

4. Notes

1. The importance of keeping the animal warm before, during and after surgery cannot be overemphasized. This can be best achieved using a heated table or a heated underblanket available from several commercial suppliers.
2. Intubation is carried out with the aid of a metal guide wire (such as those available from human cardiac catheterisation) and a fiber-optic light placed over the throat region to illuminate the entrance to the trachea. We have found that the use of the guide wire aids greatly with the correct placement of the catheter in the trachea.
3. Following ligation of the coronary artery, the chest should be left open for 15 min to allow manual manipulation of the heart during any subsequent arrhythmias that occur after myocardial infarction (MI); usually 7–14 min after MI. These arrythmias can often be prevented by gentle application of a moistened cotton tip to the surface of the heart.
4. Heart failure in the experimental models is usually characterized using a range of methods to demonstrate left-ventricular dysfunction and/or remodelling. One or more of the following are usually applied using several of the following measurements (a) echocardiography, (b) infarct size and histological cardiac dimension measurement, (c) heart: body weight ratio, (d) expression of hypertrophic markers, e.g., the ratio of alpha: beta myosin heavy chain (beta chain being upregulated in hypertrophic myocardium), or atrial natriuretic peptide.

References

1. McMurray, J. J., Ray S. G. Abdullah, I., Dargie, H. J., and Morton, J. J. (1992) Plasma endothelin in chronic heart failure. *Circulation* **85**, 1374–1379.
2. Wei, C. M., Lerman, A. Rodehoffer R. J., and Burnett, J. J. (1994) Endothelin in human congestive heart failure. *Circulation* **89**, 1580–1586.
3. Pacher, R., Stanek, B., and Hulsmann, M. (1996) Prognostic impact of big-endothelin-1 plasma concentrations compared with invasive hemodynamic evaluation in severe heart failure. *J. Am. Coll. Cardiol.* **27**, 633–641.
4. Love, M. P., Haynes, W. G., Gray, G. A., Webb, D. J., and McMurray, J. J. V. (1996) Endothelin in chronic heart failure: the therapeutic potential of converting enzyme inhibition and receptor blockade. *Circulation.* **94**, 2131–2137.

5. Love, M. P., Haynes, W. G., Webb, D. J., and McMurray, J. J. V. (2000) Venous endothelin receptor function in patients with chronic heart failure. *Clin. Sci.* **98**, 65–70.

6. Kiowski, W., Sutsch, G., and Hunziker, P. (1995) Evidence for endothelin-1 mediated vasoconstriction in severe chronic heart failure. *Lancet* **346**, 732–736.

7. Cowburn, P. J., Cleland, J. G. F., McArthur, J. D., MacLean, M. R., McMurray, J. J. V., Dargie, H. J., and Morton, J. J. (1999) Endothelin(B) receptors are functionally important in mediating vasoconstriction in the systemic circulation in patients with left ventricular systolic dysfunction. *J. Am. Coll. Cardiol.* **33**, 932–938.

8. Sakai, S., Miyauchi, T., and Sakurai, Y. (1996) Inhibition of myocardial endothelin pathway improves long-term survival in heart failure. *Nature* **384**, 353–355.

9. Mylona, P. and Cleland, J. G. F. (1999) Update of REACH-1 and MERIT-HF clinical trials in heart failure. *Eur. J. Heart Failure* **1**, 197–200.

10. Schaper, W., ed. (1998) Spotlight on Animal Models and Human Cardiovascular Disease. *Cardiovasc. Res.* **39**, 1–260.

11. Arnolda, L. F., Llewellyn-Smith, I. J., and Minson, J. B. (1999) Animal models of heart failure. *Aust. New Zealand J. Med. 29,* 403–409.

12. Sakai, S., Miyauchi, T., and Yamaguchi, I. (2000) Long-term endothelin receptor antagonist administration improves alterations in expression of various cardiac genes in failing myocardium of rats with heart failure. *Circulation* **101,** 2849–2853.

13. Gray, G. A., Mickley, E. J., Webb, D. J., and McEwan, P. E. (2000) Localisation and function of ET-1 and ET receptors in small arteries post-myocardial infarction: Upregulation of smooth muscle ET_B receptors that modulate contraction. *Br. J. Pharmacol.* **130**, 1735–1744.

14. Smith, P. J. W., Ornatsky, O., Stewart, D. J., Picard, P., Dawood, F., Wen, W. H., et al. (2000) Effects of estrogen replacement on infarct size, cardiac remodelling, and the endothelin system after myocardial infarction in ovariectomized rats. *Circulation* **102**, 2983–2989.

15. Mulder, P., Richard, V., Derumeaux, G., Hogie, M., Henry, J. P., Lallemand, F., et al. (1997) Role of endogenous endothelin in chronic heart failure- Effect of long-term treatment with an endothelin antagonist on survival, hemodynamics, and cardiac remodelling. *Circulation* **96**, 1976–1982.

16. Mulder, P., Boujedaini, H., Richard, V., Derumeaux, G., Henry, J. P., Renet, S., et al. (2000) Selective endothelin-A versus combined endothelin-A/endothelin-B receptor blockade in rat chronic heart failure. *Circulation* **102,** 491–493.

17. Docherty, C. C. and MacLean, M. R. (1998) Endothelin (B) receptors in rabbit pulmonary resistance arteries: Effect of left ventricular dysfunction. *J. Pharmacol. Exp. Therap.* **284**, 895–903.

18. Cannan, C. R., Burnett, J. C., and Lerman, A. (1996) Enhanced coronary vasoconstriction to endothelin-B-receptor activation in experimental congestive heart failure. *Circulation* **93**, 646–651.

19. Arai, M., Yoguchi, A., Iso, T., Takahashi, T., Imai, S., and Suzuki, T. (1995) Endothelin and its binding sites are upregulated in pressure-overload cardiac hypertrophy. *Am. J. Physiol.* **37,** H2084–H2091.

20. Iwanaga, Y., Kihara, Y., Hasegawa, K., Inagaki, K., Yoneda, T., Kaburagi, S., et al. (1998) Cardiac endothelin-1 plays a critical role in the functional deterioration of left ventricles during the transition from compensatory hypertrophy to congestive heart failure in salt-sensitive hypertensive rats. *Circulation* **98,** 2065–2073.

21. Bolger, G. T., Berry, R., Liard, F., Garneau, M., and Jaramillo, J. (1992) Cardiac responses and binding sites for endothelin in normal and cardiomyopathic hamsters. *J. Pharmacol. Exp. Therap.* **260,** 1314–1322.

22. Friedrich, E. B., Muders F., Luchner, A., Dietl, O., Riegger, G. A. J., and Elsner, D. (1999) Contribution of the endothelin system to the renal hypoperfusion associated with experimental congestive heart failure. *J. Cardiovasc. Pharmacol.* **34,** 612–617.

23. Tojo, T., Tsunoda, Y., Nakada, S., and Tomoike, H. (2000) Effects of long-term treatment with nonselective endothelin receptor antagonist, TAK-044, on remodelling of cardiovascular system with sustained volume overload. *J. Cardiovasc. Pharmacol.* **35,** 777–785.

24. Seta, Y., Kanda, T., Yokoyama, T., Arai, M., Sekiguchi, K., Tanaka, T., et al. (2000) Therapy with the nonpeptide endothelin receptor antagonist 97-139 in a murine model of congestive heart failure - Reduction of cardiac mass and myofiber hypertrophy. *Jap. Heart J.* **41,** 79–85.

25. Miyauchi, T. and Masaki, T. (1999) Pathophysiology of endothelin in the cardiovascular system. *Ann. Rev. Physiol.* **61,** 391–415.

26. Selye, H., Oemar, B. S., and Siebenmann, R. (1960) Simple technique for the surgical occlusion of coronary vessels in rats. *Angiology* **11,** 398–407.

27. Pfeffer, M. A., Pfeffer, J. M., and Fishbein, M. C. (1979) Myocardial infarct size and ventricular function in rats. *Circ. Res.* **44,** 503–512.

28. Pfeffer, M. A., Lamas, G. A., Vaughan, D. E., Parisi, A. F., and Braunwald, E. (1988) Effect of captopril on progressive ventricular dilatation after anterior myocardial infarction. *New Engl. J. Med.* **68,** 525–533.

29. McEwan, P. E., Valdenaire, O., Sutherland, L., Webb, D. J., and Gray, G. A. (1998) A non-radioactive method for localisation of ET receptor mRNA *in situ.* *J. Cardiovasc. Pharmacol.* **31,** S443–S447.

14

Local Forearm Vasoconstriction to Endothelin-1 Measured by Venous Occlusion Plethysmography In Vivo

Fiona E. Strachan and David J. Webb

1. Introduction

As a consequence of its potent vasoconstrictor and growth promoting properties, endothelin-1 (ET-1) has been implicated in the pathophysiology of diseases such as hypertension, heart failure and renal failure *(1,2)*. This has lead to the rapid development of endothelin receptor antagonists as potential vasodilator treatments for cardiovascular disease *(3)*, with some of these compounds currently being investigated in clinical trials *(4–6)*. The previous chapters describe a number of in vitro and in vivo techniques employed in preclinical studies investigating the physiology and pathophysiology of the endothelin system. The current chapter describes the application of venous occlusion plethysmography and local intra-arterial infusion to assess the vascular effects of the endothelin system in healthy volunteers in vivo.

Venous occlusion plethysmography is a well-validated technique used to assess changes in forearm resistance vessels in vivo *(7)*. When coupled with brachial artery infusion, this technique provides a valuable method for the assessment of pharmacological and physiological, vasoactive properties of locally active doses of potentially vasoactive compounds. The use of locally active, sub-systemic doses allows assessment of the direct vascular effects of these compounds in intact vessels exposed to normal physiological conditions *(7)*, without the confounding effects on other organs such as the brain, heart and kidneys and consequent neurohumoral reflexes, associated with systemic drug administration. Vasoconstriction of the forearm vascular bed to local intra-arterial infusion of ET-1 has previously been demonstrated by venous

From: *Methods in Molecular Biology, vol. 206: Peptide Research Protocols: Endothelin*
Edited by: J. Maguire and A. Davenport © Humana Press Inc., Totowa, NJ

occlusion plethysmography *(8–10)* and inhibition of this response has been used to assess the efficacy of endothelin receptor antagonists in early clinical trials *(6,11)*. The importance of ET-1 as an endogenous mediator of vascular tone has also been confirmed by forearm vasodilatation in response to local infusion of endothelin receptor antagonists *(6,10,12)*. Assessment of the local response to endothelin agonists and antagonists in patient groups has provided important information on the role of the endothelin system in the pathophysiology of cardiovascular disease *(13,14)*.

The characteristically slow onset of and sustained vasoconstriction to ET-1 *(8,9)* precludes the construction of a full dose response curve on a single visit. This is due to the undesirable increase in the length of infusion required to allow development of the maximum response for each dose and the possibility of an accumulation of effect with subsequent increases in dose level. When investigating local vascular effects, we have used a single dose of ET-1, either in the presence or absence of an endothelin receptor antagonist *(6,11)* or in comparisons between patient groups and healthy matched control subjects *(13,14)*. The current chapter describes the method used to investigate local vasoconstriction in response to brachial artery infusion of ET-1, at the localy active dose level of 5 pmol/min, in healthy men. This method has been used as a model *(15)* in proof of concept studies assessing the effects of endothelin receptor antagonists against ET-1 mediated tone in healthy volunteers *(6,11,16)* and to compare responses between patients with heart failure *(17)* and renal failure *(13)* with healthy control subjects.

2. Materials

1. Intra-arterial needle, lignocaine 1% (*see* **Note 1**).
2. Infusion equipment and infusion device (*see* **Note 2**).
3. Venous occlusion plethysmography equipment comprising upper arm and wrist cuffs, cuff inflators, air source, strain gauges, plethysmograph, computer (PC or Mac), MacLab or PowerLab and Chart software or equivalent (*see* **Note 3**).
4. Saline 0.9% solution (Baxter Healthcare Ltd, Thetford, UK) for baseline infusion.
5. ET-1 infusate: ET-1 (Clinalfa, Nottingham, UK) diluted in 0.9% saline on the day of the study to a concentration of 5 pmol/mL (12.5 ng/mL) for infusion at 1 mL/min (*see* **Note 4**).
6. Microsoft Excel or equivalent data handling program.

3. Methods

1. Obtain approval from local ethics review committee and recruit study subjects in advance of the study start (*see* **Note 5**).
2. On the day of the study, set air conditioning in the clinical study area to heat to 23–25°C (*see* **Note 6**). Switch on air source and open chart file (*see* **Note 7**), and dilute ET-1 for infusion (*see* **Note 4**).

3. Ask the volunteer to lie supine (*see* **Note 6**); apply the upper arm cuffs, wrist cuffs, strain gauges, and blood pressure cuff (*see* **Note 8**).

4. Check blood pressure to ensure that the volunteer still meets the study inclusion criteria and ensure that the volunteer has complied with all the study restrictions (*see* **Note 5**).

5. Carry out test recording to check equipment and allow the volunteer to become familiar with recording procedure. For each forearm blood flow (FBF) recording, the wrist cuffs are inflated to 220 mm Hg for 3 min while the upper arm cuffs are intermittently inflated to 40 mm Hg for 10 s and deflated for 5 s, approximately, within the 3-min recording period (*see* **Note 9**).

6. Cannulate the brachial artery of the nondominant arm (*see* **Note 10**) and start infusion of saline 0.9% for baseline assessment of forearm blood flow (FBF). Infuse saline for at least 30 min at a rate of 1 mL/min and record FBF at 10-min intervals. Record blood pressure (BP) and pulse after each FBF recording (*see* **Note 11**). Start ET-1 (5 pmol/min) infusion after third satisfactory FBF baseline recording and at least 30 min baseline infusion. Infuse ET-1 for 90 min; measure FBF, BP and pulse at 10-min intervals throughout.

7. When the infusion is complete, remove arterial cannula, and apply pressure over site for at least 5 min. Before discharge home, the cannulation site should be examined for any adverse effects and limb perfusion assessed, e.g., skin color and evidence of distal pulse. It is also good practice to contact each volunteer 24 h after the study to monitor for any symptoms resulting from the cannulation procedure. Volunteers can be discharged 4 h following cannulation, provided there is no evidence of systemic effects of any study treatment or procedure. Subsequent cannulations should be at least 5–7 d after the previous cannulation.

8. After the study has been completed, plethysmographic data listings are extracted from the chart files and transferred to a template spreadsheet (Excel 5.0; Microsoft Ltd, Wokingham, UK) to calculate forearm blood flows (*see* **Note 12**). Blood flow in both forearms is obtained from the mean of the last 5 consecutive recordings of each measurement period. Recordings made in the first 60 s after wrist cuff inflation were not used for analysis because of the transient instability in blood flow that this causes *(18)*. Forearm blood flow results are expressed as the % change from baseline in the ratio of blood flow between the infused and noninfused arms *(7)* (*see* **Note 13**). Baseline blood flow is taken as the last measurement during the saline infusion, before the start of the ET-1 infusion.

4. Notes

1. The brachial artery of the nondominant arm was cannulated under local anesthesia (1% lignocaine; Astra Pharmaceuticals, Kings Langley, UK) with a 27 SWG steel needle (Coopers Needle Works, Birmingham, UK) attached to a 16G epidural catheter (Portex Ltd, Hythe, Kent, UK) (**Fig. 1**). The cannulae are provided nonsterile and are sterilized by our hospital CSSD department.

   Some centres use wider bore cannulae that are able to record arterial blood pressure *(19)*. However, we prefer the 27 SWG cannulae as they are generally less traumatic.

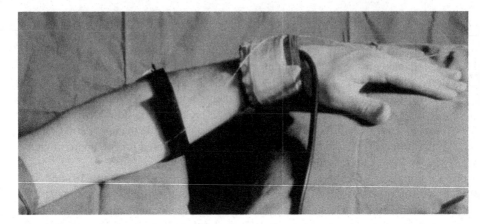

Fig. 1. Intra-arterial cannula inserted into the left brachial artery.

2. Patency is maintained by infusion of 0.9% physiologic saline via a syringe pump (IVAC P1000). Infusions are administered from 50-mL syringes (Bekton-Dickson, UK) connected directly to the epidural catheter (*see* **Note 1**). The rate of intra-arterial infusion is maintained constant at 1 mL/min throughout.
3. Venous occlusion plethysmography is performed using a dual channel strain gauge plethysmograph (Hokanson) and calibration is achieved using the internal standard of the Hokanson plethysmography unit. The voltage output is transferred from the plethysmograph to a Macintosh computer or PC using a MacLab, or PowerLab, analog-to-digital converter and Chart software (v. 3.2.8 at least; both from AD Instruments, Castle Hill, NSW, Australia).
4. Endothelin-1 (Clinalfa, Nottingham, UK) is administered by continuous infusion, via the brachial artery, for 90 min at a rate of 5 pmol/min. This dose was selected, on the basis of previous work showing, in vivo, that ET-1 at 5 pmol/min causes slow onset venoconstriction of ~60% in human skin capacitance vessels *(20)* and ~40% in human resistance vessels *(10)*. A single dose of ET-1 is advised in individual studies because the slow onset and long lasting action of the endothelin isopeptides precludes the use of repeated doses in a single study to examine conventional dose-response relationships *(8)*.
ET-1 is diluted in 0.9% saline (Baxter Healthcare Ltd, Thetford, UK) from sterile stock solutions on the day of the study. In order to minimize the effects of differences between drug batches, the same batch of ET-1 should be used for all volunteers included in the study. We infuse the ET-1 infusate on the day of dilution, *see* supplier for further details on product stability and sterility.
Concerns over the binding of ET-1 to infusion lines and syringes and subsequent loss of activity have been raised, prompting dilution of ET-1 in colloid solutions by some investigators *(21)*. However, our standard method *(6,9–11)* is to dilute ET-1 in saline and have shown responses to be sustained and reproducible *(15)*.
5. Clinical studies can only be conducted with the approval of the local research ethics committee and with the written informed consent of each subject. Volun-

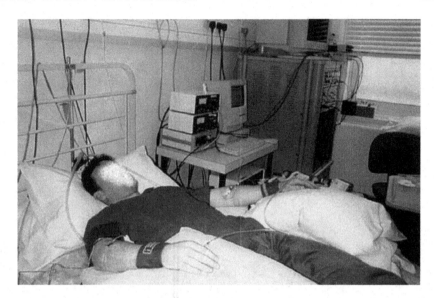

Fig. 2. Venous occlusion plethysmography experimental set up. The volunteer lies supine with his arms supported above the level of the heart.

teers with significant medical history, including asthma, allergies and epilepsy should be excluded from this type of study. All subjects should be instructed to abstain from vasoactive medication in the 2 wk before each study and from alcohol, caffeine-containing drinks, and tobacco from at least 12 h before each study. Each subject should fast for at least 3 h before any measurements are taken.

6. The room temperature must be maintained constant (varying <1°C) between 23–25°C. It is important that volunteers are relaxed and still throughout the infusion. Explain all procedures to the volunteers before the study. Practice recordings are useful both to check equipment and to familiarize the volunteer with the recording procedure.

7. We use Chart software to record FBF, and record on two channels: Channel 1 for the noninfused arm and Channel 2 for the infused arm.

8. Subjects rest recumbent throughout each study. Pressure cuffs (Hokanson) are applied to upper arms, wrists and mercury-in-silastic strain gauges (Hokanson) are securely applied to the widest part of each forearm (**Fig. 2**).

9. The response to intra-arterial infusion is assessed by measurement of FBF in both the infused and noninfused forearms. The noninfused arm acts as a contemporaneous control for the infused arm.

   As the blood flow to the hands is largely made up of skin blood flow, the hands are excluded from the circulation during each FBF recording through inflation of wrist cuffs to 220 mm Hg. Upper arm cuffs are intermittently inflated to 40 mm Hg for the first 10 s in every 15 s to temporarily prevent venous outflow from the forearm and thus obtain plethysmographic recordings (**Fig. 3**). Recordings of forearm blood flow are made over 3 min periods at 10-min intervals.

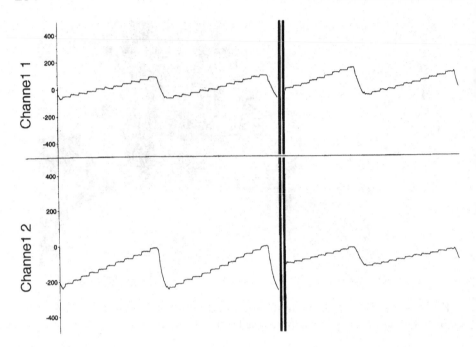

Fig. 3. Traces obtained during forearm blood flow measurements, noninfused arm data are shown on Channel 1 and infused arm data on Channel 2. The left hand section was recorded during baseline saline infusion, the right hand section was recorded during infusion of ET-1. Vasoconstriction is indicated by the reduction in the gradient of the slope of the traces on Channel 2 (the infused arm).

10. To insert the cannula: palpate the brachial artery and identify site where pulse is strongest, as an indicator of appropriate site for cannula insertion; apply local anaesthetic (lignocaine 1%) to the surrounding area by subcutaneous injection. Before insertion, ensure the cannula is patent and is connected to the epidural catheter line then prime the line. Insert the cannula under the skin at a site distal to the point where the pulse is strongest, disconnect from syringe and advance towards artery. When the cannula enters the artery, as indicated by "flashback" of arterial blood in the line, reconnect to the saline syringe and start the infusion immediately. The line should be purged immediately to prevent clotting of blood in the line. There is a risk of extravazation during the infusion and it is important to observe the cannula site and ask the volunteer to report any pain or discomfort throughout the infusion to monitor for signs of extravazation.

11. Blood pressure and pulse are measured in the noninfused arm using a well-validated semi-automated noninvasive method *(22)*. The blood pressure cuff is applied over the upper arm forearm blood flow cuff. Blood pressure is measured

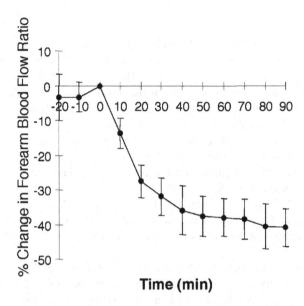

Fig. 4. Standard graph presenting FBF response to local infusion of ET-1.

immediately after forearm blood flow to avoid any effect of the venous congestion caused by this procedure on these measurements *(23)*. The measurement of
blood pressure throughout the infusion is included for safety reasons, to exclude
significant systemic effects of the infusion.
12. Our method of measurement of FBF involves transferring data from the Chart
file to an Excel spreadsheet with forearm blood flows calculated for five individual venous occlusion cuff inflations. Some investigators use programs that
automatically calculate FBF and do not require any data handling *(12,19)*.
Blood flow in both forearms is obtained from the mean of the last five consecutive recordings of each measurement period. Baseline blood flow is taken as the
last measurement during the saline infusion, before the start of the active drug
infusion. Forearm blood flow results are expressed as the % change from baseline
in the ratio of blood flow between the infused and noninfused arms *(7)*.
13. All results are generally expressed as mean ± standard error of the mean (SEM).
Blood pressure, heart rate and baseline measurements during local infusion studies are compared using the student's paired *t*-test, to assess whether there are any
changes between study visits. Forearm blood flow responses are presented as %
change from baseline (**Fig. 4**) and are examined by repeated-measures analysis
of variance (ANOVA) using statistical software package such as Excel (Microsoft
Ltd., Wokingham, UK) or equivalent. Statistical significance is accepted at the
5% level. Results can also be expressed as the area under the curve (AUC) to
present a summary statistic for the overall response.

References

1. Battistini, B., Chailler, P., D'Orleans Juste, P., Briere, N., and Sirois, P. (1993) Growth regulatory properties of endothelins. *Peptides* **14**, 385–399.
2. Haynes, W. G. and Webb, D. J. (1993) The endothelin family of peptides: local hormones with diverse roles in health and disease? *Clin. Sci.* **84**, 485–500.
3. Strachan, F. E. and Webb, D. J. (1998) The endothelin system: a novel therapeutic target in cardiovascular disease. *Emerging Drugs* **3**, 95–112.
4. Freed, M. I., Wilson, D. E., Thompson, K. A., Harris, R. Z., Ilson, B. E., and Jorkasky, D. K. (1999) Pharmacokinetics and pharmacodynamics of SB 209670, an endothelin receptor antagonist: effects on the regulation of renal vascular tone. *Clin. Pharmacol. Ther.* **65**, 473–482.
5. Weber, C., Schmitt, R., Birnboeck, H., Hopfgartner, G., vanMarle, S. P., Peeters, P. A. M., et al. (1996) Pharmacokinetics and pharmacodynamics of the endothelin-receptor antagonist bosentan in healthy human subjects. *Clin. Pharmacol. Ther.* **60**, 124–137.
6. Haynes, W. G., Ferro, C. F., O'Kane, K. P. J., Somerville, D., Lomax, C. C., and Webb, D. J. (1996) Systemic endothelin receptor blockade decreases peripheral vascular resistance and blood pressure in humans. *Circulation* **93**, 1860–1870.
7. Webb, D. J. (1995) The pharmacology of human blood vessels *in vivo*. *J. Vasc. Res.* **32**, 2–15.
8. Clarke, J. G., Benjamin, N., Larkin, S. W., Webb, D. J., Davies, G. J., and Maseri, A. (1989) Endothelin is a potent long-lasting vasoconstrictor in men. *Am. J. Physiol.* **257**, H2033–H2035.
9. Haynes, W. G., Strachan, F. E., and Webb, D. J. (1995) Endothelin ETA and ETB receptors cause vasoconstriction of human resistance and capacitance vessels in vivo. *Circulation* **92**, 357–363.
10. Haynes, W. G. and Webb, D. J. (1994) Contribution of endogenous generation of endothelin-1 to basal vascular tone. *Lancet* **344**, 852–854.
11. Ferro, C. J., Haynes, W. G., Johnston, N. R., Lomax, C. C., Newby, D. E., and Webb, D.J. (1997) The peptide endothelin receptor antagonist, TAK-044, produces sustained inhibition of endothelin-1 mediated arteriolar vasoconstriction. *Br. J. Clin. Pharmacol.* **44**, 377–383.
12. Verhaar, M. C., Strachan, F. E., Newby, D. E., Cruden, N. L., Koomans, H. A., Rabelink, T. J., and Webb, D. J. (1998) Endothelin-A receptor antagonist mediated vasodilatation is attenuated by inhibition of nitric oxide synthesis and by endothelin-B receptor blockade. *Circulation* **97**, 752–756.
13. Hand, M. F., Haynes, W. G., and Webb, D. J. (1999) Reduced endogenous endothelin-1-mediated vascular tone in chronic renal failure. *Kidney Int.* **55**, 613–620.
14. Love, M. P., Haynes, W. G., Gray, G. A., Webb, D. J., and McMurray, J. J. (1996) Vasodilator effects of endothelin-converting enzyme inhibition and endothelin ETA receptor blockade in chronic heart failure patients treated with ACE inhibitors. *Circulation* **94**, 2131–2137.

15. Strachan, F., Newby, D., Sciberras, D., McCrea, J., Goldberg, M., and Webb, D. (1998) Reproducibility of forearm vasoconstriction to intra-arterial endothelin-1. *Br. J. Clin. Pharmacol.* **45,** 194P–195P.

16. Strachan, F. E., Newby, D. E., Sciberras, D. G., McCrea, J. B., Goldberg, M. R., and Webb, D. J. The effect of the nonselective endothelin receptor antagonist L-753,037 on forearm vasoconstriction to endothelin-1. *Br. J. Clin. Pharmacol.,* in press.

17. Love, M. P., Ferro, C. J., Haynes, W. G., Webb, D. J., and McMurray, J. J. (1996) Selective or nonselective endothelin receptor blockade in chronic heart failure? *Circulation* **94,** 2899–2900.

18. Kerslake, D. M. (1949) The effect of the application of an arterial occlusion cuff to the wrist on the blood flow in the human forearm. *J. Physiol.* **108,** 451–457.

19. Stroes, E. S., Koomans, H. A., de Bruin, T. W. A., and Rabelink, T. J. (1995) Vascular function in the forearm of hypercholesterolaemic patients off and on lipid-lowering medication. *Lancet* **346,** 467–471.

20. Haynes, W. G. and Webb, D. J. (1993) Endothelium dependent modulation of responses to endothelin-1 in human veins. *Clin. Sci.* **84,** 427–433.

21. Kiowski, W., Luscher, T. F., Linder, L., and Buhler, F. R. (1991) Endothelin-1 induced vasoconstriction in humans: reversal by calcium-channel blockade but not by nitrovasodilators or endothelium-derived relaxing factor. *Circulation* **83,** 469–475.

22. Wiinberg, N., Walter-Larson, S., Eriksen, C., and Nielsen, P. E. (1988) An evaluation of semi-automatic blood pressure manometers against intra-arterial blood pressure. *J. Ambulatory Monitoring* **1,** 303–309.

23. Patterson, G. C. and Shepherd, J. T. (1954) The blood flow in the human forearm following venous congestion. *J. Physiol. (Lond)* **125,** 501–507.

Index

Printed in the United States
by Baker & Taylor Publisher Services